HYDROGELS

Design, Synthesis and Application in Drug Delivery and Regenerative Medicine

HYDROGELS

Design, Synthesis and Application in Drug Delivery and Regenerative Medicine

Editors

Thakur Raghu Raj Singh
Senior Lecturer in Pharmaceuticals
School of Pharmacy
Queens University Belfast
Belfast
UK

Garry Laverty
Lecturer in Pharmaceuticals
School of Pharmacy
Queens University Belfast
Belfast
UK

Ryan Donnelly
Chair in Pharmaceutical Technology
School of Pharmacy
Queens University Belfast
Belfast
UK

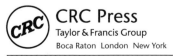

CRC Press
Taylor & Francis Group
Boca Raton London New York

CRC Press is an imprint of the
Taylor & Francis Group, an **informa** business

A SCIENCE PUBLISHERS BOOK

Cover Credit
Cover illustrations reproduced by kind courtesy of Drs. Sina Naficy and Geoffrey M. Spinks (authors of Chapter 3) and Drs. Nicola J. Irwin, Colin P. McCoy and Johann L. Trotter (authors of Chapter 5)

CRC Press
Taylor & Francis Group
6000 Broken Sound Parkway NW, Suite 300
Boca Raton, FL 33487-2742

First issued in paperback 2021

ISBN-13: 978-0-367-78144-6 (pbk)
ISBN-13: 978-1-4987-4861-2 (hbk)

Library of Congress Cataloging-in-Publication Data

Names: Singh, Thakur Raghu Raj, editor. | Laverty, Garry, editor. | Donnelly, Ryan F., editor.
Title: Hydrogels : design, synthesis and application in drug delivery and regenerative medicine / editors, Thakur Raghu Raj Singh, Lecturer in Pharmaceuticals, School of Pharmacy, Queens University Belfast, Belfast, UK, Garry Laverty, Lecturer in Pharmaceuticals, School of Pharmacy, Queens University Belfast, Belfast, UK, Ryan Donnelly, Chair in Pharmaceutical Technology, School of Pharmacy, Queens University Belfast, Belfast, UK.
Description: Boca Raton, FL : CRC Press/ Taylor & Francis Group, [2017] | Includes bibliographical references and index.
Identifiers: LCCN 2017021438| ISBN 9781498748612 (hardback : alk. paper) | ISBN 9781498748629 (e-book)
Subjects: LCSH: Colloids in medicine.
Classification: LCC R857.C66 H88 2017 | DDC 615.1/9--dc23
LC record available at https://lccn.loc.gov/2017021438

Visit the Taylor & Francis Web site at
http://www.taylorandfrancis.com

and the CRC Press Web site at
http://www.crcpress.com

Preface

Hydrogels are three-dimensionally cross-linked polymeric networks that are capable of absorbing and retaining huge amounts of water without leaking it. The half liquid-like and half solid-like characteristics of hydrogels impart many interesting properties that are not found in either a pure solid or a pure liquid. Therefore, hydrogels are commonly used in clinical practice and experimental medicine for a wide range of applications, including drug delivery, tissue engineering and regenerative medicine, diagnostics, cellular immobilization, separation of biomolecules or cells, and barrier materials to regulate biological adhesions.

This book will cover the design and synthesis of hydrogels and its application in the area of drug delivery and regenerative medicine. Firstly, we have reviewed basics of hydrogels, so as to provide a sound background to the use of hydrogels in a number of applications, namely, structure and dynamics of water, thixothrophic behavior, polymer network parameters, and mechanism of drug release from hydrogels. Secondly, we have provided extensive review of hydrogel applications such as in the coating of medical devices to enhance its clinical performance, bone regeneration, wound management, imaging, sensing, diagnostics, and tissue engineering. Finally, we have also presented leading strategies that are being employed in engineering hydrogel-based materials with molecular control, increased complexity, tuneable functionality, and 3D cell culture. We have reviewed each chapter in detail to elucidate the underlying concepts and principles that drive continued innovation. Furthermore, we have also covered key case studies, so that it will allow detailed discussions and critical analysis of the existing research carried out to date, in each chapter. We are indebted to the contributors for their hard work, openness to suggestions for directions of their Chapters and prompt delivery of the Chapters. Editing this text took considerable time and we would like to thank our families for their patience and support throughout the project. We also like to thank the publisher, CRC Press/ Taylor & Francis Group, for considerable help and encouragement as we completed this project.

Thakur Raghu Raj Singh
Garry Laverty
Ryan Donnelly

Contents

CHAPTER 1

Microarchitecture of Water Confined in Hydrogels

Rolando Barbucci,[1,*] *Vincenza Spera,*[2] *Emilia Armenia*[3]
and *Vincenzo Quagliariello*[3]

Introduction

When looking at, or holding a hydrogel you get the impression that the gel is a state that is neither completely liquid nor completely solid. The half liquid-like and half solid-like characteristics cause many interesting properties that are not found in either a pure solid or a pure liquid. A hydrogel, as definition, is a three-dimensionally cross-linked polymeric network that is capable of absorbing and retaining huge amounts of water without leaking it. Schematically we can divide the hydrogels into physical and chemical hydrogels according to their constitution as shown in Fig. 1.

In the first case, even if the term physical is not particularly appropriate, the polymer chains are held together by physical interactions such as hydrophobic interactions, hydrogen bonds, electrostatic interactions, and entanglements among chains. The physical hydrogels are reversible under specific conditions causing shape instability and are generally harder than the chemical hydrogels. Alginate is a well-known example of a polymer that forms a hydrogel by ionic interactions (Gacesa 1988). The polymer is a polysaccharide with mannuronic and glucuronic acid residues and can be crosslinked by calcium ions.

[1] Institute for Polymers, Composite and Biomaterials (IPCB), National Research Council of Italy, Mostra d'Oltremare, Padiglione 20, Viale J.F. Kennedy 54 80125, Napoli, Italy.
[2] Glaxosmithkline (GSK), Località Bellaria di Rosia, 53018 Sovicille. Siena, Italy.
[3] Department of Anesthesiological, Surgical and Emergency Sciences, Second University of Naples, Via Costantinopoli 16, 80138, Naples, Italy.
* Corresponding author: rolando.barbucci@ipcb.cnr.it

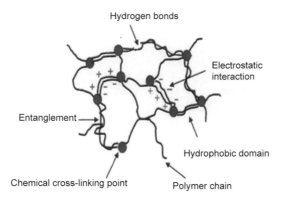

Fig. 1. Schematic representation of hydrogel with different interactions (Adapted from Barbucci 2013).

Hydrophobic interactions have also been exploited to design physical gels. They are generally obtained from multiblock copolymers or graft copolymers. The latter can be composed of a water-soluble polymer backbone, for example, a polysaccharide, to which hydrophobic units are attached, or hydrophobic chains containing water-soluble grafts.

Hydrogen bonding interactions can also be used to form physically gel-like structures. Mixtures of two or more natural polymers can display rheological synergism, meaning that the viscoelastic properties of the polymer blends are more gel-like than those of the constituent polymers measured individually (Gupta et al. 2006). Blends of, for example, gelatin–agar, starch–carboxymethyl cellulose, and hyaluronic acid–methylcelluloses form physically gel-like structures that are injectable. Crystallization of polymers has also been used to form physically gels. When aqueous solutions of poly(vinyl alcohol) (PVA) undergo a freeze–thawing process, a strong and highly elastic gel is formed. Gel formation is ascribed to the formation of PVA crystallites that act as physical sites in the network (Yokoyama et al. 1986) as shown in Fig. 2.

The ubiquitous non-covalent interactions in biological systems are also being used to generate hydrogels with unique, dynamic functions (Mohammed and Murphy 2009). Biological systems are dominated by non-covalent interactions, which can be defined as intermolecular interactions, in which there is no change in either chemical bonding or electron pairing (Kollman 1977). These interactions provide an excellent mechanism for dynamically regulating the assembly and function of biological systems. The formation of coiled-coil aggregates of the terminal domains in near-neutral aqueous solutions triggers the formation of a three-dimensional polymer network, with the polyelectrolyte segment retaining solvent and preventing precipitation of the chain.

In the second case, covalent bonds among the polymer chains are formed. Obviously physical interactions can also be present in the chemical hydrogels. The network shows good mechanical strength and the covalent bonds prevent dissolution of the network in aqueous environment. Chemically crosslinked gels can be obtained by radical polymerization of low-molecular-weight monomers in the presence of a cross-linking agent.

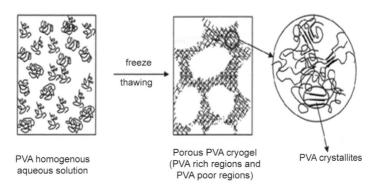

PVA homogenous aqueous solution

Porous PVA cryogel (PVA rich regions and PVA poor regions)

PVA crystallites

Fig. 2. Formation of PVA crystallites from a homogeneous PVA solution by freeze thawing technique (Adapted from Jinchen 2013).

Aside from radical polymerization of mixtures of vinyl monomers, chemically crosslinked hydrogels can also be obtained by radical polymerization of polymers derivatised with polymerizable groups (macromonomers). If polymers have pendant functional groups (e.g., OH, COOH, and NH2), covalent linkages between polymer chains can be established by the reaction of functional groups with complementary reactive groups such as an amine-carboxylic acid or an isocyanate-OH/NH2 reaction, or by Schiff base formation Fig. 3.

A novel hydrogel concept based on enzymatic reaction has also been reported. A tetrahydroxy PEG was functionalized with glutaminyl groups (PEG-Qa). PEG networks were then formed by the addition of transglutaminase to an aqueous solution of PEG-Qa and poly(lysine-co-phenylalanine) (Sperinde and Griffith 1997).

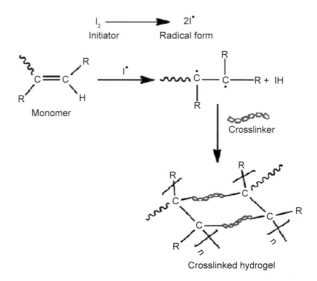

Fig. 3. Crosslinked gel obtained by radical reaction of a low MW monomer and I_2 as initiator with a crosslinking agent (Adapted from Dipankar and Sagar 2015).

High-energy radiation, such as gamma (γ) and electron beam radiation can be used to polymerize unsaturated compounds. Photo-crosslinkable NIPAAm copolymers with a UV-reactive benzophenone (BP) conjugated comonomer have been designed (Matsukuma et al. 2006). The photo-cross-linking was carried out by making use of the photochemistry of the BP groups, the photochemically produced triplet state which can abstract hydrogen atoms from almost any polymer, thus generating radicals.

The Properties of Water and its Role in the Hydrogel

A gel can hold an extraordinary amount of water even 99%. Thus the hydrogel is essentially water. It holds together the polymeric materials and water nicely although slightly wet. Thinking of the mechanical properties coming solely from the polymeric matrix does not seem reasonable. The overall behaviour and the technological performance of hydrogels are determined, to a large extent, by the amount, structure and properties of water as well the characteristics assumed by it in contact and interacting with the solid polymeric network (Fig. 4).

As a whole, water is a typical substance with unusual properties (Wiggins 2008; Chaplin 2000). For instance, the boiling point of water is too high in comparison with hydrides of B, C, N, F, S, Se, and Te due to much stronger hydrogen bonding. Extrapolation of the relationship between the boiling points of hydride compounds and their molecular weights gives an expected boiling point for water of about 75°C. There are many other unusual properties of water such as too high melting and critical points, surface tension, viscosity, heat of vaporization, short NMR spin-lattice relaxation time at low temperatures, a wider variety of stable (and metastable) crystals and amorphous structures of solid water than other materials; faster freezing of hot water than cold water (Mpemba effect); anomalously fast mobility of protons and hydroxide ions under an electric field; high dielectric constant, etc. (Chaplin 2000) up to 72 anomalies.

Water can be thought of as a structure where extensive connectivity of different regions is established by the hydrogen bonds. There are changes in time with a constantly varying local structure arising from the rearrangement of the local

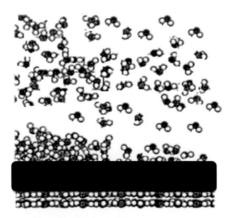

Fig. 4. The disposition of water in the bulk and interacting with the surface.

network while still retaining the essential connectivity within the network. Transient hydrogen bonded clusters are permanently formed and broken and very few free water molecules are present, as confirmed by IR experiments (Maréchal 1996). In most simulations, water appears as a three-dimensional network of randomly distributed hydrogen bonds with a local tetrahedral geometry. One of the main questions still open regarding water structure is the way in which hydrogen bonds fluctuate to enable the structural changes to occur. It then seems, as stated by Dore (Dore 2000), that "our fundamental understanding of the disordered hydrogen-bonded network is still at a fairly rudimentary stage".

The presence of a solid interface in water, here represented by the polymeric network, clearly represents a major perturbation to the hydrogen-bond network. There are several methods used to determine the characteristics of interfacial water (Matricardi et al. 2016):

a) Measurements of attractive or repulsive forces between two surfaces distant one from another. On this respect Israelachvili and colleagues (Israelachvili and Adams 1978) measured the force required to displace solvents sandwiched between parallel mica surfaces. The closer the surfaces got, the higher the force required. The force-separation relation was not purely monotonic, but a series of regularly spaced peaks and valleys of force were observed. The surfaces have the capacity to organize solvent into at least 10–12 layers (Fig. 5).
b) Contact angle method
c) Differential scanning calorimetry
d) Thermally stimulated depolarization current (TSDC) (Gun'ko et al. 2005)
e) Dielectric relaxation spectroscopy
f) Temperature-programmed desorption (TPD)
g) FTIR and Raman spectroscopies

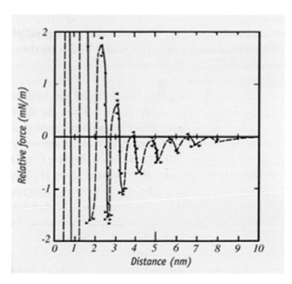

Fig. 5. Organization of the solvent in 10–12 layers as described by the force separation relation (Israelachvili 1978).

h) Rheology
i) 1H NMR spectroscopy with layer-by-layer freezing-out of bulk and interfacial water
j) XRD and neutron diffraction
k) Adsorption, surface charge density and zeta-potential
l) As well as other chemical, biochemical and biophysical methods (Chaplin 2000).

Close to the surface, the hydrogen bond network is distorted as hydrogen bonds among water molecules are partially substituted by bonds between water and surface. All the experiments and simulation results seem to provide a rather coherent picture of the behaviour of interfacial and confined water near hydrophilic surfaces. The mobility of molecules directly adsorbed on the hydrophilic surface is reduced by more than one order of magnitude, whereas for full hydration water molecules at a longer distance from the surface exhibit short diffusion coefficients close to that of the bulk.

On hydrophilic substrates, water was usually found to have a higher density than in the bulk, and its structure and dynamics have sometimes been compared to those of supercooled water and amorphous ice. Table 1 summarizes many differences (Clegg and Drost-Hansen 1991).

Water adsorbed on polymer surfaces is distinct and behaves differently from predictions based on bulk water. Using a hydrogel, Gerald H. Pollack (Pollack 2001) plunked a piece into a chamber and suffused it with an aqueous suspension of microspheres. As soon as the liquid suspension met the gel, the microspheres began moving away from the gel's surface leaving a microsphere-free zone just under 100 micron wide. Water remained in that zone but microspheres did not. Microspheres of all kinds were excluded; they ranged in size from 10 microns down to 0.1 microns and were fabricated from diverse substances. Even red blood cells, several strains of many sizes and bacteria were excluded. The protein albumin was excluded, as were various dyes with MW's as low 100 Da, only a little larger than common salt. The experiments showed that the free zone close to the gel surface (Exclusion Zone, EZ) (Pollack 2013) rather broadly excludes substances of many sizes from very small to very large and once formed, the zone remained intact. Almost any hydrophilic surface can generate an EZ, and the EZ excludes almost anything suspended or dissolved in the water. Many experiments showed that the water in the exclusion zone differs in

Table 1. Comparisons of pure and vicinal water properties.

Comparison of some properties of pure and vicinal water		
Property	Bulk	Vicinal
Density (g/cm^3)	1.00	0.97
Specific heat (cal/Kg)	1.00	$1.25+/-0.05$
Thermal expansion coefficient ($^\circ$C^{-1}) (adiab.)	250×10^{-6} (25°C)	$300–700\times10^{-6}$
Compressibility coefficient (Atm^{-1})	45×10^{-6}	$60–100\times10^{-6}$
Excess sound absorption (cm^{-1} x s^2)	7×10^{-17}	Circa 35×10^{-17}
Heat conductivity ((cal/sec)/cm^2/$^\circ$C/cm)	0.0014	Circa 0.01–0.05
Viscosity (çP)	.089	2–10
Energy of activation ionic conduction (Kcal/mol)	Circa 4	5–8
Dielectric relaxation frequency (Hz)	19×10^9	2×10^9

character from the water beyond the exclusion zone and the differences are appreciable. EZ water is more viscous and more stable than bulk water, its molecular motions are more restricted, its light-absorption spectra differ in the UV-visible light range, as well in the infrared range, and it has a higher refractive index. These multiple differences imply that EZ water fundamentally differs from bulk water. The EZ hardly resembles liquid water and thus an unexpected feature of water has been identified. Next to hydrophilic surfaces, water molecules organize into liquid crystalline arrays building EZ honeycomb layers, which can project unexpectedly far from their nucleating surfaces. Like crystals of ice, these liquid crystals exclude many substances ranging in size from macroscopic colloidal particles to submicroscopic solutes. Those EZ layers can slide past one another if sufficient shearing force is applied, but ordinarily the planes stick to one another, creating what is seen macroscopically as the EZ (Fig. 6).

On hydrophobic surface (Lee et al. 1984) the orientation of water molecules near the surface is biased so that hydrogen bonding groups tend to avoid a direction toward the nonpolar material, which cannot itself participate in hydrogen bonding. Water thus maintains a hydrogen bonding interaction, which is comparable to that in the bulk. The liquid structure nearest the surface is characterized by "dangling" hydrogen bonds, i.e., a typical water molecule at the surface has one potentially hydrogen-bonding group oriented toward the hydrophobic surface. The density extends at least 10 Å into the liquid, and significant molecular orientation preferences extend at least 7 Å into the liquid. Still it appears that whatever the substrate, the spatial range at which water structure is perturbed is rather limited, less than 15 Å from the surface.

In both hydrophilic (Cicero et al. 2005) and hydrophobic cases (Lee et al. 1984), the properties of the confined water become more like those of the bulk with increasing distance from the surfaces. Moreover all the macromolecules are characterized by alternate hydrophilic and hydrophobic moieties with different characteristics. Therefore, one can assume that unusual water observed at mosaic hydrophobic/hydrophilic surfaces of solid materials can be found in different macromolecules. Water bound at the hydrophilic/hydrophobic interfaces can be assigned to several structural types as weakly and strongly associated waters, which can be also weakly or strongly bound to the macromolecules.

Not only the polymer that forms the skeleton of the hydrogel, but also the arms that binding the polymeric chains determine the characteristics of the network of the hydrogel, considering these cross-linking agents also show hydrophilic/hydrophobic moieties. Thus the cross-linking density and the functionality of crosslinker must be taken into account to get a complete representation of hydrogel. For instance it is clear

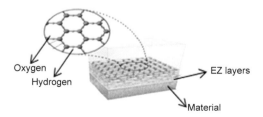

Fig. 6. Liquid crystalline water arrays forming EZ honeycomb structure on a surface (Adapted from Pollack 2013).

hexafunctional crosslinkers generate more rigidly crosslinked polymer networks, compared with tetrafunctional or bifunctional crosslinkers. When a hydrophilic cross-linking agent is employed, the hydrogel behaves with a high affinity towards water and when the crosslinker is replaced with a more hydrophilic one, the swelling of the hydrogel is enhanced. For instance by replacing bisacrylamide with more hydrophilic glyoxalbis (diallyacetal) (GLY) as crosslinker, the swelling of the crosslinked N-isopropylacrylamide (NIPAAm) hydrogel is enhanced (Xue and Hamley 2002). Of course a pronounced increase of the polymer–water interaction parameter is also observed with increasing GLY content. The swelling degree of the hydrogel, here considered a parameter to measure the hydrophilicity of hydrogel, is obviously reduced as the amount of crosslinker increases. The degree of swelling is observed to decrease with the crosslink density at exponent of 0.5 (Alvarez-Lorenzo and Concheiro 2002). However, at low crosslink density, the increase in amount of hydrophilic crosslinker may increase the degree of swelling. The poly(2-hydroxyethyl methacrylate) hydrogels show an exceptionally large increase of swelling with increasing the amount of crosslinker tripropylene glycoldiacrylate at pH 12.0 (Ferreira et al. 2000). Moreover the structure and elasticity of the hydrogels depend on the nature of cross-linking agent as well as on the cross-linking degree. The polymeric network differs from that of the less-crosslinked one so that we can say the two hydrogels are completely different despite having the same cross-linking agent and the same polymer.

Another parameter to be taken into account is represented by the different cross-linking methods, which can distinctly influence the polymer network structure (Martens and Anseth 2000). Cross-linking by γ-ray irradiation randomly introduces the crosslinks in the hydrogels, whereas generally the chemically crosslinked hydrogels exhibit inhomogeneous distribution of cross-linking points due to the difference in the reactivity ratios of monomers and crosslinkers (Pradas et al. 2001). The small angle neutron scattering studies demonstrate that the poly(NIPPAm) hydrogels crosslinked by γ-ray irradiation are more homogeneous than the hydrogels crosslinked by conventional polymerization (Norisuye et al. 2002). Nevertheless with polysaccharides, specific reactive groups in the polymer skeleton have been utilized to be crosslinked and homogeneous stoichiometry hydrogels were obtained. Hyaluronane is a straight chain polymer consisting of alternating N-acetyl-D-glucosamine and beta-D-glucuronic acid residues. The hydrogel was synthetized by using 2-chloro-1-methyl pyridinium iodide (CMP-I) as carboxylate groups activating. The CMP-I was added in a stoichiometric amount to activate 50% of the carboxylic groups of the polysaccharide. The cross-linking agent was an alkyldiamine, which underwent a nucleophilic attack on the carboxylic group (Fig. 7) (Barbucci et al. 2000).

The hydrogel was then analyzed by potentiometric and NMR techniques. Both the results were close to the theoretical result—those obtainable from the amount of CMP-I added to the solution, i.e., 50% of the carboxylic groups present in the polysaccharide. By NMR studies a homogeneous structure of the Hyal hydrogel was obtained with a regular alternated crosslinked arm in the backbone (Barbucci et al. 2006a) (Fig. 8).

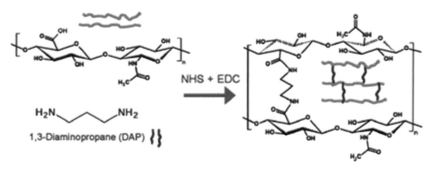

Fig. 7. Reaction scheme for the formation of the Hyal Hydrogel. The reaction involves the formation of an amide bond between the carboxylic groups of the polymer and the amine group of the diamine by using EDC and NHS as chemical activators (Adapted from Barbucci et al. 2000).

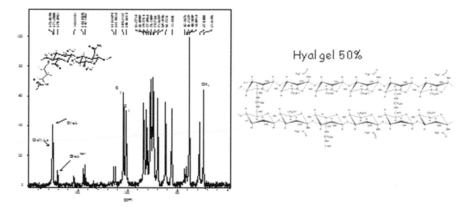

Fig. 8. NMR spectrum of the Hyal hydrogel with the figure of the homogeneous structure with alternating crosslinked arm (Adapted from Barbucci et al. 2006).

Organization of Water and Polymer-water Interactions

It is well known, that equilibrium water content as well as state of water, influence the properties of the hydrogel. In fact, as we have already said, given the paucity of the amount of solid material, polymer and cross-linking agent, present in a hydrogel which is also less than 5% of the mass, the properties and characteristics of a hydrogel depend on the organization of water. The characteristics of water in the hydrogel are primarily determined by specific polymer–water interactions and by geometrical confinement of water in the walls of the hydrogel.

A better understanding of these topics is of fundamental importance for improving our knowledge on the structure–property relationships in hydrogels. Water in hydrogels has very often been divided, on the basis of the different experimental techniques, into different classes, such as freezable and non-freezable water, mobile, immobile and clustered water, and free and bound water (Khalid et al. 2002). The classification depends, however, qualitatively and quantitatively, on the experimental technique employed and the analysis of data. The most accredited classification considers that water in the hydrogels exists in three physical states (Fig. 9):

1. The free water which is not intimately bound to the polymer chain and behaves like bulk water, freezing at the usual freezing point (at 0°C).
2. The intermediate or interstitial water, which is weakly, bound to the polymer chain or interacts weakly with the bound water. It freezes at temperature lower than the usual freezing point.
3. The bound water (non freezing water), which is strongly associated with the hydrophilic segments of polymers and does not freeze at the usual freezing point.

The content of the bound, non-freezing water is affected by the polymer and crosslinker nature as well as their density in the hydrogels. Various hydrogels are reported to have quite different contents of non-freezing water, for example, the 23% non-freezing water in the chitosan–PEO hydrogel (Khalid et al. 2002), the 24–28% non-freezing water in a chitosan hydrogel (Qu et al. 2000), the 35% non-freezing water in the HEMA hydrogels and as high as the 43% non-freezing water in the 2,3-dihydroxy propyl methacrylate (DHPMA) hydrogels (Gates et al. 2003). The molecules of non-freezing water are hydrogen bonded to the hydrophilic groups of the polymer. Therefore, the content of non-freezing water increases with the increase of the ratio of hydrophilic groups (Katime et al. 2000) and decreases with the increase of the ratio of hydrophobic groups (Kim et al. 2003). All that means the hydrogel characteristics

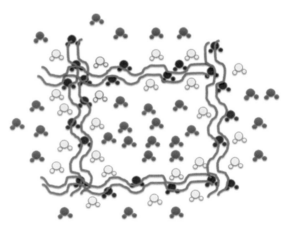

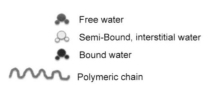

Free water

Semi-Bound, interstitial water

Bound water

Polymeric chain

Fig. 9. The three physical states of water in the hydrogels.

depend on both the quantity of not-freezing water as well as the interstitial water and on the types of interactions occurring among them and the solid network. Obviously, the proportion of free water becomes preponderant as the swelling ratio increases but it is not influential on the properties of hydrogel. For instance, the main fraction of water in macropores corresponds to non-bound, practically bulk water, and bound water ($<1\%$ of total amount of water in initial hydrogel) is weakly bound by the polymer. The latter is due to the absence of narrow nanopores in the macropore structures. Thus the main portion of water in macroporous hydrogels can be attributed to bulk water located in macropores.

Furthermore, other factors known as kosmotropic (structure-makers)/chaotropic (water-structure breakers) effects, dependent on the structure of polymeric groups (Wiggins 2008) and lead to changes in the water structure. On this regard, the chaotropiccations such as $N(CH_3)_4^+ > NH_4^+ > Cs^+ > Rb^+ > K^+$ and anions $ClO_4^- > NO_3^- > I^- > Br^- > Cl^-$ are accumulated in LDW and kosmotropic cations such as $Al^{3+} > Mg^{2+} > Ca^{2+} > H^+ > Na^+$ and anions $C_6H_5O_7 > SO_4^{-2} > PO_4^{-3}$ accumulated in HDW (Chaplin 2015). In fact according to NMR studies, water is described in terms of a two-state mixture model including high-density water (HDW with collapsed (condensed) structure, under standard conditions) and low-density water (LDW with expanded structure) being in the dynamic equilibrium. However, this equilibrium shifts toward a certain state due to the effects of chaotropic and kosmotropic solutes or surface functionalities, also ionic charges or contra-ions, of hydrogel.

In view of this organization of water molecules in the hydrogel, divided into three layers, bound water, interstitial and free water, the experiments and Pollack's hypothesis, i.e., the EZ's ordered structure (Pollack 2013), could participate in the first two layers since these water molecules being closest to the polymer surface and strictly organized, are those that can remove almost anything suspended or dissolved in the water. Water dipoles would stack one upon another, forming a honeycomb layer projecting farther and farther from the surface until the disruptive forces of "thermal" (Brownian) motion limit further ordered growth. The lattice is extremely tight and therefore highly exclusive of solutes.

This brief review reveals the complex structure and dynamics of interstitial and bound water, which exhibits strongly modified properties when compared to bulk water. Part of the difficulty arises from the fact that no current theory is capable of precisely predicting water interaction with a surface, even when the surface structure is well characterized.

The Presence and Functionality of Pores within the Hydrogels

A hydrogel is composed of statistically distributed microchannels or fluctuating pores created by the mobility of the polymer segments within an interpenetrating network, in the presence of a solvent (Fig. 10).

At a given site in the network, these pores are formed and removed as a result of thermal motion of the chain. The presence of pores in the hydrogels is particular relevant for one of the hydrogel applications: tissue regeneration (Migliaresi and Motta 2014; Pollack 2001) because the pore dimension strongly affects the capability of cells to adhere and proliferate (Fig. 11).

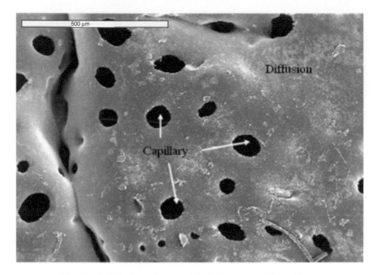

Fig. 10. SEM of a hydrogel with different pore dimensions.

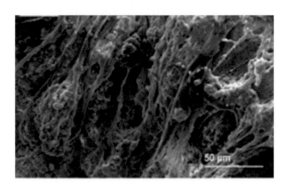

Fig. 11. Fibroblast cells attached on a scaffold surface of an alfa-Elastin hydrogel (Adapted from Annabi et al. 2010).

There are two kinds of porosity within a hydrogel; micro-porosity consists of the pores among individual polymer chains. This porosity is a result of the solvation of the hydrophilic polymer by water, which induces the polymeric chains to swell. The length scale of microporosity is on the order of 10 nm to 100 nm, which is sufficient for the diffusion of water, oxygen, salts, and low molecular weight metabolites. Macro-porosity is on the length scale of 1 μm to 100 μm. Tissue engineered scaffolds require macro-porosity to permit rapid protein diffusion, cellular migration, and ingress of microvessels from surrounding tissue (Fig. 12).

Experiments demonstrated the optimum pore size of 5 μm for neovascularization, 5–15 μm for fibroblast ingrowth, 20–125 μm for regeneration of adult mammalian skin, 100–350 μm for regeneration of bone, 40–100 μm for osteoid ingrowth, and 20 μm for the ingrowth of hepatocytes (Whang et al. 1999). Fibrovascular tissues also require pore sizes greater than 500 μm for rapid vascularization and survival of transplanted cells.

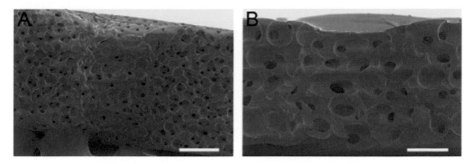

Fig. 12. Porous poly(HEMA) gels with macroporosity (A) 62 μm and (B) 147 μm (Adapted from Annabi 2010).

Several techniques (Wake et al. 1993) have been used to obtain macroporous materials, for instance rapid prototyping techniques (e.g., 3D printing and stereolithography) use software to plot the porous networks which are precisely sculpted in three dimensions by a method suitable to the polymer of interest (Yang et al. 2002) or the use of a particulate leeching strategy such as leeching of salt crystals or microspheres from crosslinked polymer scaffolds (Mikos et al. 1994). The freeze-drying is one of the most widely used methods (Cho et al. 2008). This technique produces matrices with porosity greater than 90% and the pore sizes depend on the growth rate of ice crystals during the freeze-drying process (Dore 2000; Gun'ko et al. 2005). A new technique was developed starting from the already synthesized hydrogel and guaranteeing control of the size of the pores (Barbucci and Leone 2004) (Fig. 13). The porous structure was obtained by stratifying the hydrogels into a cell culture strainer with a defined and controlled drilling. The filter was placed on a beaker containing a porogen salt ($NaHCO_3$) at the bottom. By adding a 0.1 M HCl solution a violent effervescence was produced. The formation of CO_2 bubbles and their passage through the filter, first, and the matrix of hydrogel, second, induced the hydrogel to assume a porous morphology (Table 2).

The degree of porosity generally has a substantial effect on the mechanical properties, with the stiffness of the scaffold decreasing as porosity increases (Gerecht et al. 2007), and the mechanical characteristics varying greatly with fluid flux caused by deformation (Martin et al. 2000). On the contrary the microporous polysaccharide hydrogels obtained starting from the preformed hydrogel, shows a decreased water

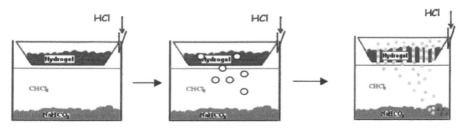

Fig. 13. Disposal and mechanism for the formation of porous hydrogel starting from a preformed hydrogel (Barbucci and Leone 2004).

Table 2. Parameters relative to pores obtained starting from Alginate (AA) Carboxymethylcellulose (CMC) and Hyaluronate crosslinked hydrogels (Barbucci and Leone 2004).

	Materials								
	AA **No pores**			**CMC** **Distance between Laminae:** **76 ± 13 µm**			**Hyal** **No pores**		
Native Hydrogel	**Diameter (µm)**	**Density (pores/mm^2)**	**Thickness (µm)**	**Diameter (µm)**	**Density (pores/mm^2)**	**Thickness (µm)**	**Diameter (µm)**	**Density (pores/mm^2)**	**Thickness (µm)**
Cell strainer (Ø 40 µm)	13 ± 4	5.0 ± 1.5	2.2 ± 1.1	14 ± 4	2.0 ± 0.5	2.7 ± 0.9	15 ± 3	3.0 ± 0,5	1.8 ± 0.9
Cell strainer (Ø 70 µm)	30 ± 2	1.5 ± 0.5	2.4 ± 0.9	30 ± 4	1.50 ± 0.03	2.3 ± 1.4	35 ± 2	1.00 ± 0.01	2.7 ± 0.8
Cell strainer (Ø 100 µm)	40 ± 4	1.5 ± 0.3	2 ± 1	40 ± 9	1.00 ± 0.01	3.7 ± 2.1	40 ± 4	0.50 ± 0.02	0.70 ± 0.05

uptake in comparison with the corresponding native matrices. In fact crossing the hydrogel, the CO_2 bubbles mechanically provoke the approach of the polymeric chains of the hydrogel. Furthermore the acidic CO_2 bubbles crossing the matrix induce a local lowering of pH and provoke the protonation of COO-, with the consequent hydrogen bonds formation (Fig. 14). As a consequence the rheological properties of the porous hydrogels are enhanced compared to the hydrogels without pores (Leone et al. 2004).

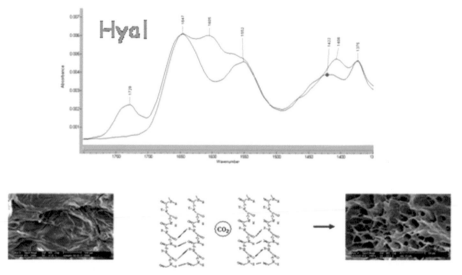

Fig. 14. Infrared spectra of the porous Hyal gel in comparison with that of the native Hydrogel. A new band at 1729 cm⁻¹ appears, ascribed to the protonated carboxylic groups hydrogen bonded Infrared spectra of the porous Hyal gel in comparison with that of the native Hydrogel. A new band at 1729 cm⁻¹ appears ascribed to the protonated carboxylic groups hydrogen bonded (Leone et al. 2004).

The analysis of the porous structure of hydrogels in a freeze-dried state can be carried out by the Confocal Laser Scanning Microscopy (CLSM) which provides information on changes in the hydrogel structure during and/or after drying (Savina et al. 2011) (Fig. 15). Fluorescein isothiocyanate (FITC) stained Poly 2-hydroxyehylmetacrylate-allylglycidylether (HEMA-AGE) gel was freeze-dried and CLSM image of the dried sample was compared with that obtained for hydrated hydrogel. This comparison shows that changes in the porous structure of the gel after freeze-drying were insignificant.

Mechanism of Swelling

In the dried state the hydrogels are a composite of a solid material (polymers and crosslinkers), small amount of water, mainly due to bound water, and air present in the pores, as shown in Fig. 16.

While the swelling capacity of hydrogels is the sole function of the solid content of the composite, the mechanical properties are a function of all elements—solid, liquid,

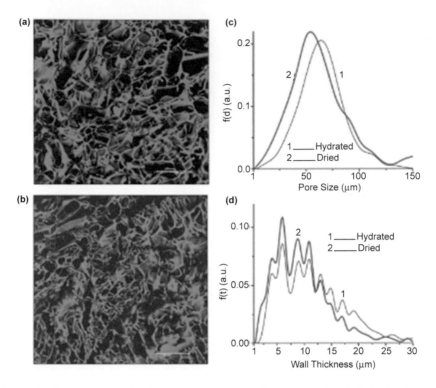

Fig. 15. Confocal Laser Scanning Microscopy images of HEMA-AGE hydrogels in hydrated (a) and dried (b) states with the distribution of pore size (c) and wall thickness (d) (Savina et al. 2011).

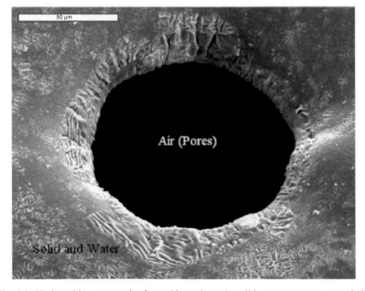

Fig. 16. Hydrogel is a composite formed by polymeric solid component, water and air.

and gas. The solid part provides mechanical property; the liquid and the gaseous parts of the composite weaken the properties by reducing the intermolecular interaction of the polymer chains, which are the only source for the mechanical strength. Higher molecular weight polymers provide better hydrogels swelling and higher mechanical properties.

Considering the hydration process, when the dry hydrogel comes in contact with water, the latter attacks the polymer surface of hydrogel, hydrates the polar groups starting to make up the bound water layer (Barbucci and Pasqui 2013). As soon as the polar groups are hydrated, the network starts to swell, i.e., starts expanding, allowing other solvent molecules to penetrate within the hydrogel network. The polymer chains change their conformation leading to increase the water mobility, while the hydrophobic groups will begin to aggregate among them finding a hostile environment, which is the aqueous one. After this first process where not all the polar groups are hydrated, the network will absorb a further amount of water, due to osmotic pressure that pushes the polymer chains to an infinite dilution. This water goes to hydrate other naked polar groups, forming other bound water layers, and to fill the space between the already hydrated with bound water polymeric chains. This process creates the interstitial water layer. The swelling is opposed by the covalent and physical crosslinks, which give rise to the elastic force. The interstitial water puts both the water and the hydrogel in contact with the external environment because it links the free water, which keeps the characteristics of the water in the bulk. At last, at the equilibrium where the elasticity and osmotic forces are balanced, there is no additional swelling.

Increasing the number of ionic groups in the skeleton of the polymer increases the swelling capacities of hydrogel. This is due to the simultaneous increase of the number of counter-ions inside the gel, which produces an additional osmotic pressure that swells the gel (Flory 1953). Furthermore the ionic polymers lead to a hydrogel with a swelling dependence on ionic strength, inferior mechanical properties, and brittleness in dry and swollen states. The swelling can be suppressed with increasing salt concentration in the external solution, which decreases the concentration difference of the counterions between the inside and outside the gel phase. Figure 17 illustrates the typical swelling behaviour of ionic PAAm hydrogels of various charge densities in water and in aqueous NaCl solutions (Durmaz and Okay 2000). The ionic comonomer used in the hydrogel preparation is 2-acrylamido-2-methylpropane sulfonic acid (AMPS). AMPS sodium salts dissociate completely over the entire pH range so that AMPS Na containing hydrogels exhibit pH-independent swelling. Increase of the AMPS Na content from 0 to 80 mol % results in a 27-fold increase in the hydrogel volume in water. In 1.0 M NaCl solution, the swelling ratio is almost independent on the ionic group content due to screening of charge interactions within the hydrogel.

Several investigations concern the behaviour of no-charged hydrogels such as polyvinyl alcohol (PVA), Guar Gum (GG), polyethylene glycol (PEG), etc. (Gun'ko et al. 2005). It was revealed the clear hydrophilic character of these polymers manifests in the formation of polymer-water hydrogen bonds and in the preferential solvation by water (Varghese et al. 2000). The analysis of hydrogen bond lifetimes has shown that the solvent dynamics near the polymer is slower than in the bulk. This is correlated to the number of hydrogen bonds, which typically increases in the vicinity of the no-charged polymer. Nonionic hydrogels show low to medium pH-independent swelling, less swelling dependency on salt, and good mechanical properties (Xue and Hamley 2002).

Despite the fact that functional groups and ions mainly determine the swelling balance of a hydrogel, the amount and type of crosslinker critically affect the swelling properties (Castelli et al. 2000). For a hydrogel with a given hydrophilic/hydrophobic balance value, fewer crosslinkers result in high swelling. The addition of more crosslinks offsets the driving forces for the swelling, and the hydrogel eventually disintegrates at very high crosslinker concentration. This feature has been utilized in making superdisintegrants, which are used to disintegrate tablet and capsule pharmaceutical dosage forms. Swelling is improved with bifunctional crosslinkers as opposed to tri or more functional crosslinkers. As cross-linking and functionality increases, the hydrogels become more stiff and rigid. While the solid part of the composite controls the swelling forces and pressure, the other two phases, water and air, significantly improve the swelling kinetics.

The water component in the dry composite is bound water that comes from the synthesis step. Generally, the amount of the bound water is about 1–5% and cannot be removed during the drying process; however, freeze-drying the hydrogels can minimize the water. Water can affect the composite properties positively by plasticizing the polymer, which expedites the initial swelling or diffusion process. A negative effect of water is that it reduces the molecular interactions between the polymer chains and the rigidity of the composite. Water can also facilitate hydrolysis and oxidation reactions during hydrogels storage. The air component in the composite facilitates the diffusion of external materials into the polymer structure by reducing the intermolecular interactions between the polymer chains. As shown in Fig. 18 with highly porous superabsorbent hydrogels the interconnected pores provide a rapid diffusion by increasing the capillary action of the transport process.

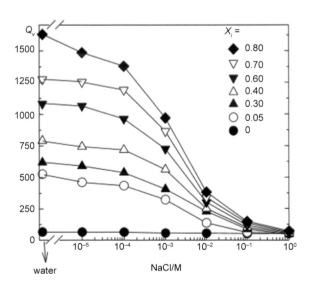

Fig. 17. Swelling of the ionic PAAm hydrogels of various charge densities and in different aqueous NaCl solutions (Durmaz and Okay 2000).

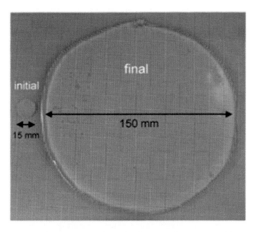

Fig. 18. The typical behaviour of a superadsorbent hydrogel. The native gel is a disk of 15 mm diameter, in water the diameter is 10 times that of the previous one.

Pores are important for purification or any other processes for which a faster mass transport (such as drying) is desired (Arndt et al. 2009; Omidian and Park 2010). Physical and chemical stability of a hydrogel decreases at higher pore concentration. Pores can lose their structural integrity during storage depending on the water content of the hydrogels, the storage temperature, and the relative humidity of the storage environment. The porosity of hydrogel may be divided into four main classes; non-porous, micro-porous, macro-porous and super-porous hydrogels (Dorkoosh et al. 2002). Non-porous gels show molecular size pores equal to the macromolecular correlation length (10–100 A), while micro-porous (100–1000 A) and macro-porous (0.1–1 μm) hydrogels have larger pores. The size of pores in super-porous hydrogels (SPHs) is usually in the range of several hundred micrometers, which are connected to form the open channel system and act as a capillary system, causing a rapid uptake of water into the aqueous solution to equilibrium state in a matter of a minute regardless of their size (Hammer et al. 2013) (Fig. 19). We must always take into account how crucial the dimension of walls between the pores is for the response time. Porous gels swell or shrink very fast compared with nonporous gels of the same size.

Achilleos et al. have developed a technique for the real-time visualization of dynamic deformation profiles during gel swelling processes (Achilleos et al. 2000). The system, which is based on caged photo-activated fluorophores covalently attached to the gel network, can provide quantitative information on transport fields such as polymer deformation and concentration. Based on this technique and other simulations (Kojima et al. 1998), it is obvious that swelling is not a continual process.

On the other hand, in the hydrating hydroxypropylcellulose (HPC) tablet, the growth of the gel layer can clearly be seen, the size of the dry core decreased as more of the table became hydrated. In addition, as shown in Fig. 20 an interface layer between the dry core and the gel layer is clearly recognized (Kojima et al. 1998). It was confirmed through images of MRI that there three moieties: gel layer, interface layer and dry core in the hydrating HPC tablet. One of the very important features of hydrogel swelling is the rate of swelling or swelling kinetics. Osmotic pressure

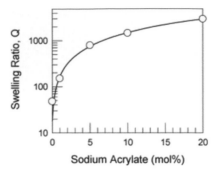

Fig. 19. Swelling ratio (mass of swollen gel/mass of dry sample) of DMAA-SA gels as a function of the sodium acrylate.

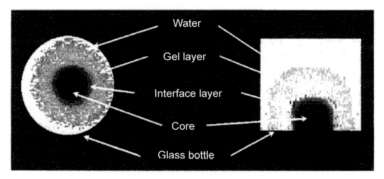

Fig. 20. Hydrating hydroxypropylcellulose (HPC) an interface between the dry core and the gel layer is evident (Adapted from Kojima et al. 1998).

forces, electrostatic forces and viscoelastic restoring forces are the three main forces governing the swelling behaviour of hydrogels. This process is determined, as we said, by several physicochemical factors particularly the sample/particle size, porosity extent and the type of the porous structure.

The diffusion into the hydrogel can be described as a diffusion of different species. A solvent (the swelling agent) has to diffuse into the hydrogel network, meeting the polymeric chains. Their mobility aids the penetration of water inside, through the pores. The relation between the relative rate of penetrant diffusion and relaxation of the polymer chain can be used to distinguish different types of time-dependences of degree of swelling (Q) even if the rate of the hydrogel swelling is mainly determined by how fast polymer chains can relax: Alfrey Jr. et al. have proposed three models for the swelling process (George et al. 2004).

1. Case I or Fickian diffusion: The diffusion is significantly slower than the rate of relaxation of the polymer chains. The change of the degree of swelling is determined by the diffusion of the swelling agent. The mass uptake is proportional to the square root of diffusion time, $Q \sim t^{1/2}$.

2. Case II diffusion: The rate of penetrant diffusion is higher than the relaxation rate of polymer chains. This case is characterized by a mass solvent uptake that is proportional to the time, $Q \sim t$. All that results in a continuous renewable interface between the swollen hydrogel region and the internal not hydrated polymer network (glassy core). This interface moves continuously from the external region to the internal core as the solvent uptake proceeds till to the formation of a fully swollen hydrogel. Generally, more a hydrogel is crosslinked, lower its water uptake is. The absorption process in highly crosslinked hydrogels resembles that occurring for metal mesh. It works like a single diffusion process as the high crosslink density limits polymer chain movement.

3. Case III or anomalous diffusion: Both rates are comparable, $Q \sim t^a$. The exponent of the time dependence amounts between 0.5 and 1.

We must admit a lot of papers discussed this topic and other mathematical formulas were used too, but here we emphasized the different factors regulating the rate of the swelling process in a simple schematic way.

Mechanism of Dehydration

As in the swelling process, the de-swelling mechanism occurs through three different steps, the loss of free water, the loss of interstitial water and at last and only partially the loss of the bound water (Barbucci and Pasqui 2013; Okano 1998) (Fig. 21).

The de-swelling process provokes dehydration with a consequent shrinking of the hydrogel even if complete removal of water molecules doesn't ever occur. By heating

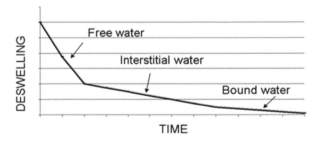

Fig. 21. Typical deswelling of hydrogel versus time graph.

or lyophilizing the hydrogel a further reduction of volume occurs for the further loss of the solvent, mainly from the interstitial and bound layers.

Free water evaporates first from the hydrogel, the interstitial water then begins to evaporate, and the hydrogel transforms into an intermediate state between that of a gel and a glass. When the water content is reduced to less than a boundary level, the hydrogel transforms into a glassy state, with a trace of bound water remaining in the dried polymer. The relative amount of the three types of water varies according

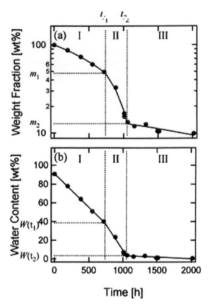

Fig. 22. Weight fractions (a) and fraction of water content (b) of PDMAA hydrogel versus time during the dehydration.

to the water content (Takushi et al. 1990; Koshoubu et al. 1993) and depends on the structure of the polymer network (Fig. 22). Sekine and Ikeda-Fukazawa (Sekine and Ikeda-Fukazawa 2009) analyzed the changes in the Raman scattering spectra of poly-N,N-dimethylacrylamide (PDMAA) hydrogel with natural drying and showed the process of structural changes of water and polymer network with dehydration.

They found that the strength of the hydrogen bonds formed by water decreases with decreasing water content. The bound water in the PAA hydrogel is isolated from the surrounding water, and it primarily forms four strong hydrogen bonds with hydrophilic groups in the side chain of PAA. In contrast, the water in the PDMAA hydrogel coheres and forms a networked structure with weak hydrogen bonding (Fig. 23). It was therefore concluded that the water structure depends on the structure of the functional groups in the polymer side chains, and the effect of the functional groups structure is an important factor for determining the properties of the gel materials.

Using differential scanning calorimetry (DSC) (Ikeda-Fukazawa et al. 2013) it was also observed that the melting temperature of the water in PDMAA hydrogel decreased as the water content decreased Tanaka and Kishi (Tanaka and Mochizuki 2010; Kishi et al. 2009) investigated the thermal properties of several hydrated polymers, including poly(2-methoxyethyl acrylate) and poly(ethylene glycol), and found that the melting temperature of water depended on the molecular species. Furthermore, Kitano (Kitano et al. 2006) analyzed the Raman spectra of amphoteric random copolymers of methacrylic acid (MA) and N-[3-(dimethylamino)propyl] methacrylamide (DMAPMA) with varying ratios of MA and DMAPMA, and found that the water structure changes with the components of the copolymer. These results

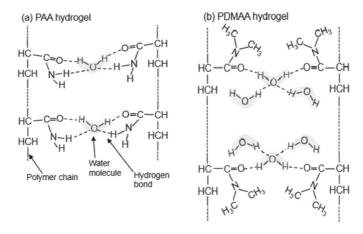

Fig. 23. Structure of PAA and PDMAA with bound water.

confirm that the water structure in hydrogels is sensitive to the polymer species. When the dry hydrogel is reswollen in water, the opposite process occurs, starting from the hydration of the polymeric chains forming the bound water layer and subsequently the establishment of interstitial and free water layers. The composition and disposition of waters inside the polymeric network changes in comparison with those found in the previous process. The uptake of water takes place starting from a dry hydrogel which does not resemble the previous dry hydrogel, of departure. The relocation of

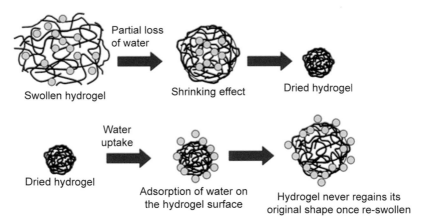

Fig. 24. Sequence of dehydration and rehydration of hydrogel.

the water molecules occurs on a different structural coil. In fact the final volume of the hydrogel results different from that previously seen. The conformation of the polymeric chains, their entanglements and physical interactions are different and the reswelling process occurs differently whenever we rehydrate a dried gel (Fig. 24).

This means that any process of swelling, deswelling, reswelling, while always taking on the same polymeric structure by a chemical point of view, will take place on coils having different conformations, entanglements, interactions and bond strengths of both polymers and crosslinkers.

Drug Entrapment

Intimately connected with the process of swelling/deswelling is the mechanism of drug loading which is particularly important for what is one of the most important applications of hydrogels: drug delivery. Here we will discuss mainly the factors that govern the uptake of the drug into the hydrogel, and omit the issues related to the release of the drug from the same matrix. Drugs can be incorporated into hydrogel matrices by two ways (Lin and Metters 2006) (Fig. 25):

In the post-loading method the hydrogel matrix has been already formed. Generally the hydrogel, in the dry state, comes in contact with a solution containing the drug. The concentration of the solution becomes determinant. A high concentration of drug in solution increases its viscosity and delays the drug diffusion within the hydrogel. For an inert hydrogel system diffusion is the major force for drug uptake and depends on the gel swelling rate or the time it takes to reach equilibrium.

In the *in situ* loading, a polymer precursor solution is mixed with drug or drug-polymer conjugates with or without a crosslinker and allowed to polymerize, trapping the drug within the matrix (Kim et al. 1992). Hydrogel network formulation and drug encapsulation are accomplished simultaneously. The polymerization conditions may have deleterious effects on drug properties and the difficulties in device purification and polymers.

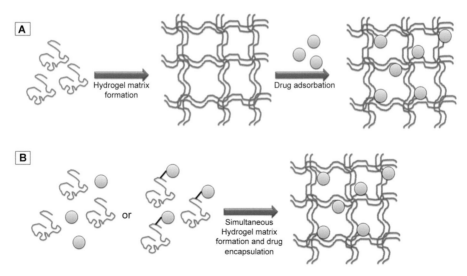

Fig. 25. Schematic representation of (A) post loading and (B) *in situ* loading of drugs into hydrogel network.

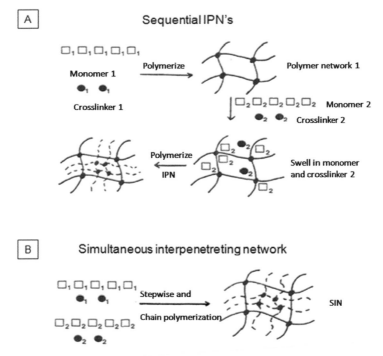

Fig. 26. Two methods of IPN synthesis: (A) sequential and (B) simultaneous (Adapted From Sperling 2011).

A particular class of compounds of this uptake method is represented by the Interpenetrating polymer networks (IPNs), which are capable to show a more efficient drug loading compared to conventional hydrogels. An interpenetrating polymer network is formed when a second hydrogel network is polymerized within an already synthesized hydrogel. Immersing a pre-polymerized hydrogel into a solution of monomers and a polymerization initiator typically does this. IPNs can be formed either in the presence of a cross-linker to produce a fully interpenetrating polymer network (full IPN) or in the absence of a cross-linking mechanism to generate a network of embedded linear polymers entrapped within the original hydrogel (semi-IPN), as illustrated in Fig. 26.

IPN is defined as polymer comprising two or more networks, which are at least partially interlaced on a molecular scale but not covalently bonded to each other and cannot be separated unless chemical bonds are broken (Sperling 1981; Donatelli et al. 1981). The main advantages of IPNs are that relatively dense hydrogel matrices can be produced which feature stiffer and tougher mechanical properties, more widely controllable physical properties, and more efficient drug loading. Drug loading is often performed in conjunction with the polymerization of the interpenetrating hydrogel phase (Mohamadnia et al. 2007). As an example, a lightly crosslinked chitosane-PNIPAM interpenetrating network significantly increased the loading capacity of diclofenac compared to a pure PNIPAM hydrogel (Alvarez-Lorenzo et al. 2005).

Variables Affecting Drug Entrapment

Drug loading is dependent on many variables, such as the molecular weight and charge density of both the drug and hydrogel, degree of cross-linking, nature of the solvent, and mixing conditions. Drug loading (D.L.) range per unit mass of a polymer can be estimated from the following simple relationship:

$$(Vs/Wp)xCo = D.L.limit$$

Where: Vs is the adsorbing solvent,Wp is the dried polymer weight, Co is the drug concentration in solution (Kim et al. 1992).

Cross-linking Degree

Generally as the cross-linking degree increases, the drug loading and release rate decreases due to the reduced effective diffusion coefficient in the post loading method. On the contrary in the *in situ* loading method, higher the concentration of cross-linking agent then higher will be the entrapment efficiency. The higher amount of glutaraldehyde appears to favor the cross-linking reaction, obtained with an increase in loading efficiency.

Interactions

Also the interaction between drug and polymer contributes to increasing loading efficiency (Chuang et al. 2000). Charge interactions between ionic polymers and charged drugs have frequently been employed to increase the strength of the interactions between the gel and a target drug and to improve drug entrapment. Phosphate-functionalized polymers are effective because of their multivalent anionic charge. Phosphate-containing soft contact lenses can bind the cationic drug naphazoline in quantities directly proportional to the phosphate content (Sato et al. 2005). Similarly, the uptake of cationic lysozyme into N-isopropylacrylamide-based hydrogels functionalized with polyoxyethyl phosphate-containing comonomer is significantly enhanced compared to non-functionalized PNIPAM hydrogels (Nakamae et al. 2004). Amino functional groups can similarly be applied to uptake anionic drugs. For example, copolymerization of 4-vinylpyridine or N-(3-aminopropyl) methacrylamide increased the loading of non steroidal anti-inflammatory drugs (NSAID) into a poly(hydroxyethylmethacrylate) hydrogel by more than one order of magnitude (Andrade-Vivero et al. 2007). Both anionic and cationic functional groups typically found in carbohydrate-based polymers can have significant effects on increasing the loading of a drug of opposite charge (Rodriguez et al. 2003). On the other hand, if hydrophobic interaction is a dominant force between the drug and the polymer, relatively hydrophobic polymers are more advantageous in increasing loading efficiency.

Solubility

Using small-molecule as hydrophilic drugs having high solubility's in both the hydrophilic hydrogel matrix and the aqueous solvent, it is relatively simple to load a high quantity of drug into a hydrogel by simple partitioning from a concentrated aqueous drug solution. However, this process is relatively inefficient in the case of large macromolecule drugs (e.g., proteins, nucleic acids, etc.), which have diffusive limitations to their partitioning into a hydrogel phase, or hydrophobic drugs, which are sparingly soluble in both the aqueous and the hydrogel phases. Macromolecular drug uptake is typically restricted by the diffusion of the macromolecular drug payload through the hydrogel network and thus can be addressed at least partially by engineering the pore size of hydrogels.

The problem with hydrophobic drugs is in many respects a more difficult problem given the inherent incompatibility of the hydrophilic hydrogel network and the hydrophobic drug. Thus, the problem of hydrophobic drug use is twofold: how to load the hydrophobic drug into the gel matrix and, once present, how to effectively release the drug into the aqueous gel environment. A variety of strategies have been used to improve hydrophobic drug loading into hydrogels. One simple approach is to form a solid molecular dispersion of a poorly soluble drug, exploiting the enhanced solubility of many hydrophobic compounds in the amorphous state rather than the crystalline state (Zahedi and Lee 2007). By this strategy, drugs are loaded into hydrogels in an appropriate solvent and bind strongly to the polymer chains in the hydrogel via hydrogen bonding interactions, preventing drug recrystallization when the hydrogels are exposed to water and enhancing release of the hydrophobic drug. However, drug recrystallization typically occurs over time, limiting the commercial use of solid molecular dispersions. Instead a variety of strategies for introducing hydrophobic domains directly into otherwise hydrophilic hydrogel networks have permitted significant improvements in the loading of hydrophobic drugs. These strategies foresee random copolymerization of a hydrophobic monomer, grafting of hydrophobic side chains, incorporation of cyclodextrin (Dupinder and Seema 2013).

Furthermore an electrochemistry method for inducing a greater loading of drugs with low affinity to the hydrophilic gel, such as large hydrophobic molecules or macromolecules consists of exploiting the presence of charges on the skeleton of the drug. In this case the gel while being hydrophilic must be non-ionic. The non-ionic hydrogel is pasted on the electrode carrying a charge opposite to that of drug. The electrode is then immersed in the solution and submitted to electrical stimulus (Fantozzi et al. 2010). The drug is convinced to enter into the hydrogel in a substantial amount. By changing the polarity of the electrode a substantial delivery of the drug can be also obtained. The Guar Gum hydrogel, a polysaccharide non ionic hydrogel was used as a drug scaffold that remains inert to the current flow and permits the migration of the ionic drug, bleomycin. However all of these classes of drugs are becoming increasingly important clinically as a result of improved understanding of the molecular basis of disease and the more frequent application of molecular design approaches.

References

Achilleos, E.C., R.K. Prud'homme, K.N. Christodoulou, K.R. Gee and I.G. Kevrekidis. 2000. Dynamic deformation visualization in swelling of polymer gels. Chem. Eng. Sci. 55(17): 3335–3340.

Alvarez-Lorenzo, C. and A. Concheiro. 2002. Reversible adsorption by a pH- and temperature-sensitive acrylic hydrogel. J. Controlled Release. 80(1): 247–257.

Alvarez-Lorenzo, C., A. Concheiro, A.S. Dubovik, N.V. Grinberg, T.V. Burova and V.Y. Grinberg. 2005. Temperature-sensitive chitosan-poly(N-isopropylacrylamide) interpenetrated networks with enhanced loading capacity and controlled release properties. J. Controlled Release. 102(3): 629–641.

Andrade-Vivero, P., E. Fernandez-Gabriel, C. Alvarez-Lorenzo and A. Concheiro. 2007. Improving the loading and release of NSAIDs from pHEMA hydrogels by copolymerization with functionalized monomers. J. Pharm. Sci. 96(4): 802–813.

Arndt, K.F., F. Krahl, S. Richter and G. Steiner. 2009. Swelling-related processes in hydrogels. Hydrogel Sensors and Actuators. 69–136.

Barbucci, R., R. Rappuoli, A. Borzacchiello and L. Ambrosio. 2000. Synthesis, chemical and rheological characterization of new hyaluronic acid-based hydrogels. J. Biomater. Sci. Polym. Ed.11(4): 383–399.

Barbucci, R. and G. Leone. 2004. Formation of defined microporous 3D structures starting from cross-linked hydrogels. J. Biomed. Mater. Res. B Appl. Biomater. 68(2): 117–126.

Barbucci, R., G. Leone, A. Chiumiento, M.E. Di Cocco, G. D'Orazio, R. Gianferri et al. 2006a. Low- and high-resolution nuclear magnetic resonance (NMR) characterisation of hyaluronan-based native and sulfated hydrogels. Carbohydr. Res. 341(11): 1848–1858.

Barbucci, R., G. Leone and S. Lamponi. 2006b. Thixotrophy property of hydrogels to evaluate the cell growing on the inside of the material bulk (Amber effect). J. Biomed. Mater. Res. B Appl. Biomater. 76(1): 33–40.

Barbucci, R. and D. Pasqui. 2013. Hydrogels: characteristics and properties. *In*: Migliaresi, C. and A. Motta (eds.). Scaffolds for Tissue Engineering: Biological Design, Materials and Fabrication. Pan Stanford Publishing, Singapore.

Castelli, F., G. Pitarresi and G. Giammona. 2000. Influence of different parameters on drug release from hydrogel systems to a biomembrane model. Evaluation by differential scanning calorimetry technique. Biomater. 21(8): 821–833.

Chaplin, M.F. 2000. A proposal for the structuring of water. Biophysical Chemistry. 83(3): 211–221.

Cho, C.H., J.F. Eliason and H.W. Matthew. 2008. Application of porous glycosaminoglycan-based scaffolds for expansion of human cord blood stem cells in perfusion culture. J. Biomed. Mat. Res A. 86(1): 98–107.

Chuang Y., M.K. Yen and C.H. Chiang. 2000. Formulation factors in preparing BTM-chitosan microspheres by spray drying method. Int. J. Pharm. 242: 239–242.

Cicero, G., J.C. Grossman, A. Catellani and G. Galli. 2005. Water at a hydrophilic solid surface probed by ab initio molecular dynamics: inhomogeneous thin layers of dense fluid. J. Am. Chem. Soc. 127(18): 6830–6835.

Clegg, J.S. and W. Drost-Hansen. 1991. On the biochemistry and cell physiology of water. Hochachka and Mommsen (eds.). Biochem. Mol. Biol. Fishes. Vol. 1, ed. Elsevier, N.Y.

Das Dipankar and Sagar Pal. 2015. Modified biopolymer dextran based crosslinked hydrogels: application in controlled drug delivery. RSC Adv. Issue 32,5.

Donatelli, A.A., L.H. Sperling and D.A. Thomas. 1976. Interpenetrating Polymer Networks Based on SBR/PS. 1. Control of Morphology by level of Cross-linking. Macromol. 9(4): 671–675.

Dore, J. 2000. Structural studies of water in confined geometry by neutron diffraction. Chem. Phys. 258(2): 327–347.

Dorkoosh, F.A., J.C. Verhoef, G. Borchard, M. Rafiee-Tehrani, J.H.M. Verheijden and H.E. Junginger. 2002. Intestinal absorption of human insulin in pigs using delivery systems based on superporous hydrogel polymers. Int. J. Pharm. 247(1): 47–55.

Dupinder, Ki. and S. Seema. 2013. Variables effecting drug entrapment efficiency of microspheres: a review. Int. Res. J. Pharm. App. Sci. 3(3): 24–28.

Durmaz, S. and O. Okay. 2000. Acrylamide/2-acrylamido-2-methylpropane sulfonic acid sodium salt-based hydrogels: synthesis and characterization. Polym. 41(10): 3693–3704.

Fantozzi, F., E. Arturoni and R. Barbucci. 2010. The effects of the electric fields on hydrogels to achieve antitumoral drug release. Bioelectrochem. 78(2): 191–195.

Ferreira, L., M.M. Vidal and M.H. Gil. 2000. Evaluation of poly(2-hydroxyethyl methacrylate) gels as drug delivery systems at different pH values. Int. J. Pharm. 194(2): 169–180.

Flory, Paul J. 1953. Principle Polym. Chem. Cornell University Press.

Gacesa, P. 1988. Alginates. Carb. Polym. 8: 161–182.

Gates, G., J.P. Harmon, J. Ors and P. Benz. 2003. 2, 3-Dihydroxypropyl methacrylate and 2-hydroxyethyl methacrylate hydrogels: gel structure and transport properties. Polym. 44(1): 215–222.

George, K.A., E. Wentrup-Byrne, D.J. Hill and A.K. Whittaker. 2004. Investigation into the diffusion of water into HEMA-co-MOEP hydrogels. Biomacromol. 5(4): 1194–1199.

Gerecht, S., S.A. Townsend, H. Pressler, H. Zhu, C.L. Nijst, J.P. Bruggeman et al. 2007. A porous photocurable elastomer for cell encapsulation and culture. Biomater. 28(32): 4826–4835.

Gun'ko, V.M., V.V. Turov, V.M. Bogatyrev, V.I. Zarko, R. Leboda, E.V. Goncharuk et al. 2005. Unusual properties of water at hydrophilic/hydrophobic interfaces. Adv. Colloid Interface Sci. 118(1): 125–172.

Gupta, D., C.H. Tator and M.S. Shoichet. 2006. Fast-gelling injectable blend of hyaluronan and methylcellulose for intrathecal, localized delivery to the injured spinal cord. Biomater. 27(11): 2370–2379.

Hammer, J., L.H. Han, X. Tong and F. Yang. 2013. A facile method to fabricate hydrogels with microchannel-like porosity for tissue engineering. Tissue Eng. Part C: Methods. 20(2): 169–176.

Ikeda-Fukazawa, T., N. Ikeda, M. Tabata, M. Hattori, M. Aizawa, S. Yunoki et al. 2013. Effects of crosslinker density on the polymer network structure in poly-N, N-dimethylacrylamide hydrogels. J. Polym. Sci. B: Polym. Phys. 51(13): 1017–1027.

Israelachvili, J.N. and G.E. Adams. 1978. Measurement of forces between two mica surfaces in aqueous electrolyte solutions in the range 0–100 nm. J. Chem.Soc., Faraday Trans. 1: Phys. Chem. Cond. Phas. 74: 975–1001.

Jinchen Sun and T. Huaping. 2013. Alginate-based biomaterials for regenerative medicine applications. Mater. 6: 1285–1309.

Katime, I., E. Díaz de Apodaca, E. Mendizábal and J.E. Puig. 2000. Acrylic acid/methyl methacrylate hydrogels. I. Effect of composition on mechanical and thermodynamic properties. J. Macromol. Sci. Pure Appl. Chem. A37: 307–321.

Khalid, M.N., F. Agnely, N. Yagoubi, J.L. Grossiord and G. Couarraze. 2002. Water state characterization, swelling behavior, thermal and mechanical properties of chitosan based networks. Eur. J. Pharm. Sci. 15(5): 425–432.

Kim, S.W., Y.H. Bae and T. Okano. 1992. Hydrogels: swelling, drug loading, and release. Pharm. Res. 9(3): 283–290.

Kim, S.J., S.J. Park and S.I. Kim. 2003. Synthesis and characteristics of interpenetrating polymer network hydrogels composed of poly(vinyl alcohol) and poly(N-isopropylacrylamide). React. Funct. Polym. 55(1): 61–67.

Kishi, A., M. Tanaka and A. Mochizuki. 2009. Comparative study on water structures in polyHEMA and polyMEA by XRD-DSC simultaneous measurement. J.Appl.Polym. Sci. 111(1): 476–481.

Kitano, H., K. Takaha and M. Gemmei-Ide. 2006. Raman spectroscopic study of the structure of water in aqueous solutions of amphoteric polymers. Phys. Chem. Chem. Phys. 8(10): 1178–1185.

Kojima, M., S. Ando, K. Kataoka, T. Hirota, K. Aoyagi and H. Nakagami. 1998. Magnetic resonance imaging (MRI) study of swelling and water mobility in micronized low-substituted hydroxypropylcellulose matrix tablets. Chem. Pharm. Bull. 46(2): 324–328.

Kollman, P.A. 1977. Noncovalent interactions. Acc. Chem. Res. 10: 365–371.

Koshoubu, N., H. Kanaya, K. Hara, S. Taki, E. Takushi and K. Matsushige. 1993. Variations of mechanical properties in egg white during gel-to-glasslike transition. Jpn. J. Appl. Phys. 32(9R): 4038.

Lee, C.Y., J.A. McCammon and P.J. Rossky. 1984. The structure of liquid water at an extended hydrophobic surface. J. Chem. Phys. 80(9): 4448–4455.

Leone, G., R. Barbucci, A. Borzacchiello, L. Ambrosio, P.A. Netti and C. Migliaresi. 2004. Preparation and physico-chemical characterisation of microporous polysaccharidic hydrogels. J. Mater. Sci. Mater. Med. 15(4): 463–467.

Lin, C.C. and A.T. Metters. 2006. Hydrogels in controlled release formulations: network design and mathematical modelling. Adv. Drug Del. Rev. 58(12): 1379–1408.

Lorenzo, C. and A. Concheiro. 2003. Interactions of ibuprofen with cationic polysaccharides in aqueous dispersions and hydrogels: rheological and diffusional implications. Eur. J. Pharm. Sci. 20(4): 429–438.

Maréchal, Y. 1996. Configurations adopted by H_2O molecules: results from IR spectroscopy. Faraday Discuss. 103: 349–361.

Martens, P. and K.S. Anseth. 2000. Characterization of hydrogels formed from acrylate modified poly(vinyl alcohol) macromers. Polym. 41(21): 7715–7722.

Martin, I., B. Obradovic, S. Treppo, A.J. Grodzinsky, R. Langer, L.E. Freed et al. 2000. Modulation of the mechanical properties of tissue engineered cartilage. Biorheology. 37(1,2): 141–147.

Matricardi, P., F.A. Alhaique and T. Coviello. 2016. Polysaccharide Hydrogels. Pan Stanford Publishing Singapore.

Migliaresi, C. and A. Motta. 2014. Scaffolds for Tissue Engineering: Pan Stanford Publishing, Singapore. 10: 4032.

Mikos, A.G., A.G. Thorsen, L.A. Czerwonka, Y. Bao, R. Langer, D.N. Winslow et al. 1994. Preparation and characterization of poly(L-lactic acid) foams. Polym. 35: 1068–1077.

Mohamadnia, Z., M.J. Zohuriaan-Mehr, K. Kabiri, A. Jamshidi and H. Mobedi. 2007. pH-sensitive IPN hydrogel beads of carrageenan-alginate for controlled drug delivery. J. Bioact. Compat. Polym. 22(3): 342–356.

Mohammed, J.S. and W.L. Murphy. 2009. Bioinspired design of dynamic materials. Adv. Mater. 21(23): 2361–2374.

Nakamae, K., T. Nishino, K. Kato, T. Miyata and A.S. Hoffman. 2004. Synthesis and characterization of stimuli-sensitive hydrogels having a different length of ethylene glycol chains carrying phosphate groups: loading and release of lysozyme. J. Biomater. Sci., Polym. Ed. 15(11): 1435–1446.

Norisuye, T., N. Masui, Y. Kida, D. Ikuta, E. Kokufuta, S. Ito et al. 2002. Small angle neutron scattering studies on structural inhomogeneities in polymer gels: irradiation cross-linked gels vs. chemically cross-linked gels. Polym. 43(19): 5289–5297.

Okano, T. (ed.). 1998. Biorelated Polymers and Gels: Controlled Release and Applications in Biomedical Engineering. Academic Press, Boston.

Omidian, H. and K. Park. 2010. Engineered high swelling hydrogels. pp. 351–374. Biomedical Applications of Hydrogels Handbook. Springer, New York.

Pollack, G. 2001. Cells, Gels and the Engines of Life. Ebner and Sons Publisher. Switzerland.

Pollack, G.H. 2013. The Fourth Phase of Water: Beyond Solid, Liquid, and Vapor. Ebner and Sons Publishers.

Pradas, M.M., J.G. Ribelles, A.S. Aroca, G.G. Ferrer, J.S. Antón and P. Pissis. 2001. Porous poly (2-hydroxyethyl acrylate) hydrogels. Polym. 42(10): 4667–4674.

Qu, X., A. Wirsen and A.C. Albertsson. 2000. Novel pH-sensitive chitosan hydrogels: swelling behavior and states of water. Polym. 41(12): 4589–4598.

Rodriguez, R., C. Alvarez-Lorenzo and A. Concheiro. 2003. Interaction of ibuprofen with cationicpolysaccharides in aqueos dispersion and hydrogels. Rheological and diffusional implication. Eur. J. Pharm. Sci. 20(4-5): 429–438.

Sato, T., R. Uchida, H. Tanigawa, K. Uno and A. Murakami. 2005. Application of polymer gels containing side-chain phosphate groups to drug-delivery contact lenses. J. Appl. Polym. Sci. 98(2): 731–735.

Savina, I.N., V.M. Gun'ko, V.V. Turov, M. Dainiak, G.J. Phillips, I.Y. Galaev et al. 2011. Porous structure and water state in cross-linked polymer and protein cryo-hydrogels. Soft Matter. 7(9): 4276–4283.

Sekine, Y. and T. Ikeda-Fukazawa. 2009. Structural changes of water in a hydrogel during dehydration. J. Chem. Phys. 130(3): 034501.

Sperinde, J.J. and L.G. Griffith. 1997. Synthesis and characterization of enzymatically-cross-linked poly(ethylene glycol) hydrogels. Macromol. 30(18): 5255–5264.

Sperling, L.H. 2011. History of interpenetrating polymer networks starting with Bakelite-based compositions. ACS Sym. Ser. 1080.

Sperling, L.H. 1981. Interpenetrating Polymer Networks and related Materials. Plenum Press, New York, pp. 1–30.

Takushi, E., L. Asato and T. Nakada. 1990. Edible eyeballs from fish. Nat. 345: 298.

Tanaka, M. and A. Mochizuki. 2010. Clarification of the blood compatibility mechanism by controlling the water structure at the blood–poly(meth)acrylate interface. J. Biomater. Sci., Polym. Ed. 21(14): 1849–1863.

Thewlis, J. 1962. Oxford Encyclopaedia Dictionary of Physics, Oxford Pergamon Press.

Varghese, S., A.K. Lele and R.A. Mashelkar. 2000. Designing new thermoreversible gels by molecular tailoring of hydrophilic-hydrophobic interactions. J. Chem. Phys. 112(6): 3063–3070.

Wake, M.C., C.W. Patrick, Jr. and A.G. Mikos. 1993. Pore morphology effects on the fibrovascular tissue growth in porous polymer substrates. Cell Transpl. 3(4): 339–343.

Whang, K., K.E. Healy, D.R. Elenz, E.K. Nam, D.C. Tsai, C.H. Thomas et al. 1999. Engineering bone regeneration with bioabsorbable scaffolds with novel microarchitecture. Tissue Eng. 5(1): 35–51.

Wiggins, P. 2008. Life depends upon two kinds of water. PLoS One. 3(1): 1406.

Xue, W. and I.W. Hamley. 2002. Thermoreversible swelling behaviour of hydrogels based on N-isopropylacrylamide with a hydrophobic comonomer. Polym. 43(10): 3069–3077.

Yang, S., K.F. Leong, Z. Du and C.K. Chua. 2002. The design of scaffolds for use in tissue engineering. Part II. Rapid prototyping techniques. Tissue Eng. 8(1): 1–11.

Yokoyama, F., I. Masada, K. Shimamura, T. Ikawa and K. Monobe. 1986. Morphology and structure of highly elastic poly(vinyl alcohol) hydrogel prepared by repeated freezing-and-melting. Colloid Polym. Sci. 264(7): 595–601.

Zahedi, P. and P.I. Lee. 2007. Solid molecular dispersions of poorly water-soluble drugs in poly(2-hydroxyethyl methacrylate) hydrogels. Eur. J. Pharm. Biopharm. 65(3): 320–328.

CHAPTER 2

The Fate of Thixotropy in Hydrogels

Rolando Barbucci,[1,]* *Emilia Armenia*[2] *and*
Vincenzo Quagliariello[2]

Introduction

Thixotropy is one of the oldest documented rheological phenomena in colloid science even if a general rheological model capable of fully describing the different features of thixotropy has not yet been developed (Barnes 1997). One of the many definitions of thixotropy is reported by Oxford Encyclopedic Dictionary of Physics, *"Thixotropy: Certain materials behave as solids under very small applied stresses but under greater stresses become liquids. When the stresses are removed the material settles back into its original consistency"* (Thewlis 1962).

In 1923, Schalek and Szegvari showed that aqueous iron oxide gels have the remarkable property of becoming completely liquid through gentle shaking alone, to such an extent that the liquified gel is hardly distinguishable from the original sol (Schalek and Szegvari 1923). This characteristic is the basis for the explanation made by Garlaschelli et al. of the famous S. Gennaro miracle in Naples (Garlaschelli et al. 1991). In that case, the Cardinal of Naples applies a shear stress, in the typical blood-liquefaction ceremony; the act of checking whether liquefaction has occurred comprises of repeatedly inverting the glass-walled portable relic case (Fig. 1). Normally our approach to this kind of a

[1] Institute for Polymers, Composite and Biomaterials (IPCB), National Research Council of Italy. Mostra d'Oltremare, Padiglione 20, Viale J.F. Kennedy 54 80125, Napoli, Italy.
[2] Department of Anesthesiological, Surgical and Emergency Sciences, Second University of Naples, Via Costantinopoli 16, 80138, Naples, Italy.
* Corresponding author: rolando.barbucci@ipcb.cnr.it

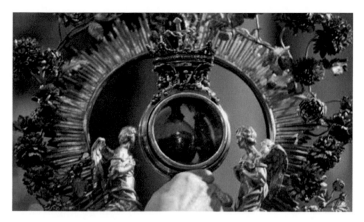

Fig. 1. Reliquary containing the blood of S. Gennaro, which is shown to the faithfuls during the ceremony of blood liquefaction.

phenomena is very skeptical and we try to explain any miracle with science, but in the particular case of san Gennaro's miracle, there isn't any scientific evidence that refutes the miracle. In fact, the ampoule is moved very slowly, and sometimes the phenomenon does not happen even with shaking, and, instead, sometimes the phenomenon happens so fast that is impossible to show it to the faithfuls.

There are several examples of thixotropic materials, including; clays and soil suspensions, creams, drilling muds, flour dough's, flour suspensions, fiber greases, jellies, paints, starch pastes, etc. All these examples are composed of mixtures containing two or more components, in which one has the duty of breaking the network of the second component. This property can be associated with seemingly compact materials such as certain colloids, which form gels when left to stand, but become sols when stirred or shaken. This effect appears in weakly crosslinked or physical gels. The bonds are weak enough to be broken by the mechanical stresses that occur during flow. The result is that during flow, the network breaks down into separate flocs, which can decrease further in size when the strain rate is increased. Reducing the shear rate causes a growth of the flocs, as arresting the flow will allow the particulate network to rebuild. In short, all liquids with microstructure can show thixotropy, because thixotropy only reflects the finite time taken to move from any one state of microstructure to another and back again, whether from different states of flow or to or from rest. A competition between breakdown due to flow stresses and build-up due to in-flow collisions and Brownian motion occurs (Mewis and Wagner 2009).

During the mechanical stress we can observe:

- Alignment of particles in the flow direction
- Loss of junctions in polymers
- Rearrangement of microstructure
- Breakdown of flocs.

On a microscale, we can imagine the picture presented in Fig. 2, where the effect of the mechanical stress on a typical thixotropic material is presented. We start from a

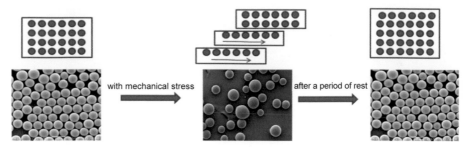

Fig. 2. Schematic drawing that shows the typical reversible behavior of a material with thixotropic properties under a mechanical stress, then after a period of rest (Adapted from Barbucci 2013).

point where the seemingly solid material is made by particles linked among them by the other liquid component of the mixture, i.e., water. Then if the shear rate is applied progressively and sufficient time is allowed for a high enough shear rates to develop; the particles are separated from each other by the breaking of weak interactions of the mixture. In other cases where the thixotropic material is a flocculated suspension, the shear rate determines a floc size decreasing, until at a determined shear stress value the flocs disintegrate completely into their constituent primary particles and become liquid. The capability of polysaccharide-based hydrogels to absorb a large amount of water makes them similar to highly viscous solutions and is the basis of the thixotropic behavior that characterizes some of them. When an appropriate stress is applied (by a rheometer or by squeezing the hydrogel through a syringe), some of the interactions present in the hydrogel break, generating flocs that slide on the water that connects them, with a laminar flux. The system undergoes a reversible gel–sol isothermal transition. Once the stress is removed, the gel structure slowly recovers as a consequence of the Brownian motion of particles (Frendlich and Juliiusberg 1935) and the three-dimensional form of the material is restored. The same phenomenon is observed by squeezing the hydrogel through a syringe (Fig. 3). Figure 4 shows the typical trend of a stress sweep test performed on a polysaccharide-based hydrogel. For low values of oscillation stress, the storage modulus (G') is higher than the viscous one (G"), indicating the gel-like nature of the material. Over the cross-point (i.e., the oscillation stress at which G' and G" have the same value) G" becomes higher than G', which is a characteristic behavior of a liquid. This implies a gel–sol transition of the material. The thixotropic nature of the hydrogel is demonstrated by a double rheological graph, obtained by putting together an increasing and decreasing shear curve. The two curves do not overlap, meaning that the material morphology has changed after the stress sweep test for the breaking of some interactions and the formation of gel flocs. The area within the two curves is called the hysteresis loop and it represents the energy dissipated in the sol–gel transition. Its presence confirms the thixotropic nature of a hydrogel. By increasing and decreasing the applied stress cyclically on the same sample we observe that at the end of the second step the G' and G" values are lower than those at the first step. The same curves and G' and G" values remain in the subsequent stress cycles (Fig. 5). These processes determinate a change in the overall structure of the hydrogel without affecting its chemistry, as demonstrated by NMR and

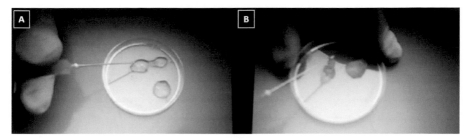

Fig. 3. (A) The hydrogel exits from the syringe needle in liquid form, (B) after few minutes of rest the hydrogel is transformed back into gel and can be lifted from the petri dish.

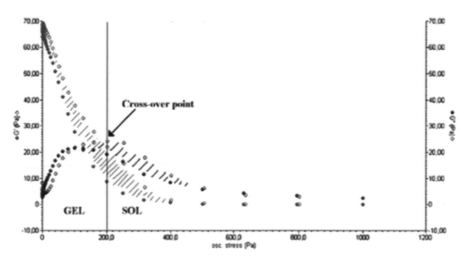

Fig. 4. Elastic (G', red) and viscous (G", blue) moduli versus oscillation stress for a CMC hydrogel in the stress sweep test. The cross over point (G' = G") represents the point at which the sol-gel transition occurs. At the beginning G' > G" and the hydrogel is present in a gel state, after the cross point, G' > G" and the hydrogel is transformed into liquid (Adapted from Camponeschi et al. 2015).

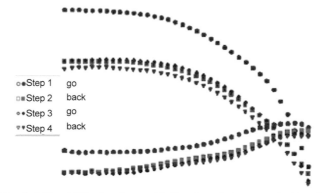

Fig. 5. Typical trend of G' and G" values from oscillation stress during sweep test in a rheometer cycle, performed on a polysaccharide-based hydrogel. The figure shows the G' and G" value versus oscillation stress from each step of the tests (Pasqui et al. 2012).

FT-IR studies. Furthermore the swelling is higher for the squeezed or stressed hydrogel than for the native one. Upon application of a shear stress, such as the passage from a syringe needle, the strength of the interactions present in the hydrogel decreases, making the hydrogel softer. Basically, a different arrangement of water molecules from a bound state to the interstitial state occurs, as ascertained by the curve-fitting analysis of the FT-IR spectra of the swollen polysaccharide hydrogel, leading to a decrease in the mechanical properties of the hydrogels. With native-based hydrogel, the polymer-water interactions occurring via hydrogen bonds are quite strong, and are responsible for the higher values of G' and G" when compared with the same hydrogel squeezed (Pasqui et al. 2012) (Fig. 6). Table 1 highlights the storage modulus and elastic modulus of some polysaccharide hydrogels before and after the passage through the needle of a syringe. Some examples are represented by carboxymethylcellulose (CMC), hyaluronane (Hyal), alginic acid amidated (AAA), carboxymethylcellulose amidated (CMCA) and chitosan hydrogels (Barbucci et al. 2006; Fini et al. 2008; Leone et al. 2008). These properties highlight the injectable nature of these hydrogels, which is a very useful property for biomedical applications. A medical application for the osteoarthritis therapy was envisaged using polysaccharide hydrogels loaded with an anti-inflammatory drug, ibuprofen. The fact that such polysaccharide hydrogels, thanks to their thixotropic properties, can be easily injected *in situ* makes the matter easier. Animals treated with the injection of the Hyal hydrogel-Ibuprofen in the knee joints revealed a repairing mechanism relieving the pain for the patient (Barbucci et al. 2005).

The hysteresis loop is also present in another polysaccharide: Guar Gum, a non-ionic hydrophilic compound extracted from the endospermic seed of a plant (Barbucci et al. 2008). The loop demonstrates the thixotropic nature of the hydrogel. Furthermore, in order to verify visible morphological changes in the structure of the polysaccharide hydrogel and an eventual rearrangement of the structure, SEM analysis were performed before and immediately after the mechanical stress. The native structure of the Guar Gum hydrogel is compact; on the contrary after the mechanical stress the gel shows a porous structure. After four days of settling the gel regained its typical compact native structure (Fig. 7).

AFM analysis was also performed on the same hydrogel to obtain high-resolution images of small areas. The morphology of the native hydrogel is typical of a soft material with different non-homogeneous areas. The morphology of the same Guar Gum hydrogel after being subjected to a shear rate of 700 s^{-1} is completely different.

Table 1. Storage modulus (G') and elastic modulus (G") for 3 different polysaccharide hydrogels in the native form and after being squeezed (Camponeschi et al. 2015).

Hydrogel	State	G' (Pa)		G" (Pa)	
Carboxymethylcellulose	Native	550	±30	25	±1
	Squeezed	240	±20	20	±2
Hyaluronic acid	Native	970	±25	65	±10
	Squeezed	340	±20	45	±5
Chitosan	Native	4350	±650	165	±45
	Squeezed	3460	±150	230	±15

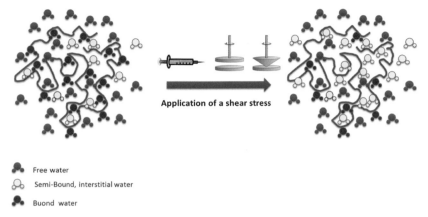

Free water

Semi-Bound, interstitial water

Buond water

Fig. 6. Schematic drawing showing the arrangement of water molecules inside a polysaccharide-based hydrogel in the native state and after a mechanical stress (like a syringe or rheometer). It shows the different arrangement of some water molecules passing from a bound water state to a semi-bound water state (Adapted from Pasqui et al. 2012).

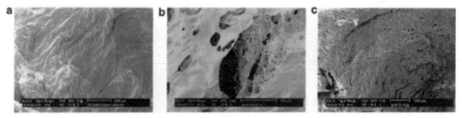

Fig. 7. SEM images of (a) the native GG hydrogel, (b) the GG hydrogel after mechanical stress and (c) the GG hydrogel after 4 days of setting (Barbucci et al. 2008).

The presence of nanoparticles (overall diameter of 27 nm) is observed all over the surface of the gel. Leaving the hydrogel in a quiescent condition for 2, 3 and 24 hr, the particle diameter increases (52 nm) as time elapsed and the particles interpenetrate each other, moving the hydrogel back to its original morphology. After 24 hr, the nanoparticles are present only in a few parts of the surface, while the major parts of the surface are completely rearranged into a homogeneous structure (Fig. 8).

Applications

Interpenetration Hydrogels (IPH)

A new class of hydrogels can be developed, formed by two different thixotropic hydrogels and called Inter Penetrating Hydrogels (IPH) (Barbucci et al. 2011). The preparation procedure is simple because it does not use chemical reactions. Exploiting their thixotropic properties, two hydrogels must be converted to liquid using two independent syringes, so as to mix them mechanically in the liquid form. Another method consists in putting the two hydrogels in the same syringe and then, by moving the piston up and down, avoiding the release of the gels, exerting an adequate pressure

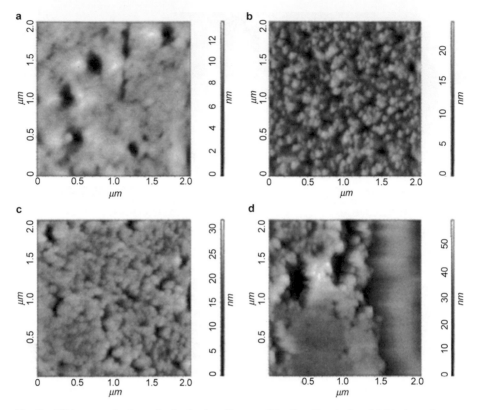

Fig. 8. AFM topography (scan size 2 x 2 micron²) scans of the Guar Gum hydrogel (a) in the native state (b) after 30 min (c) after 2 hr (d) after 24 hr of the steady state flow test. The area analyzed is the same (Barbucci et al. 2008).

on the two gels by the piston in order to allow the contemporaneous transformation of both of them into liquid. Once this transformation has been obtained the liquid escapes from the syringe. After a period of rest the two hydrogels are transformed into a new gel. The gel obtained shows different mechanical, biological and physicochemical properties from the native gels.

The native thixotropic hydrogels used were carboxymethylcellulose (CMC), chitosan (CHT), guar gum (GG) and hyaluronan (Hyal), while the IPHs were CMC-CHT, CMC-GG and CMC-Hyal. Specifically a positively charged hydrogel such as CHT with a negatively charged CMC or two negatively charged hydrogels as CMC and Hyal were mixed. A hydrogel by mixing CMC with a neutral hydrogel (GG) was also prepared. The rheological analysis showed the G' values higher than those of the native hydrogels in the case of the system CMC-CHT, because hydrogels have two opposite charges. The percentage composition that gave the highest G' value was 50%. When hydrogels carrying the same negative charge, such as Hyal and CMC were mixed, the G' values were always lower than those of the native compounds. In contrast the G' value of the CMC-GG IPH continuously decreased as the percentage of GG in

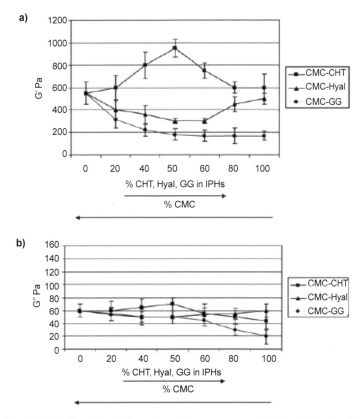

Fig. 9. (a) G' and (b) G'' plotted in relation to the relative percentage of each native hydrogel in the IPHs (Barbucci et al. 2011).

the composition of the hydrogel increased (Fig. 9). The IR spectra of the IPHs show some differences present in the CMC-CHT spectrum with respect to the spectra of each native component. This evidence suggests an interaction between the negatively charged carboxylate groups of CMC and the positively charged amine groups of CHT. On the contrary the spectra of both CMC-Hyal and CMC-GG IPHs containing two negatively charged native hydrogels and a negatively charged polysaccharide CMC with a neutral hydrogel GG respectively, can be considered the sum of the individual spectra of the native hydrogels, indicating the absence of any chemical interaction between the two native components (Barbucci et al. 2011).

If we look now at the behavior of cells on the IPHs, comprised with the native hydrogels, the growth trend of the NIH 3T3, endothelial and fibroblast cells cultured on native and IPH hydrogels was monitored. Figure 10 shows the number of fibroblast cells increased with time with all the IPHs and was constantly higher than that of all the native hydrogels at each time. Cells cultured on the CMC-GG IPH showed the lowest cell proliferation while the CMC-CHT and CMC-Hyal IPHs were the best scaffolds. Of the different compositions of IPHs those containing 50% of each hydrogel component were tested.

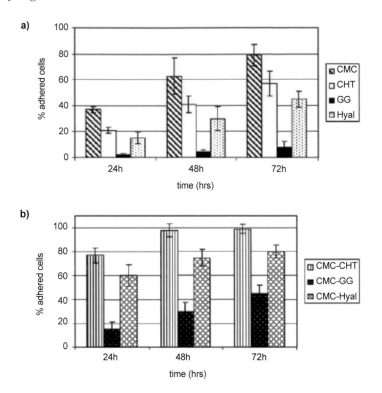

Fig. 10. Percentage of fibroblasts versus time for (a) the native hydrogels and (b) for IPHs (Barbucci et al. 2011).

Hybrid hydrogels with magnetic nanoparticles

Modern science has recently learned how to synthesize a bewildering array of artificial materials with structures engineered at the atomic scale. The smallest particles contain tens or hundreds of atoms, with dimensions on the scale of nanometers, hence nanoparticles (NP). They have the ability to enter, translocate within, and damage living organisms. This ability depends primarily on their small size, which allows them to penetrate physiological barriers and travel within the circulatory systems. Moreover, for several years while nanoparticles have been studied as therapeutic tools, magnetic nanoparticles (MNPs) were applied extensively for local delivery of pharmaceuticals via magnetic drug targeting and via attachment of high affinity ligands. The rationale in cancer treatment for magnetic micro- and nanoparticle based targeting lies in the potential to reduce or eliminate the side effects of chemotherapy drugs by reducing their systemic distribution as well as the possibility of administering lower but more accurately targeted doses of the cytotoxic compounds used in these treatments.

Recently, significant advances have been achieved in the development of magnetic hydrogels, i.e., the combination of hydrogels with micro- and/or nanomagnetic particles that can quickly respond to an external magnetic field, enabling their enhanced controllability. In fact, various biomimetic hydrogels have been employed to mimic the native hydrated microenvironment and to engineer thin or avascular tissues such as skins, cartilages and bladders. Thus the development of magnetic hydrogels holds great potential applications in tissue engineering and cell/drug delivery.

Various chemotherapeutic agents embedded in magnetic hydrogels can target pathological sites via magnetic drug targeting. For example, alginate hydrogels have been embedded with MNPs (iron oxide) to control drug and cell release both *in vitro* and *in vivo* by inducing large deformation and volume changes (over 70%) using an external MF (Zhao et al. 2011).

There are several methods to obtain magnetic nanoparticles entrapped inside hydrogels; MNPs can be directly introduced into the matrix of a preformed hydrogel or they can be added during the gel formation synthesis or alternatively they can be used as crosslinkers among the polymer chains (Fig. 11). For both *in situ* precipitation and the blending method, there are no covalent bonds between the MNPs and the hydrogel networks.

Saslawski et al. reported the preparation of alginate–strontium ferrite microspheres and Liu et al. (Saslawski et al. 1998; Liu et al. 2009) prepared some hydrogel beads with alginate gel cores and shells of magnetic nanoparticles. Liu et al. synthesized magnetic γ-Fe_2O_3 alginate microspheres (Liu et al. 2010) and Brule et al. prepared magnetic microbeads encapsulating a concentrated magnetic fluid composed of iron oxide NPs (diameter 8 nm) with a magnetic core into alginate (Brule et al. 2011).

All these methods share the lack of a specific interaction between the NPs and the polymer matrix allowing the movement of the NPs inside the hydrogels. Moreover the NPs can attract each other with the consequent formation of big aggregates, which

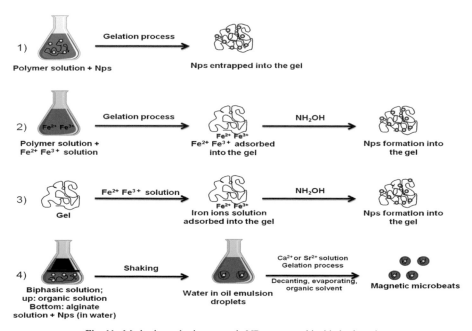

Fig. 11. Methods to obtain magnetic NPs entrapped inside hydrogels.

inhibit the magnetic properties of the gel. In some cases, depending on the size of the NPs and the gel mesh size, magnetic NPs can lift out the hydrogel when exposed to an external magnetic field (Galicia et al. 2009). Thus, the stability of MNPs dispersed within the hydrogels cannot be guaranteed (Burke et al. 2002). These numerous problems can be overcome by using the grafting-onto method. With the grafting-onto method, covalent bonds are formed between polymer network and the MNPs by grafting some functional groups onto the surface of the MNPs, which work as nano-crosslinkers to form a covalent hydrogel.

Yanzhao Zhu et al. (Yanzhao et al. 2012) prepared a novel magnetic hydrogel (ferrohydrogel) based on a thermodynamically stable Pickering emulsion (PE) droplets containing Fe_2O_3 nano-particles based on a work done by Sacanna et al. (Sacanna et al. 2007). They successfully made several stable oil-in-water Pickering Emulsions (PEs) with decent monodispersed nanodroplets. Such emulsions find a way around in homogeneous distribution. The uniform distribution of crosslinking points in the ferrohydrogel network was confirmed by SEM and DTS characterization (Fig. 12).

Dissolution experiments showed that the crosslinking in the ferrohydrogels originated from the siloxane-based shell hydrolyzed from 3-methacryloxypropyl trimethoxysilane (TPM). Ferronano-modified TPM droplets acted as individual, multifunctional crosslinkers in the hydrogel and, therefore, conferred the hydrogel high resistance to relatively harsh environments without a loss of ferronanos and fracturing of the 3D network structure. The microscopic characterization of the gel structure suggested a well-defined network structure, which resulted in its fabulous

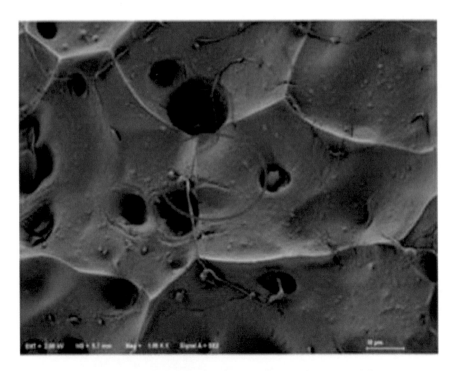

Fig. 12. SEM graph of the Pickering Emulsion (PE) gel (Yanzhao et al. 2015).

mechanical properties. Over and above the effort to make magnetic hydrogels for the drug release shed light on the embedding of MNPs into the hydrogel (Fig. 13). This process includes the following steps:

1. Synthesis of the MNP hydrogel and characterization
2. Encapsulation of drugs in the MNP hydrogel
3. Intravenous injection of the magnetic hydrogel (this point becomes very easy if the hybrid magnetic hydrogels are thixotropic)
4. Targeting to the pathological site via an applied static magnetic field (SMF) gradient
5. Release of drug from magnetic hydrogel via alternating magnetic field (AMF).

Magnetic hybrid hydrogels with functionalized $CoFe_2O_4$ MNPs covalently bonded to a carboxymethylcellulose (CMC) polymer were prepared (Barbucci et al. 2011). The $CoFe_2O_4$ MNPs were modified with an aminopropyl silane to introduce amino groups onto the surface of metal oxide NPs as nano-crosslinkers, which were also bound to the carboxylic groups of the CMC polymer via amide bonds (Fig. 14). The injectability of the hydrogel through a syringe is a witness of its thixotropic nature, this characteristics facilitates the introduction of such materials at the site of application. Steady state flow tests were performed on the hydrogels before and after the passage through a syringe. The yield stress represents the stress that is necessary to overcome the rigidity of the structure, namely to initiate flow. During the steady state flow test, the sample is subjected to an increasing shear stress. In Fig. 15, the shear rate is plotted as a function of the shear stress. The results of the test are reported for the native hybrid hydrogel, for the hydrogel immediately after being squeezed and for the squeezed hydrogel after one hour of rest. A decrease in the yield stress for the hydrogel immediately after squeezing compared to that of the native one was observed. After 1 hr of rest, the squeezed hydrogel showed the same yield stress of the native one. This demonstrates that the material recovers the initial characteristics after a suitable period of time, even maintaining the chemical structure after the passage through the syringe.

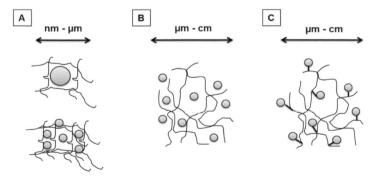

Fig. 13. Combination of nanoparticles and hydrogel to form new functional materials. Three structural designs: (a) micro- or nano sized hydrogel particles stabilizing inorganic or polymer nanoparticles, (b) nanoparticles non covalently immobilized in a hydrogel matrix, and (c) nanoparticles covalently immobilized in hydrogel matrix.

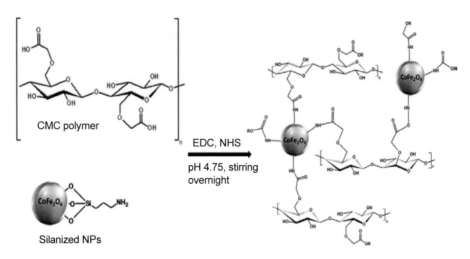

Fig. 14. Reaction for the formation of the CMC-NP hybrid hydrogel. The reaction involves the formation of an amide bond between the carboxylic groups of the polymer and the amine groups of the NP-NH$_2$ (the crosslinker agent) in the presence of N-(3-dimethylaminopropyl)-N-ethylcarbodiimide hydrochloride (EDC) and N-hydroxysuccinimide (NHS) (Barbucci et al. 2011).

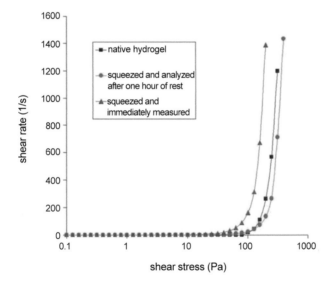

Fig. 15. Steady state flow test of native CMC–NP hydrogel, squeezed and immediately measured, squeezed and analyzed after one hour of rest (Barbucci et al. 2011).

Stress sweep test analyses were also performed to measure the elastic (G') and viscous (G") moduli of the CMC–NP hydrogel. The CMC–NP hydrogel showed a value of the storage modulus G' (1050 Pa) which is higher than the loss modulus G" (80 Pa), demonstrating the gel like nature of the hydrogel formed by using MNPs as crosslinkers. The material was then squeezed again through a syringe needle and once squeezed, showed a value of G' (190 Pa) which was higher than G" (20 Pa) confirming that the sample maintained gel-like characteristics even if both moduli are lower than those of the native hydrogel (Fig. 16). Furthermore, the stress sweep measurements obtained increasing (step 1 and step 3) and decreasing (step 2 and step 4) the applied oscillation stress showed for low values of oscillation stress (between 15 mPa and 400 mPa) the storage modulus is higher than the viscous one (G'>G"). For step 1 a crosspoint (i.e., the oscillation stress at which G' and G" assume the same value) of 70 Pa was found. Above this value the viscous modulus is higher than the storage modulus, a characteristic trend of a liquid. By decreasing the oscillation stress (step 2), G' and G" show lower values than those found during the increase in oscillation stress. At the end of step 2, the G' value is slightly lower than that of the hybrid hydrogel at the beginning of the test. By repeating several times the same sequence of steps (that is increasing and decreasing in the oscillation stress) on the same sample, G' and G" values always follow the same trend of step 2.

Since the chemical structure was not changed by mechanical stress the observed rheological thixotropic behavior was attributed to the movement of water molecules bound to the polymer chains (Barbucci et al. 2011). In particular, the presence of water molecules organized near the polymeric chains (bound water) influences the rheological properties of the hydrogels, making the materials tougher. Under mechanical stress, a partial removal of bound water molecules occurs, making the hydrogel softer (Fig. 6).

In order to verify whether the hybrid hydrogel is capable of working as a drug carrier and depot, some samples were immersed in a water solution containing toluidine blue as a drug model. Once the hydrogel had become blue, it was washed several times with water until no release of dye was observed in the washing water.

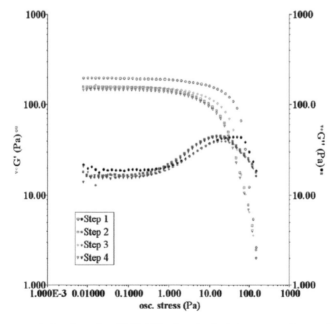

Fig. 16. Stress sweep test performed on CMC–NP hydrogels after being squeezed by a syringe. The figure reports the G' and G" value vs. oscillation stress for each step of the test (Barbucci et al. 2011).

Then the hybrid hydrogel was squeezed through a syringe with the aim of testing its injectability and its capability of keeping the drug inside the hydrogel once injected. Figure 17 shows the hydrogel loaded with toluidine blue after the passage through a syringe in an aqueous solution. It is apparent that the hydrogel is still blue, meaning that the drug is not released when the hydrogel is squeezed through the syringe.

Moreover, a test was carried out to verify the capacity of the hybrid hydrogel to be guided by the use of a magnet capable of producing a magnetic field of 0.4 T, placed outside the beaker. The hydrogel loaded with the drug moves according to the position of the magnet without any release of NPs or dye in the solution. These results show the possible use of the hybrid hydrogel as a drug carrier thanks to its thixotropy, and consequently injectability.

Now the use of an alternating magnetic field (AMF) can be used as a strategy for drug release. As shown in Fig. 18, when AMF (1 mT or 2 mT at 40 kHz) is applied on the system the amount of methylene blue (MB) released from the CMC-MNP is

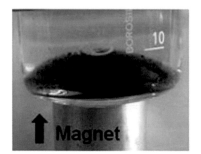
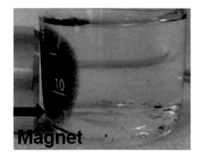

Fig. 17. Images showing the attraction of CMC–NP hydrogels loaded with toluidine blue after being squeezed through a syringe. The magnet is capable to attract the material from the center to the wall of the beaker (Barbucci et al. 2011).

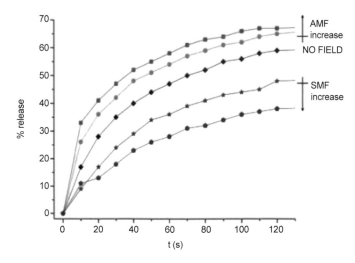

Fig. 18. Release of methylene blue from carboxymethylcellulose-CoFe$_2$O$_4$ with the application of static or alternating magnetic field (Uva et al. 2014).

greater than that released by the same CMC-MNP not exposed to magnetic stimuli. On the contrary by applying a static magnetic field (0.23 T or 0.48 T), the release of the MB is slowed down compared to that obtained without the application of any magnetic field. This system shows the ability to control an increase or a decrease in the release of methylene blue dye using the same hydrogel.

By a cyclic sequence of AMF and SMF applications, it is possible to achieve a modulation of the drug release. Figure 19 shows the release trend of methylene blue from CMC-NP 50 hydrogel under the application of SMF and AMF in sequence (Camponeschi et al. 2015). Furthermore hydrogels with magnetic (Fe_3O_4) NPs used as crosslinkers of polysaccharide chains were investigated for the release of the antitumor DOXO drug (Uva et al. 2015). Using an AMF can significantly enhance the drug release from the hydrogel. On the contrary, the application of a static magnetic field (0.5 T) does not affect the release properties of the CMC-NP (Fe_3O_4) hydrogel.

The release of any molecule from a magnetic hybrid hydrogel depends on the structural modifications occurring in the hydrogel as a consequence of the application of Static Magnetic Field (SMF) or Alternating Magnetic Field (AFM). Field Emission Scanning Electron Microscopy (FE-SEM) analysis of the hydrogels showed a more packed structure with some rough protuberances when a SMF was applied to the hydrogel in comparison to the smooth surface of the native hydrogel (Fig. 20). On the contrary the formation of several pores, cracks and unraveling on the hydrogel surface was observable after the application of AMF.

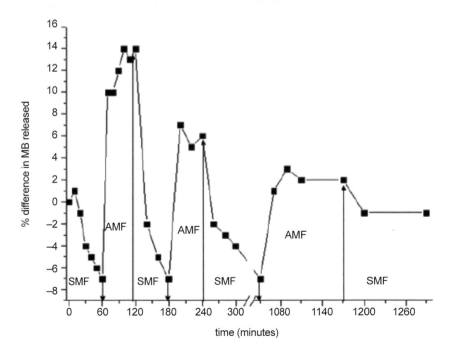

Fig. 19. Release curve of methylene blue from CMC-($CoFe_2O_4$) NP in 0.15 M NaCl under the SMF (0.5 T) and AMF (0.5 T, 4 Hz) applied in sequence (Camponeschi et al. 2015).

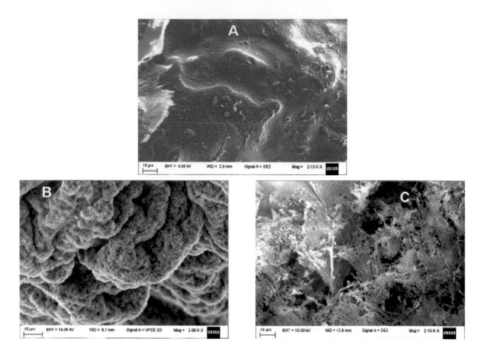

Fig. 20. FE-SEM images of (a) freeze-dried CMC-CoFe$_2$O$_4$ NP, (b) with application of SMF and (c) after AMF (Uva et al. 2014).

The SMF determines a lengthening and thinning of the CoFe$_2$O$_4$ NP hydrogel with the consequent reduction in the pore diameters, thus hindering the release of the drug (Fig. 21). In contrast, AMF determines the formation of fissures and pores, allowing an easier release of the drug. Unexpectedly but strictly consequential, a similar trend for the water uptake of the two hybrid CoFe$_2$O$_4$ NP hydrogels, measured under SMF and AMF, was observed. The water uptake of both the MNP hydrogels under AMF was in fact larger than in the absence of any magnetic field. The water uptake without the application of the magnetic field was, in turn, greater than the value obtained under SMF.

The MNPs in the CMC hydrogel exhibits a hysteretic behavior at room temperature, thus absorbing power from the AMF at any frequency and inducing torques on the NPs, which are transmitted to the polymer strands to which the NPs are covalently bound. This effect only occurs because the MNPs act as crosslinkers, i.e., as nodes of the polymeric network (Fig. 22). The torques induce a strong destruction of the hydrogel morphology. A different trend was observed with Fe$_3$O$_4$ NP hydrogel, where the influence of SMF is null and the line of DOXO release lays on that without any magnetic field (Fig. 23) (Uva et al. 2014). That behavior might be due to the partial strong aggregation of the nanoparticles in the hydrogel, as revealed by FESEM image, which does not allow any modification of the hydrogel material subjected to SMF.

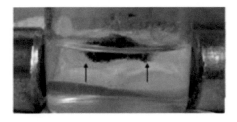
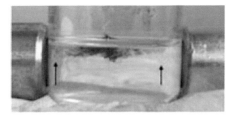

Fig. 21. CMC-NP hydrogel between two opposing permanent magnets at the beginning of the test (to the left) and after some hours (to the right).

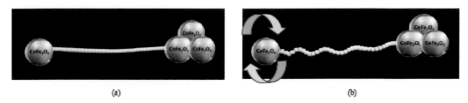

(a)   (b)

Fig. 22. Schematic drawing of a polymer chain with crosslinked nanoparticles (a) without application of AMF and (b) with application of AMF (Uva et al. 2014).

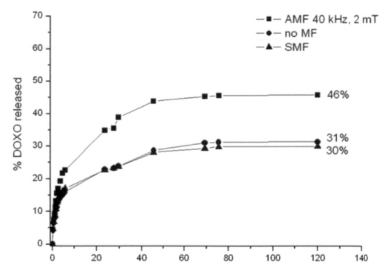

Fig. 23. Release trends of DOXO from CMC-(Fe_3O_4)NPs in NaCl 0.15 M (circles) in the presence of AMF (squares) and with SMF (triangles) (Uva et al. 2015).

Obstacle to Clinical Applications

Although magnetic hydrogels can control pulsatile release of drugs remotely via an external MF, it is currently difficult to delivery drugs to regions within deep tissues as the targeting efficiency depends on the distance between the tumor and the magnets.

In addition, the cytotoxicity and biodegradability of magnetic hydrogels and the long-term fate of embedded MNPs *in vivo* also need to be considered. Even though there are no universal criteria to predict this important aspect of magnetic hydrogels due to their different physicochemical properties, two steps should take place during the clearance of the embedded MNPs, they include:

1. The release of MNPs embedded in hydrogels can be achieved as the hydrogels biodegrade and the cells secrete their own ECM (Xu et al. 2012).
2. The elimination of MNPs out of the body is also required.

Up to now there is little knowledge or discussion on the effect of nanoparticles on organs such as the liver, kidneys, spleen, etc. However, one can speculate that as long as there is translocation to and accumulation of nanoparticles in these organs, potentially adverse reactions and cytotoxicity may lead to disease. For instance, particle debris has been found in the liver of patients with worn orthopedic prosthesis (Milosev et al. 2006) and the injection of magnetic nanoparticles smaller than 100 nm into the tongue and facial muscles of mice resulted in synaptic uptake (Oberdörster et al. 2005). Therefore nanoparticles used by themselves or as crosslinkers of polymers, exploited as beneficial to destroy cancer cells may cause harmful effects elsewhere in the body.

The United States Food and Drug Administration (FDA) has approved the use of MNPs in several clinical applications such as the magnetic resonance imaging (MRI), and these should be rapidly eliminated through the known pathways for Fe metabolism by the reticuloendothelial system (RES), particularly by the liver (LaConte et al. 2005). However, further studies of the biodistribution and elimination of metallic and bimetallic MNPs *in vivo* are needed for more clinical applications. In the case of magnetic hydrogels with MNP as crosslinkers, the MNP will never be found naked but they will appear more frequently wrapped by pieces of polymers, which have not undergone a complete degradation. Thus the process becomes more complicated to study. Surface coatings can render noxious particles nontoxic, while less harmful particles can be made highly toxic. Nickel-ferrite particles, with and without surface oleic acid, show different cytotoxicity (Yin et al. 2005). Spherical gold nanoparticles with various surface coatings are not toxic to human cells, despite the fact that they are internalized (Connor et al. 2005; Goodman et al. 2004). Quantum dots of CdSe can be rendered nontoxic when appropriately coated (Derfus et al. 2004).

The viability and functions of various cell types (stromal cells such as fibroblasts and potential target cells such as endothelial or tumor cells) in the presence of the MNP hybrid hydrogels and the *in vivo* biocompatibility of the hydrogels when implanted subcutaneously in mice were studied, considering the potential use of delivery system for antitumor and vascular targeting drugs (Finetti et al. Unpublished results). On the whole, the results for CMC gel alone, CMC gel + Fe_3O_4 NPs (50%), CMC gel + $CoFe_2O_4$ NPs (50%) and CMC gel + $CoFe_2O_4$ NPs (70%), documented a high biocompatibility of the biomaterials tested with the appearance of toxic effect only by gels containing the higher concentration of nanoparticles which, at the end of the incubation, were retrieved attached on and inside the cells (Fig. 24). In addition tumour cells were shown to be more sensitive, when compared to the other cell lines, to higher concentrations of NPs, thus indicating a potential selective effect toward cancer cells. In the subcutaneous implants (0.5 mg/sample) all the biomaterials were well tolerated.

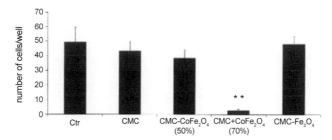

Fig. 24. Endothelial cell number after 7 days incubation with MNP hydrogels (Finetti et al. Unpublished results).

No signs of infection or rejection were observed in the implant location during the 7 day period of the experiment as the implants became progressively infiltrated by fibrovascular tissue. Skin that was in close proximity to all implants was noted to be normal and healthy.

This *in vivo* data document that hybrid hydrogels are processed biologically: although the CMC scaffold is degraded, the MNPs remain in the subcutaneous tissue where they induce inflammatory cell infiltrate at the site of implantation. The use of a low concentration of MNPs embedded in CMC gels could reduce their *in vivo* toxicity. Considering the nature of MNPs, Fe_3O_4 showed a better safety profile, probably due to the slow prolonged release of Co ions from cobalt-ferrite MNPs. This data clearly indicates the possibility of clinical exploitation of CMC hydrogel containing low percentage of MNPs.

References

Barbucci, R., M. Fini, L. Martini, P. Torricelli, R. Giardino, S. Lamponi et al. 2005. Hyaluronic acid hydrogel added with ibuprofen-lysine for the local treatment of chondral lesions in the knee *in vitro* and *in vivo* investigations. Journal of Biomedical Materials Research: Part B—Applied Biomaterials. 75B: 42–48.

Barbucci, R., G. Leone, A. Chiumiento, M.E. Di Cocco, G. D'Orazio, R. Gianferri et al. 2006. Low and high resolution Nuclear Magnetic Resonance (NMR) characterisation of Hyaluronan based native and sulphated hydrogels. Carbohydrate Research 341: 1848–1858.

Barbucci, R., D. Pasqui, R. Favaloro and G. Panariello. 2008. A thixotropic hydrogel from chemically cross-linked guar gum: synthesis, characterization and rheological behaviour. Carbohydrate Research. 343: 3058–3065.

Barbucci, R., D. Pasqui, G. Giani, M. De Cagna, M. Fini, R. Giardino et al. 2011. A novel strategy for engineering hydrogels with ferromagnetic nanoparticles as crosslinkers of the polymer chains. Potential applications as a targeted drug delivery system. Soft Matter. 7: 5558.

Barbucci, R., R. Giardino, M. De Cagna, L. Golini and D. Pasqui. 2011. Inter-penetrating hydrogels (IPHs) as a new class of injectable polysaccharide hydrogels with thixotropic nature and interesting mechanical and biological properties. Soft Matter. 6: 3524–3532.

Barbucci, R. and D. Pasqui. 2013. Hydrogels: characteristics and properties. pp. 337–369. *In*: Migliaresi, C. and A. Motta (eds.). Scaffolds for Tissue Engineering: Biological Design, Materials and Fabrication. Pan Stanford Publishing, Singapore.

Barbucci, R., E. Spera, E. Armenia and V. Quagliariello. submitted for publication. CRC Press. Barnes, Howard A. 1997. Thixotropy a review. J. Non-Newtonian Fluid Mech. 70: 1–33.

Brule, S., M. Levy, C. Wilhelm, D. Letourneur, F. Gazeau, C. Menager et al. 2011. Doxorubicin release triggered by alginate embedded magnetic nanoheaters: a combined therapy. Adv. Mater. 23: 787–790.

Burke, N.A.D., H.D.H. Stover and F.P. Dawson. 2002. Magnetic nanocomposites: preparation and characterization of polymer-coated iron nanoparticles. Chem. Mater. 14: 4752.

Camponeschi, F., A. Atrei, G. Rocchigiani, L. Mencuccini, M. Uva and R. Barbucci. 2015. New Formulations of Polysaccharide-Based Hydrogels for Drug Release and Tissue Engineering. Gels 1: 3–23.

Connor, E.E., J. Mwamuka, A. Gole, C.J. Murphy and M.D. Wyatt. 2005. Gold nanoparticles are taken up by human cells but do not cause acute cytotoxicity. Small. 1(3): 325–7.

Derfus, A.M., W.C.W. Chan and S.N. Bhatia. 2004. Probing the cytotoxicity of semiconductor quantum dots. Nano Lett. 4: 11.

Dong, Y. and S.S. Feng. 2005. Poly(d,l-lactide-co-glycolide)/montmorillonite nanoparticles for oral delivery of anticancer drugs. Biomaterials. 26: 6068.

Fini, F¹, G. Micheletti, L. Bernardi, D. Pettersen, M. Fochi and A. Ricci. 2008. An easy entry to optically active alpha-amino phosphonic acid derivatives using phase-transfer catalysis (PTC). Chem. Commun. (Camb); (36): 4345–7. doi: 10.1039/b807027j. Epub 2008 Jul 21.

Finetti, F., E. Terzuoli, S. Donnini, R. Barbucci, M. Ziche and L. Morbidelli. Biological characterization of biohydrogels with paramagnetic nanoparticles as crosslinkers, unpublished results.

Frendlich, H. and S. Juliiusberg. 1935. Thixotropy, influenced by the orientation of anisometric particles in sols and suspensions. Trans Faraday Soc. 31: 920–921.

Fuhrer, R., E.K. Athanassiou, N.A. Luechinger and W.J. Stark. 2009. Crosslinking metal nanoparticles into the polymer backbone of hydrogels enables preparation of soft, magnetic field-driven actuators with muscle-like flexibility. Small. 5: 383.

Galicia, J.A., F. Cousin, E. Dubois, O. Sandre, V. Cabuil and R. Perzynski. 2009. Static and dynamic structural probing of swollen polyacrylamide ferrogels. Soft Matter. 5: 2614–2624.

Gao, D., H. Xu, M.A. Philbert and R. Kopelman. 2008. Bioeliminable nanohydrogels for drug delivery. Nano Lett. 8: 3320.

Garlaschelli, L., F. Ramaccini and S. Della Sala. 1991. A Thixotropic mixture like the blood of Saint Januarius. Nature. 10: 353.

Goodman, C.M., C.D. McCusker, T. Yilmaz and V.M. Rotello. 2004. Toxicity of gold nanoparticles functionalized with cationic and anionic side chains. Bioconjug. Chem. 15(4): 897–900.

Grief, A.D. and G. Richardson. 2005. Mathematical modelling of magnetically targeted drug delivery. J. Magn. Mater. 293: 455–463.

Jung, C.W. and P. Jacobs. 1995. Physical and chemical properties of superparamagnetic iron oxide MR contrast agents: ferumoxides, ferumoxtran, ferumoxsil. Magnetic Resonance Imaging. 13: 661–674.

Karlsson, H.L., P. Cronholm, J. Gustafsson and L. Moller. 2008. Copper oxide nanoparticles are highly toxic: A comparison between metal oxide nanoparticles and carbon nanotubes. Chemical Research in Toxicology 21: 1726–1732.

Karlsson, H.L., J. Gustafsson, P. Cronholm and L. Moller. 2009. Size-dependent toxicity of metal oxide particles-A comparison between nano- and micrometer size. Toxicology Letters 188: 112–118.

Kim, J.I., C. Chun, B. Kim, J.M. Hong, J.-K. Cho, S.H. Lee et al. 2012. Thermosensitive/magnetic poly(organophosphazene) hydrogel as a long-term magnetic resonance contrast platform. Biomaterials. 33: 218.

LaConte, L., N. Nitin and G. Bao. 2005. Magnetic nanoparticle probes. Mater. Today 8: 32.

Ladet, S., L. David and A. Domard. 2008. Multi-membrane hydrogels. Nature 452: 76.

Leone, G., M. Fini, P. Torricelli, R. Giardino and R. Barbucci. 2008. An amidated carboxymethylcellulose hydrogel for cartilage regeneration. J. Mater. Sci. Mater. Med. 19: 2873–80.

Leone, G., P. Torricelli, A. Chiumiento, A. Facchini and R. Barbucci. 2008. Amidic alginate hydrogel for nucleus pulposus replacement. JBMR-A 84A(2): 391–401.

Liu, H., C. Wang, Q. Gao, J. Chen, B. ren, X. Liu et al. 2009. Facile fabrication of well-defined hydrogel beads with magnetic nanocomposite shells. Int. J. Pharm. 376: 92–98.

Liu, J., Y. Zhang, C. Wan, R. Xu, Z. Chen and N. Gu. 2010. Preparation and characterization of highly luminescent water-soluble CdTe quantum dots as optical temperature probes. J. Phys. Chem. C. 14: 7673–7679.

Liu, T.Y., S.H. Hu, D.M. Liu and S.Y. Chen. 2006. Magnetic-sensitive behavior of intelligent ferrogels for controlled release of drug. Langmuir 22: 5974.

Milosev I, R. Trebse, S. Kovac, A. Cör and V. Pisot. 2006. Survivorship and retrieval analysis of Sikomet metal-on-metal total hip replacements at a mean of seven years. J. Bone Joint Surg. Am. 88(6): 1173–82.

Lubbe, A.S., C. Bergemann, J. Brock and D.G. McClure. 1999. Phisiologic aspect in magnetic drug targeting. J. Magn. Mater. 194: 149–155.

Mewis Jan and J. Wagner Norman. 2009. Thixotropy. Advances in Colloid and Interface Science 147-148: 214–22.

Neuberger, T., B. Schopf, H. Hofmann, M. Hofmann and B. von Rechenberg. 2005. Superparamagnetic nanoparticles for biomedical applications: possibilities and limitations of a new drug delivery system. J. Magn. Mater. 293: 483–496.

Nicodemus, G.D. and S.J. Bryant. 2008. Cell encapsulation in biodegradable hydrogels for tissue engineering applications. Tissue Eng. Part B. 14: 149.

Oberdörster, G[1], A. Maynard, K. Donaldson, V. Castranova, J. Fitzpatrick, K. Ausman et al. 2005. ILSI Research Foundation/Risk Science Institute Nanomaterial Toxicity Screening Working Group. Principles for characterizing the potential human health effects from exposure to nanomaterials: elements of a screening strategy. Part Fibre Toxicol. 2: 8.

Pasqui, D., M. De Cagna and R. Barbucci. 2012. Polysaccharide based hydrogels: the key role of water in affecting mechanical properties. Polymers 4: 1517–1534.

Peppas, N.A., P. Bures, W. Leobandung and H. Ichikawa. 2000. Hydrogels in pharmaceutical formulations. Eur. J. Pharm. Biopharm. 50: 27.

Sacanna, S., W.K. Kegel and A.P. Philipse. 2007. Spontaneous oil-in-water emulsification induced by charge-stabilized dispersions of various inorganic colloids. Langmuir 23: 10486.

Sacanna, S., W.K. Kegel and A.P. Philipse. 2007. Thermodynamically stable pickering emulsions. Phys. Rev. Lett. 98.

Saslawski, O., C. Weigarten, J.P. Benoit and P. Couvreur. 1988. Magnetically responsive microspheres for the pulsed delivery of insulin. LifeSci. 42: 1521–1528.

Schalek, E. and A. Szegvari. 1923. Ueber eisen oxydgallerten. Kolloid-Z. 32: 318–9.

Sun, C., J.S.H. Lee and M. Zhang. 2008. Magnetic nanoparticles in MR imaging and drug delivery. Adv. Drug Delivery Rev. 60: 1252.

Thewlis, J. 1962 (ed.). Oxford Encyclopedia Dictionary of Physics. Pergamon Press, Oxford.

Uva, M., D. Pasqui, L. Mencuccini, S. Fedi and R. Barbucci. 2014. Influence of alternating and static magnetic fields on drug release from hybrid hydrogels containing magnetic nanoparticles. J. Biomater. Nanobiotechnol. 5: 116–127.

Uva, M., L. Mencuccini, A. Atrei, C. Innocenti, E. Fantechi, C. Sangregorio et al. 2015. On the mechanism of drug release from polysaccharide hydrogels cross-linked with magnetite nanoparticles by applying alternating magnetic fields: the case of DOXO. Delivery Gels 1: 24–43.

Xu, F., F. Inci, O. Mullick, U.A. Gurkan, Y. Sung, D. Kavaz et al. 2012. Release of magnetic nanoparticles from cell-encapsulating biodegradable nanobiomaterials. ACS Nano. 2012 Aug 28 6(8): 6640–9. doi:10.1021/nn300902w. Epub 2012 Jul 27.

Yanzhao Zhu, Zhongkui Wu, Hanmin Lu and Zhi Yue. 2012. High-mechanical-strength ferrohydrogels with a magnetically dispersed phase as multifunctional crosslinkers. J. Appl. Polym. 132: 41950.

Yin, H., H.P. Too and G.M. Chow. 2005. The effects of particle size and surface coating on the cytotoxicity of nickel ferrite. Biomaterials 26(29): 5818–26.

Zhao, X., J. Kim, C.A. Cezar, N. Huebsch, K. Lee, K. Bouhadir et al. 2011. Active scaffolds for on-demand drug and cell delivery. Proc. Natl. Acad. Sci. USA. 108: 67.

CHAPTER 3

Hydrogel Network Parameters

Sina Naficy and Geoffrey M. Spinks*

Introduction

Hydrogels are polymeric networks swollen in aqueous media. They encompass a varied group of crosslinked polymeric materials with hydrophilic structures that render them capable of holding large amounts of water within their three-dimensional networks. The hydrogel network can be prepared from monomers and/or polymers via creating covalent or physical crosslinking. Because of this three-dimensional structure, hydrogels exhibit rubber like behaviour, where the network has been diluted with solvent molecules. The final mechanical and diffusive properties of hydrogels are, then, determined by their network structure and the degree of swelling. By tuning the network parameters, hydrogels can be tailored to fulfil most requirements needed for a wide range of different applications. Hence, as the first step in synthesizing new hydrogel materials, it is essential to consider the impact of network parameters on the final performance of the hydrogels. The most important parameters that determine the network structure are directly related to the characteristics of the crosslinks that connect polymer chains together. The concentration of elastically active polymer chains between crosslinking points, the length of these polymer chains, the density of crosslinking points and the distribution of crosslinking points are all network parameters that collectively define the nature of crosslinking. In this chapter, the effects of each of these factors on the mechanical properties, diffusive properties and swelling behaviour of hydrogels are reviewed.

Mechanical Properties of Polymer Networks

A hydrogel can be pictured as a swollen three-dimensional network composed of long polymer chains connected together at crosslinking points. Because of the plasticizing

Innovation Campus, University of Wollongong, NSW, Australia, 2500.
* Corresponding author: gspinks@uow.edu.au

effect of the diluting solvent molecules, the polymer chains of a fully swollen network are in their rubbery state and capable of undergoing large conformational changes in response to external stress or pressure. The effect of diluting molecules on the glass transition temperature, T_g, of a polymer chain has been described with several equations such as the Fox equation:

$$1/T_g = w_s/T_{g,s} + w_p/T_{g,p} \qquad\qquad 1$$

where $T_{g,s}$ and $T_{g,p}$ are the glass transition temperatures of the solvent and dry polymer respectively and w_s and w_p are their respective weight fractions. Table 1 lists common hydrophilic polymers often used to make hydrogels along with their T_g and the amount of water calculated from Equation 1 that is required in their network to reduce the overall T_g to below the freezing point of water. Because water has a very low T_g (−137°C), even small amounts of water can decrease the hydrogel T_g to well below room temperature, causing the polymer chains to enter their rubbery state. Hence, the mechanical performance of a swollen hydrogel closely resembles that of an elastic network diluted with small solvent molecules. To understand the mechanical behaviour of swollen hydrogels and the impact of network parameters on their mechanical properties, it is best to begin with the mechanics of rubber networks.

The mechanical evaluation of a rubber network has been the subject of an extensive body of literature. Conceptually, there are two different approaches to treat mechanical properties of polymeric networks: the *phenomenological approach* and the *molecular approach*. In the latter case, statistical thermodynamics is used to establish a correlation between mechanical properties of a network and network parameters. In the former case, a purely mathematical method is employed to describe the mechanical properties of the network. Here, unlike the molecular approach, the focus is not to explain and interpret the network behaviour, but to develop an accurate mathematical model that can capture the overall mechanical behaviour of the network. Both approaches began and evolved separately, although it is possible to establish some correlation between parameters from different models.

The first comprehensive method to describe the phenomenological behaviour of an elastic structure was developed by Mooney in 1940. Mooney began with the assumptions of rubber incompressibility and Hooke's law to develop a purely mathematical explanation for the strain energy density function of an isotropic elastic network, W (Mooney 1940). The strain energy density function is used to describe the mechanical contribution of network deformation to the overall free energy. Based on

Table 1. List of some of the most commonly used hydrophilic polymers used to make hydrogels, along with their average T_g and the minimum amount of water that is required to shift the T_g of the swollen network to below the freezing point of water.

Commonly used hydrogels	T_g (°C) of dry polymer	Required water content (%) to form a rubbery network
Poly(acrylamide)	165	28
Poly(acrylic acid)	105	22
Poly(2-hydroxyethyl methacrylate)	57	15
Poly(vinyl alcohol)	85	19
Poly(N-isopropylacrylamide)	85–130	19–25

this energy contribution, network deformation can be related to the stresses required to deform that network accordingly. Figure 1 illustrates such an elastic network before and after external stresses are applied. Assuming a deformed rubber network, the extension ratio in each direction, λ_i, is defined as $\lambda_i = l_i/l_{i,o}$. Here, $l_{i,o}$ is the initial dimension of the undeformed network and l_i is the new dimension of the network after deformation (Fig. 1). The special form of the strain energy density function developed by Mooney is:

$$W(\lambda_i,\lambda_j,\lambda_k) = C_1(\lambda_i^2 + \lambda_j^2 + \lambda_k^2 - 3) + C_2(\lambda_i^{-2} + \lambda_j^{-2} + \lambda_k^{-2} - 3) \qquad 2a$$

In Equation 2, C_1 and C_2 are two elastic constants. Another common form of strain energy density function is the Neo-Hookean, which is similar to Equation 2a with $C_2 = 0$:

$$W(\lambda_i,\lambda_j,\lambda_k) = C_1(\lambda_i^2 + \lambda_j^2 + \lambda_k^2 - 3) \qquad 2b$$

A more generalized expression for strain energy density function, W, was later developed by Valanis and Landel (Valanis and Landel 1967) by separating the contribution of extension ratios:

$$W(\lambda_i,\lambda_j,\lambda_k) = w(\lambda_i) + w(\lambda_j) + w(\lambda_k) + A \ln(\lambda_i\lambda_j\lambda_k) \qquad 3$$

where $w(\lambda_i)$ is an energy function which only reflects the contribution of network deformation in the i-direction. The logarithmic term in Equation 3 accounts for network compressibility, and for incompressible networks, where $\lambda_i\lambda_j\lambda_k = 1$, this term is zero. As can be seen, both Mooney and Neo-Hookean expressions for the strain energy density function are specific forms of Equation 3. The principal stresses are then determined as:

$$\sigma_i - \sigma_j = \lambda_i dw(\lambda_i)/d\lambda_i - \lambda_j dw(\lambda_j)/d\lambda_j \qquad 4$$

By defining the strain energy density function in Equation 3 and inserting it into Equation 4, a correlation between applied stresses and the resulting network deformation is established. In addition to the expressions above, other forms of energy density functions such as Rivlin (Rivlin 1948), Ogden (Ogden 1972), Gent (Gent 1996) and Yeoh (Yeoh 1993) can be considered in Equation 4. Here, we use Mooney's expression for the strain energy density function (Equations 2a) to describe

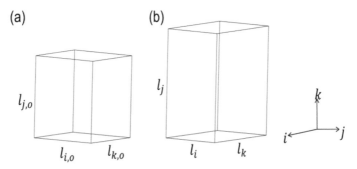

Fig. 1. A dry polymer network before (a) and after (b) deformation.

the stress-strain response of a rubber network undergoing a uniaxial deformation with a magnitude of λ, using Equation 4:

$$\sigma = [2C_1 + 2C_2\lambda^{-1}](\lambda^2 - \lambda^{-1}) \qquad \qquad 5a$$

The same treatment for the Neo-Hookean materials gives:

$$\sigma = 2C_1(\lambda^2 - \lambda^{-1}) \qquad \qquad 5b$$

As can be seen from Equations 5, regardless of the phenomenological expression used to determine the strain energy density function, the two elastic parameters C_1 and C_2 directly control the mechanical behaviour of the network. However, the physical meaning of these parameters and their connection with the network structural parameters can only be derived from the statistical mechanics. The main aim of statistical theories is to establish a relationship between the macroscopic deformation of the network and the resulting conformational changes occurring at the molecular scale.

The original work on the elasticity of polymeric networks from a statistical perspective started by Kuhn in 1936 (Kuhn 1936) and developed by others (Wall 1942; Flory and Rehner 1943; James and Guth 1943; Treloar 1943). In this approach, the Gaussian statistical theory for polymer chains is applied to determine the entropy of deformation of individual polymer chains. It is also assumed that the entropy of the network is the sum of the entropies of the individual polymer chains. Depending on the relation between network deformation and individual chain deformation, two extreme network models are obtained as *the phantom model* and *the affine model*. In both models, when the network is subject to external stresses, the polymer chains will deform accordingly. In the phantom model, however, the polymer chains are able to cross each other and the crosslinking points are allowed to fluctuate freely around their mean positions. When the network is deformed macroscopically, the positions of crosslinking points and their fluctuation domain also deform *affinely*, while the magnitude of their fluctuation remains independent of deformation. Based on these assumptions, the elastic free energy of a deformed network determined by the phantom model, W_{ph}, has the form of the strain energy density function of a Neo-Hookean material, with $C_1 = k_B T \zeta / 2V_o$:

$$W_{ph}(\lambda_i, \lambda_j, \lambda_k) = (k_B T \zeta / 2V_o)(\lambda_i^2 + \lambda_j^2 + \lambda_k^2 - 3) \qquad \qquad 6$$

where k_B is the Boltzmann constant, T is temperature and their product is the fluctuation energy unit. Also, ζ is the number of independent closed loops that construct the network, V_o is the volume of dry network and their ratio is the density of closed loops. In Equation 6, ζ is a network parameter and can be related to the number of crosslinking points, N_c, and the number of polymer chains connecting two adjacent crosslinking points together, v. For an ideal network, this relationship can be simplified as:

$$\zeta = v - N_c + 1 \qquad \qquad 7$$

Unlike the phantom model, the fluctuation of crosslinking points is totally supressed in the affine model. Still, the mean position of crosslinking points deform affinely with the macroscopic deformations. For an incompressible network, the elastic free energy defined by the affine model, W_{af}, also has the form of a Neo-Hookean strain energy density function, with $C_1 = k_B T v / 2V_o$:

$$W_{af}(\lambda_i, \lambda_j, \lambda_k) = (k_B T \upsilon / 2V_o)(\lambda_i^2 + \lambda_j^2 + \lambda_k^2 - 3) \qquad\qquad 8$$

For compressible materials, the logarithmic term in Equation 2 appears in the free energy function of the affine model (Equation 8), with A taken to be $-N_c/V_o$. Again, υ/V_o and N_c/V_o are network parameters determining the density of elastically active chains and degree of crosslinking.

While the phantom and affine models account for two extreme scenarios in which the crosslinking points are treated, other intermediate models have been developed to consider only partial constraints on the crosslinking points. Categorically, these models can be referred to as *the constrained junction affine* models. One widely used model in this category was proposed by Flory and Erman based on a phantom network in which the fluctuations of crosslinking points are spatially hindered by the adjacent chains (Flory 1977; Erman and Flory 1978; Flory 1979; Flory and Erman 1982). The strain energy density function in this case is the sum of two separate energy densities:

$$W = W_{ph} + W_c \qquad\qquad 9a$$

where,

$$W_c = (k_B T \zeta / 2V_o) \sum_n [(1 + g_n) B_n - \ln((B_n + 1)(g_n B_n + 1))] \qquad\qquad 9b$$

$$g_n = \lambda_n^2 [\kappa^{-1} + \zeta(\lambda_n - 1)] \qquad\qquad 9c$$

$$B_n = (\lambda_n - 1)(1 + \lambda_n - \zeta \lambda_n^2)(1 + g_n)^{-2} \qquad\qquad 9d$$

The term W_c in Equation 9a is the free energy contribution of spatial constraints applied to the crosslinking points of a phantom network, while W_{ph} is the free energy function of that phantom network determined by Equation 6. In Equation 9c and 9d, ζ determines the non-affine deformation of the constraint domains, and κ accounts for the extent of spatial restriction applied to the crosslinking points. Depending on how much restriction is applied on the fluctuation of these crosslinking points, the model spans from a phantom network (no restriction: $\kappa \rightarrow 0$) to an affine network (full restriction: $\kappa \rightarrow \infty$ and $\zeta \rightarrow 0$). Note that the Flory-Erman model is a specific form of the Valanis-Landel strain energy density function. The Flory-Erman model was later modified by Erman and Monnerie to apply the constraints to the center of the mass of the polymer chains rather than their crosslinking points only (Erman and Monnerie 1989; 1992).

Other versions of constraint theories have also been developed in which the topological constraints restrict the fluctuation of all units of every polymer chains within the network. The impact of these restrictions on polymer chain movement can be imagined as an uncrossable tube around the polymer strand. The random movement of the polymer segments is limited to the boundaries of these imaginary tubes, and any crossover is penalized. One example of these tube models is the Gaylord-Douglas theory (Gaylord and Douglas 1987; 1990). Similar to the Flory-Erman model, in the Gaylord-Douglas theory the elastic free energy is the summation of two terms: (1) the free energy term originated from a phantom network and (2) a free energy term accounting for tube restriction:

$$W = (k_B T \upsilon / 4V_o)(\lambda_i^2 + \lambda_j^2 + \lambda_k^2 - 3) + \gamma(\lambda_i + \lambda_j + \lambda_k - 3) \qquad\qquad 10$$

The constant γ has a nature of modulus, and determines the deviation of the Gaylord-Douglas model from the phantom model. For $\gamma \rightarrow 0$, Equation 10 reduces to the phantom model. Moreover, γ can vary with swelling ratio and also the synthesizing conditions under which the dry network has been formed.

Regardless of what models are employed to physically explain the macroscopic properties of a polymer network, the only parameters that directly relate the macroscopic deformation of a network to its structural characteristics are the density of elastically active chains, v/V_o, and the density of crosslinking points, N_c/V_o. These two terms are both connected to each other by:

$$N_c/V_o = (2/f)v/V_o \qquad\qquad 11$$

with f representing the functionality of the crosslinking units. Hence, for an ideal network, the defining structural parameters are the nature of the crosslinking points— reflected by f—and the degree of crosslinking—determined as either v/V_o or N_c/V_o. Other parameters that appear in these models, such as κ, ζ or γ remain mostly empirical, since independent information on actual status of the crosslinking points and constraints is hard to directly obtain in the molecular state. In terms of network stiffness, the elastic constant k_BTv/V_o is equivalent to the shear modulus of the dry network, G_o. By defining M_c as the number average of molecular weight of the chains between two adjacent crosslinking points, the shear modulus of a dry network can be determined from M_c and the dry network density, ρ, at any given temperature, T:

$$G_o = \rho RT/M_c \qquad\qquad 12$$

where R is the universal gas constant. In Equation 12, M_c is the only network parameter and can be controlled through the crosslinking process. As the degree of crosslinking increases, the molecular weight between two adjacent crosslink points decreases resulting in an increase in ρ/M_c and increase in network modulus.

Swelling of Polymer Networks

In the previous section, various expressions in which macroscopic deformations are related to the applied stresses have been presented. The source of dimensional deformation in all those theories is assumed to be the external stresses; with linear extension ratios are based on the dimension of the dry network. However, a crosslinked network can also undergo a dimensional deformation in the presence of a swelling agent while there is no external force is applied (swelling). The driving force for this dimension change is the interaction between solvent molecules and the long polymer chains of the network. As the network swells, the configurational entropy of the network decreases while the configurational entropy of the mixture increases. Eventually, equilibrium is reached at which the network is equilibrated in the swelling agent and its degree of swelling remains unchanged. Thermodynamically, this hypotheses has been expressed by Frenkel, Flory and Rehner as the contribution of two additive free energy terms to the overall free energy of the system: (1) the elastic free energy, ΔF_{el}, and (2) the mixing free energy, ΔF_{mix}:

$$\Delta F = \Delta F_{el} + \Delta F_{mix} \qquad\qquad 13$$

By treating the polymer network swollen in the swelling agent similar to its corresponding polymer solution of *uncrosslinked* polymer chains, ΔF_{mix} can be expressed from the classical thermodynamics model, such as the Flory-Huggins expression (Flory 1942; Huggins 1942):

$$\Delta F_{mix} = RT[n_p \ln(\varphi) + n_s \ln(1 - \varphi) + \chi n_s \varphi]$$ 14

where R is the universal gas constant, n_p and n_s are the mole number of polymer chains and solvent molecules, and φ is the volume fraction of the polymer chains. In Equation 14, χ represents the interaction between polymer chains and the solvent molecules and is called the Flory-Huggins constant. Assuming the elastic free energy term in Equation 13 is invariant to swelling, any of the free energy functions described in the previous section can be used for ΔF_{el}.

It is important to note that the same expression for entropy of deformation developed for dry elastic networks can be used for swollen networks as well. The impact of swelling on the entropy of deformation can be accounted for in the same way that any other deformation could alter the entropy term. For instance, for an affine network, the total entropy change, ΔS_t, in passing from the reference state—unstrained, dry state—to any swollen and strained states is:

$$\Delta S_t = (-k_B \upsilon/2V_o)(\lambda_{t,i}^2 + \lambda_{t,j}^2 + \lambda_{t,k}^2 - 3)$$ 15

where $\lambda_{t,n}$, $n = i, j, k$ are the total extension ratios based on the unstrained, unswollen reference dimensions. Now, considering the swelling phenomenon only, the linear extension ratios for an isotropic network in all direction are λ_s, where $\lambda_s = \varphi^{-1/3}$. Here, $1/\varphi$ is in fact the volumetric swelling ratio of the network, defined as $q = V/V_o$. The contribution of swelling to the entropy of deformation with respect to the dry reference state is:

$$\Delta S_s = (-k_B \upsilon/2V_o)(3\lambda_s^2 - 3)$$ 16

The difference between the two entropy terms in Equations 15 and 16 determines the change occurring in entropy of deformation resulted purely from the network deformation of an already swollen network when an external stress is applied:

$$\Delta S' = \Delta S_t - \Delta S_s = (-k_B \upsilon/2V_o)(\lambda_{t,i}^2 + \lambda_{t,j}^2 + \lambda_{t,k}^2 - 3\lambda_s^2)$$ 17

Now, by changing the reference state from the dry, unstrained network to the swollen, unstrained gel, new extension ratios are defined as $\lambda_n = \lambda_{t,n}/\lambda_s$, $n = i, j, k$. Hence, the entropy of deformation per unit volume of a swollen gel, with respect to the new reference state is:

$$\Delta S = \varphi \Delta S' = (-k_B \upsilon/2\lambda_s V_o)(\lambda_i^2 + \lambda_j^2 + \lambda_k^2 - 3)$$ 18

The factor φ that appears before $\Delta S'$ in Equation 18 is to normalize the entropy change per unit volume and accounts for the diluting effect of swelling. The corresponding strain energy density function for the swollen network is:

$$W = -T\Delta S = (k_B T \upsilon/2\lambda_s V_o)(\lambda_i^2 + \lambda_j^2 + \lambda_k^2 - 3)$$ 19

Comparing Equation 19 with Equation 8, it is important to remember that the reference states are different: while in Equation 8, the extension ratios are based on the dry network dimensions, in Equation 19 the undeformed but swollen network is the reference state. The impact of swelling on the mechanical properties of a swollen gel is highlighted by the $1/\lambda_s$ factor in Equation 19. While the modulus of the dry network is $G_o = k_B T \upsilon / V_o$, the swollen network has a reduced modulus of $G = k_B T \upsilon / \lambda_s V_o$. As λ_s is related to the swelling ratio of the network by $\lambda_s = q^{1/3}$, the two moduli are related to each other through the swelling ratio:

$$G = G_o / q^{1/3} \qquad 20$$

The physical meaning of Equation 20 is that swelling only has a diluting effect on the stiffness of the network. Note that the swelling ratio in Equation 20 does not need to be the equilibrium swelling ratio, Q_{eq}. The swelling ratio will reach its equilibrium value when the overall free energy is at a minimum with respect to any change in the number of solvent molecules within the swollen network:

$$\partial \Delta F / \partial n_s = 0 \qquad 21a$$

Equation 21a can be expanded using Equation 13 to obtain:

$$\partial \Delta F_{el} / \partial n_s + \partial \Delta F_m / \partial n_s - 0 \qquad 21b$$

Recalling any of the statistical models presented in the previous section, the elastic free energy term in Equation 21b can be determined as a function of network deformation. When there is no external load applied, the extension ratios resulted from the equilibrium swelling of the network is $\lambda_{s,o}$ which can be related to the free equilibrium swelling ratio of the network, $Q_{eq,o}$ by:

$$\lambda_{s,o} = (Q_{eq,o})^{1/3} \qquad 22$$

For an affine network, the elastic free energy as a function of equilibrium swelling extension ratio is:

$$\Delta F_{el} = (3 V_o / 2)(\rho RT / M_c)(\lambda_{s,o}^2 - 1) \qquad 23$$

Separately, for any swelling ratio the following relationship exists between mole number of solvent molecules per unit volume of dry network, n_s / V_o, and the molar volume of the solvent molecules, v_s:

$$q = 1 + (n_s / V_o) v_s \qquad 24$$

Equation 24 guarantees the molecular incompressibility of the system and is independent of the hypothesis presented in the form of Equation 13. At equilibrium under free swelling conditions $q \rightarrow Q_{eq,o}$ in Equation 24. Now, by inserting Equation 22 in Equation 23, and using Equation 24 to establish a correlation between $Q_{eq,o}$ and n_s, the equilibrium swelling ratio can be determined from Equation 21b and Equation 14 as:

$$\ln\left(1 - \frac{1}{Q_{eq,o}}\right) + \frac{1}{Q_{eq,o}} + \frac{\chi}{Q_{eq,o}^2} + \frac{(\rho v_s / M_c)}{Q_{eq,o}^{1/3}} = 0 \qquad 25$$

Solving Equation 25 for any given χ, v_s and ρ / M_c will give the equilibrium swelling ratio when no external stress is applied. For hydrogels swollen in water v_s is

18.03×10^{-6} m³mol⁻¹ (at 25°C). The interaction between water molecules and network polymer chains determines the value of χ. The degree of crosslinking and the nature of polymer chains determine ρ/M_c. Figure 2 plots equilibrium free swelling ratio of a hydrogel network for various degrees of crosslinking.

From Fig. 2 and Equation 25 the effect of the degree of crosslinking of a network on its equilibrium swelling ratio is clear. Separately, Equation 12 suggests that there is a direct relationship between the degree of crosslinking and the dry modulus of a network. Therefore, it is possible to relate the dry network's modulus directly to the equilibrium swelling ratio of the swollen network. This relationship is power-law in the form of:

$$G_o \sim (Q_{eq,o})^\alpha \qquad\qquad 26$$

where α depends on the polymer-solvent interaction. For a θ-solvent, in which polymer chains are inert to themselves and solvent molecules (monomer-monomer interactions are identical to the monomer-solvent interaction), α is $-8/3$. For an athermal solvent, a perfectly good solvent in which polymer chains are fully solvated, α is -1.75 (Rubinstein and Colby 2003).

It is important to remember that the free equilibrium swelling ratio, $Q_{eq,o}$, is different from the equilibrium swelling ratio of the same network subject to an external stress, Q_{eq}. Indeed, applied external stresses have a direct effect on the equilibrium swelling ratio of the network. Initially, Flory, Rehner and Gee looked at a simple tensile situation and concluded that the equilibrium swelling ratio of a polymer network under uniaxial tensile stress is higher that its free equilibrium swelling ratio: $Q_{eq,o} < Q_{eq}$ (see Flory and Rehner 1944; Gee 1946; Treloar 1950). A more general treatment of this problem was later presented by Treloar in which an homogeneous strain was assumed to act on a polymer network followed by network equilibrium in the solvent (Treloar 1975).

In general, the Flory-Rehner assumption for the total change in free energy of the network-solvent system (Equation 13) along with the molecular incompressibility assumption (Equation 24) are the starting points. In the Flory-Rehner hypothesis, the total change in free energy is the summation of network deformation (entropic)

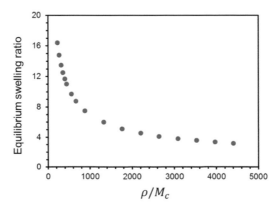

Fig. 2. Theoretical equilibrium free swelling ratio, $Q_{eq,o}$, as a function of ρ/M_c for a hydrogel network with $\chi = 0.1$.

and the contribution from polymer chains and solvent molecules mixing (entropic and enthalpic). Additionally, the external work performed by external stresses on the network-solvent system has to be taken into account. Here, we assume a general scenario in which a swollen network is in equilibrium with its surrounding and solvent molecules can freely enter or leave the network. The swollen network is subject to external stresses as shown in Fig. 3. The equilibrium swelling ratio of this network is Q_{eq}, and by addition of δn_s moles of solvent molecules to the system the network can expand further in all directions. First, we consider a situation in which the addition of δn_s results in a network dimension change only in i-direction: $\lambda_i \neq 0$ and $\lambda_j = \lambda_k = 0$. Hence, the total work done by external force acting in i-direction, f_i, is:

$$\delta W = f_i \delta l_i \qquad 27a$$

where δl_i is the absolute length change in i-direction. In Equation 27a, f_i can be related to the principal stress in i-direction by: $f_i = l_j l_k \sigma_i$, where $l_j l_k$ is the cross-sectional area on which the force is applied. Since the addition of δn_s moles of solvent molecules results in a volume change of $\delta V = v_s \delta n_s$, then $v_s \delta n_s = l_j l_k \delta l_i$. Finally, Equation 27a can be rearranged as:

$$\delta W = \sigma_i v_s \delta n_s \qquad 27b$$

Thermodynamically, for a system under equilibrium condition, any displacement from the equilibrium caused by an external force results in a small change in Helmholtz free energy, $\delta \Delta A$. Under constant temperature assumption, the change in total free energy is equal to external work: $\delta \Delta F = \delta W$. From Equation 27b, this change in total free energy in terms of partial differentiation with respect to added solvent molecules molarity is:

$$\partial \Delta F / \partial n_s = \sigma_i v_s \qquad 28a$$

and from Equation 13 and Equation 28a:

$$\partial \Delta F / \partial n_s = \sigma_i v_s = \partial \Delta F_{el} / \partial n_s + \partial \Delta F_m / \partial n_s \qquad 28b$$

The terms $\partial \Delta F_{el} / \partial n_s$ and $\partial \Delta F_m / \partial n_s$ can be defined separately from the strain energy density function of the network and the Flory-Huggins theory. By differentiating

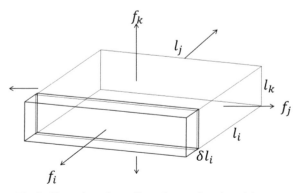

Fig. 3. Illustration of a swollen gel network under axial stress.

ΔF_{el} and ΔF_m with respect to n_s, and inserting into Equation 28b, the final result after rearranging the equation is:

$$\sigma_n = \frac{RT}{v_s}[\ln(1 - 1/Q_{eq}) + 1/Q_{eq} + \chi/Q_{eq}^2 + \lambda_n^2(\rho v_s/M_c)/Q_{eq}^{1/3}], \quad n = i, j, k \qquad 29$$

Equation 29 presents a relationship between equilibrium swelling ratio, applied stresses and extension ratios, the network parameters, M_c and ρ, and the interaction between solvent molecules and polymer chains, χ. Note that the extension ratios appear in Equation 29 are referenced to the initial unloaded dimensions of the network at its swollen state. Equation 29 can be written for all stresses applied in i, j and k direction, and by subtraction these lead to:

$$\sigma_i - \sigma_j = \left(\frac{\rho RT}{M_c}\right)\left(\frac{1}{Q_{eq}}\right)^{1/3}(\lambda_i^2 - \lambda_j^2) \qquad 30a$$

$$\sigma_i - \sigma_k = \left(\frac{\rho RT}{M_c}\right)\left(\frac{1}{Q_{eq}}\right)^{1/3}(\lambda_i^2 - \lambda_k^2) \qquad 30b$$

$$\sigma_j - \sigma_k = \left(\frac{\rho RT}{M_c}\right)\left(\frac{1}{Q_{eq}}\right)^{1/3}(\lambda_j^2 - \lambda_k^2) \qquad 30c$$

Equations 30 are valid for a swollen network at all degrees of swelling, including the equilibrium swelling condition. For a gel with a swelling ratio of q, where $q < Q_{eq}$, the Q_{eq} parameter in Equations 30 should be replaced by q. However, Equations 30 and Equation 29 should be considered together for a network equilibrated in a solvent. The combination of these equations lead to a set of three equations with seven variables: $\lambda_i, \lambda_j, \lambda_k, \sigma_i, \sigma_j, \sigma_k$, and Q_{eq}. The solution for these three equations can only determine three independent, unknown variables. Amongst the seven quantities appeared in these equations, Q_{eq} and extension ratios are interrelated. Hence, three out of seven quantities must be defined as known parameters and the rest will be determined by solving the set of equations. For instance, for a swollen network subject to known external stresses, σ_i, σ_j and σ_k, Equations 29 and 30 can be solved to determine the network deformation and swelling ratio of the network in equilibrium state. Two commonly occurring situations are uniaxial stress (either tensile or compression) and biaxial stress. In uniaxial stress $\sigma_i = \sigma$, while $\sigma_j = \sigma_k = 0$ and $\lambda_j = \lambda_k$. In biaxial stress $\sigma_i = 0$, $\sigma_j = \sigma_k = \sigma$ and $\lambda_j = \lambda_k$. By applying these conditions, simple relations can be derived between network deformation and equilibrium swelling ratio for, respectively, uniaxial and biaxial cases:

$$[\ln(1 - 1/Q_{eq}) + 1/Q_{eq} + \chi/Q_{eq}^2 + (\rho v_s/M_c)/(Q_{eq}^{1/3}\lambda_i)] = 0 \qquad 31a$$

$$[\ln(1 - 1/Q_{eq}) + 1/Q_{eq} + \chi/Q_{eq}^2 + (\tfrac{\rho v_s}{M_c})/(Q_{eq}^{1/3}\lambda_j^4)] = 0 \qquad 31b$$

The relation between equilibrium swelling ratio and network deformation can be better understood from Fig. 4, where Q_{eq} is plotted as a function of extension ratio in the direction of the applied stress. In Fig. 4, when $\lambda > 1$ the network is subject to a tensile stress and when $\lambda < 1$ the network is subject to a compression stress. By

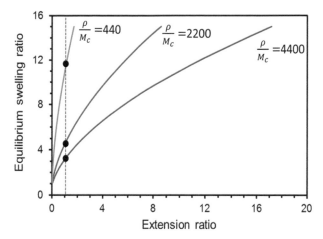

Fig. 4. Theoretical equilibrium swelling ratio, Q_{eq}, as a function of linear extension ratio for a swollen hydrogel subject to an uniaxial stress. The curves are obtained from Equation 31a for $\chi = 0.1$. The dotted line represents $\lambda = 1$ and the filled circles show the equilibrium state when no external stress is applied:
$$Q_{eq} = Q_{eq,o}.$$

increasing the magnitude of applied stress, λ goes further away from 1. Clearly, when $\lambda = 1$ there is no external force applied to the network and $Q_{eq} = Q_{eq,o}$. The dotted line in Fig. 4 represents $\lambda = 1$ and separates the tensile and compression regions. The black circles obtained at the interception of $\lambda = 1$ line with each curve show $Q_{eq,o}$ for networks with different degree of crosslinking. Here, ρ/M_c is a network parameter and is proportional to the degree of crosslinking. When an external stress is applied to a network, the equilibrium swelling ratio begins to deviate from $Q_{eq,o}$, following the curve that corresponds to that network's ρ/M_c value. Depending on whether the stress is tensile or compression, the equilibrium swelling ratio will shift to, respectively, right or left side of the curve. Also, for highly crosslinked networks, the equilibrium swelling ratio is less sensitive to the network deformation than in the case of loosely crosslinked networks.

To illustrate the impact of swelling ratio on the mechanical behaviour of swollen polymer networks, Fig. 5 presents a series of stress-extension curves for a network subject to uniaxial stresses. Three different conditions are considered here: (1) a uniaxial extension is applied to a dry network, (2) the same network is brought to contact with a swelling agent until equilibrium is reached, followed by tensile extension at a constant swelling ratio, such as can occur during fast stretching, (3) similarly, the tensile extension is performed slowly on the swollen network so that enough time is allowed to reach the new equilibrium points during the execution of the tensile test. The behaviour of the dry network under a uniaxial stress can be captured by any of the relevant equations in section two of this chapter. For the swollen network, however, the swelling ratio can vary with network deformation, as shown in Fig. 5. In reality this can happen when the mechanical deformation takes place over an extended period of time, e.g., when a very slow tensile test is undertaken. On the other hand, the swelling

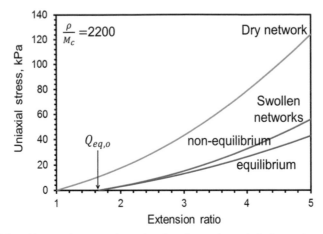

Fig. 5. Uniaxial tensile stress (true stress) as a function of extension ratio (referenced to undeformed dry network) for a polymer network in its dry state, and swollen state. For the swollen network, when the equilibrium swelling ratio is reached under no external force ($Q_{eq,o}$), the network can be subject to a fast uniaxial deformation (non-equilibrium) or a slow uniaxial deformation (equilibrium). In the former case, the swelling ratio remains unchanged during the test ($q = Q_{eq,o}$), while in the latter case at every single point of the experiment a new equilibrium swelling ratio is reached ($q = Q_{eq}$).

ratio can remain unchanged when a sudden mechanical deformation is inflicted to the network, e.g., when the tensile test is performed at high extension rates.

It is worth to note that, as the network is stretched (by swelling or mechanical deformation) the polymer chains are being extended as well. Eventually, the polymer chains are fully extended and no further deformation is possible. After this point, a sudden increase in the network's modulus is expected. Various treatments for this limited extensibility of the networks are available, such as by Gent (Gent 1996), but are not considered further here.

Mesh Size and Diffusion Coefficient

Transport properties of the hydrogels are also controlled directly by the network parameters. The rate of diffusion of small molecules through the network and the size of molecules that can pass through the network will depend on the crosslink density. These properties are important because in many hydrogel applications the polymer network is required to either swell/deswell in response to the environment or to uptake/ release small molecules. Therefore, the rate of diffusion of small molecules through the network will determine the kinetics of swelling/deswelling and uptake/release. The diffusion of molecules through the polymer network takes place through the space available between polymer chains. The length scale of this space is called the mesh size. Depending on the structure of the polymer network, the mesh size can range from a few nanometers, for homogeneously crosslinked defectless networks, up to submicrons or even larger, for heterogeneous networks with structural defects. Also, because of the topological distribution of polymer chains, there is no single value for a network's mesh size. There are various definitions for the mesh size (Fig. 6), one of which is to consider it equivalent of the correlation length in polymer solutions, ξ. In length scales smaller than ξ, monomers are mainly surrounded with solvent molecules. To reach another monomer (either as part of the same chain or an adjacent chain) the distance needs to be travelled is greater than ξ. A similar concept can be adapted for polymer networks, where ξ becomes the mesh size of that network. Based on this definition, the average mesh size of a network at any given swollen state depends on the extent of swelling, q:

$$\xi \sim q^{\beta_1} \qquad\qquad 32$$

In Equation 32, β_1 is a positive value and depends on the quality of the solvent. For polymer chains solvated in good solvents β_1 is 0.76 (Rubinstein and Colby 2003). The mesh size can also be defined as the average distance between two adjacent crosslinking points, R_c:

$$R_c \sim M_c^{1/2} q^{\beta_2} \qquad\qquad 33$$

In this case, β_2 is 0.12 and M_c is the average molecular weight between two adjacent crosslink points which is controlled by the network synthesis. Both Equations 32 and 33 establish a correlation between swelling ratio, network parameters and mesh size of a network at any given swelling state. When the swelling ratio reaches its equilibrium value, $q \to Q_{eq,o}$ for equilibrium free swelling and $q \to Q_{eq}$ for equilibrium swelling under external stresses, Equations 25 and 31 must be used to replace q in Equations 32 and 33 with, respectively, $Q_{eq,o}$ and Q_{eq}:

The magnitude of the mesh size of a network can be considered as one of the main limiting parameters by which the maximum size of molecules that can pass through the swollen network is determined. For instance, for a free swollen network in equilibrium with its surroundings, a smaller crosslink density results in larger M_c values and therefore larger swelling ratios (Equation 25), which in turn results in an increase in mesh size (either Equation 32 or Equation 33). Another indirect conclusion from the effect of external stresses on the swelling ratio is that theoretically it is possible to impact the mesh size of a swollen network through external constraints, although this effect is practically negligible.

The diffusion coefficient of small molecules passing through the swollen network can be expressed from various perspectives. In *the obstruction effect* models, the polymer network is treated as a solid intertwined network which increases the diffusion

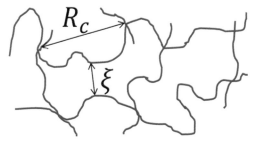

Fig. 6. Schematic representation of ξ and R_c. Depending on the definition, the mesh size can be defined by ξ or R_c. In a swollen polymer network, both parameters are directly related to the degree of swelling.

pathway of small molecules. This assumption is valid if the polymer chains' self-diffusion is much smaller than that of the diffusants. This concept was first introduced by Fricke in 1924 (Fricke 1924) and later various forms of it were developed. In general, for all obstruction effect models, the diffusion coefficient, D, of small molecules diffusing through a network swollen with a swelling agent is expressed as a function of that network's swelling ratio, q, and the diffusion coefficient of the same small molecules in the pure swelling agent, D_o:

$$\frac{D}{D_o} = F(q) \tag{34}$$

For a swollen network equilibrated in the swelling agent $q = Q_{eq}$. Now, the $F(Q_{eq})$ function in Equation 34 determines how equilibrium swelling ratio of a network — which is controlled by the network parameters—affects the diffusion process. For simplified Maxwell-Fricke model (Pickup and Blum 1989), $F(Q_{eq})$ is:

$$F(Q_{eq}) = \frac{\Psi Q_{eq}}{\Psi Q_{eq} + 1} \tag{35}$$

where Ψ is a shape factor for the diffusing molecules (ranging from 1.5 for rods to 2 for spheres). In the Mackie-Meares approach (Mackie and Meares 1955), which is based on a simple cubic lattice model, the $F(Q_{eq})$ function becomes:

$$F(Q_{eq}) = \left[\frac{1 - Q_{eq}^{-1}}{1 + Q_{eq}^{-1}} \right]^2 \tag{36}$$

In both Equations 35 and 36, the effect of diffusant size on the reduced diffusion coefficient has been neglected. Other models such as Ogston (Ogston et al. 1973), however, account for the size of diffusant by incorporating the hydrodynamic radius of the diffusing agent into the $F(Q_{eq})$ function. Another approach to define the diffusion coefficient in a swollen network is based *the hydrodynamic* theories, where the interactions between the solute, the solvent and the polymer chains are taken into account. Regardless of what model is used to determine the diffusion coefficient, however, the swelling ratio of the network always plays the central role. Therefore, any factor(s) that affect the equilibrium swelling ratio will have a direct impact on the diffusion process.

Hydrogel Toughness

Finally, the effect of network parameters on toughness is considered. Many applications for hydrogels require a reasonable degree of mechanical robustness to operate without failure when exposed to external stresses. Mechanical failure often occurs by a fracture process where a macroscopic sized crack propagates through the material causing it to separate into two or more fragments. The resistance to crack propagation through a material is the definition of a material's toughness and is quantified as the energy needed to propagate the crack by a given increase in area. Until recently, synthetic hydrogels have been considered to be very brittle materials with toughness values (or 'fracture energies') as low as $1–10$ Jm^{-2}. Newly discovered strategies to toughen hydrogels (Zhao 2014) have been very successful with several examples giving fracture energies exceeding 1000 Jm^{-2} and even approaching 10,000 Jm^{-2}. These improvements have also encouraged interest in the fundamental mechanisms involved in fracture of gels and these studies highlight the role of the network parameters (Xin et al. 2013).

The Lake-Thomas description of fracture in rubbers (Lake and Thomas 1967) provides a basis for linking network parameters to toughness. Fracture is assumed to involve a process where the network strands that span the crack plane are fully extended and subsequently broken as the crack propagates. The energy dissipated during crack growth is taken as equivalent to the energy needed to fully extend the network strands such that the strain energy per backbone bond in the network strands is equivalent to the bond dissociation energy, U. Longer strands contain more backbone bonds so they will dissipate more energy during fracture. It is important to note that while only one backbone bond actually breaks, the energy dissipated comes from entire elastic energy stored in the stretched network strand since all this energy is lost at the point of bond scission. The elastomer toughness, $G_{c,o}$, depends both on the length of the network strands between crosslinks and on the number of strands that cross the fracture plane:

$$G_{c,o} = \left(\frac{3}{8}\right)^{1/2} CdU \qquad 37$$

where U is backbone bond dissociation energy (Jmol^{-1}), C is concentration of backbone bonds in the unstrained network (molm^{-3}), and d is the unstrained width of the damage zone (m). The concentration of backbone bonds is obtained from ρ/M_o, where ρ is the dry polymer density and M_o is strand average molecular weight divided by the number of backbone bonds. The width of the fracture zone is taken as the unstrained end-end length of the strands. In a dry elastomer this length is estimated based on Gaussian strands:

$$d = n_r^{1/2} r l_r = z^{1/2} n^{1/2} b \qquad 38$$

where n_r and l_r are the number and length of rigid links per strand. The network strands have on average n backbone bonds of length b such that $z = n/n_r = l_r/b$ is the number of backbone bonds per rigid link, which is referred to as the characteristic ratio. By assuming that each strand rigid length is a cube with volume l_r^3 the strand volume is $z^2 n b^3$ with mass $n M_o/N_A$ where N_A is Avogadro's number. The number of strand units per rigid link is estimated from:

$$z = \left(\frac{M_o}{N_A \rho b^3}\right)^{1/2} \qquad 39$$

The network toughness is then given by:

$$G_{c,o} = \left(\frac{3}{8}\right)^{1/2} \frac{\rho}{M_o} Z^{1/2} b U n^{1/2} \qquad 40$$

As illustrated by Equation 40, the fracture energy of unswollen rubbers is predicted to increase with increasing strand length (n), or decreasing crosslink density.

The effect of solvent swelling on the network toughness can also be accommodated in the Lake-Thomas approach. Swelling causes a decrease in the concentration of backbone bonds ($C^* = \rho/M_oq$) and an increase in the width of the unstrained damage zone with isotropic swelling to a volumetric swelling degree of q giving:

$$d^* = z^{1/2}n^{1/2}b\left(\frac{q}{q_o}\right)^{1/3}$$ 41

q_o is the swelling ratio at which the network is synthesised and where the network strands are assumed to be in their relaxed, random coil conformations. q is the swelling ratio at which the fracture energies is measured, and may or may not be the equilibrium swelling degree (i.e., $q \leq Q_{eq,o}$). The predicted fracture energy of a solvent-swollen elastomer is then:

$$G_c = \left(\frac{3}{8}\right)^{1/2}\frac{\rho}{M_o}\left(\frac{1}{q}\right)^{2/3}\left(\frac{1}{q_o}\right)^{1/3}z^{1/2}bUn^{1/2}$$ 42

As illustrated in Fig. 7, the calculated fracture toughness for elastomers (dry and swollen) agrees closely with measured values. The figure contains data for various elastomers prepared with different crosslink densities and the required network parameters for calculating the toughness are given in Table 2. In most cases the measured values agree very closely with their predicted toughness. The measured toughness of *cis*-polyisoprene was almost 2–3 times larger than the predicted values. Since the calculated values were based on several assumptions, this level of agreement is considered excellent by previous researchers (Lake and Thomas 1967; Baumberger et al. 2006). The figure also contains two data sets from single network hydrogels. The gel toughness for polyacrylamide gels reported by Tanaka (Tanaka et al. 2000) and those by Zhang (Zhang et al. 2005) also agree within a similar accuracy with the predicted values.

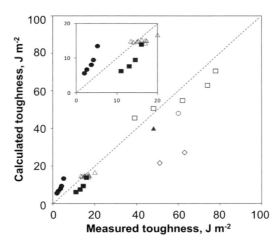

Fig. 7. Measured fracture toughness and calculated toughness values (Lake Thomas theory) for dry and swollen networks taken from literature sources: *cis*-polyisoprene [unfilled diamonds], poly(dimethyl siloxane) [unfilled squares], solvent swollen poly(dimethyl siloxane) [unfilled triangles] (Gent and Tobias 1982); polyacrylamide hydrogels [filled circles (Zhang et al. 2005) and filled squares (Tanaka et al. 2000)]; styrene-butadiene rubber [unfilled circles] neoprene rubber [filled triangles] (Bhowmick 1988). The dashed line indicates exact agreement between calculated and measured values.

Table 2. Parameters used for calculating toughness of various elastomers and gels.

	cis-polyisoprene	PDMS	Polyacrylamide	Poly(*N*-vinyl pyrrolidone)
Backbone bond energy (kJ/mol)	346[i]	367[i]	360[ii]	360
Backbone bond length (nm)	0.115[i]	0.143[i]	0.154[iii]	0.15
Dry polymer density (kg/m³)	920[i]	970[i]	1440[iv]	1160[v]
Strand unit molecular weight (kg/mol)	0.017	0.037	0.035	0.056
Backbone units per rigid link (z)	1.74[vi]	6.25[vi]	3.32[vii]	4.87[vii]

[i]Gent and Tobias1982; [ii]Webber et al. 2007; [iii]Orwoll and Chong 1999; [iv]Munk et al. 1980; [v]Guner and Kara 1998; [vi]Treloar 1958; [vii]Xin et al. 2013.

The correlation between the fracture toughness of dry and solvent-swollen networks, respectively $G_{c,o}$ and G_c, are obtained by combining the above equations:

$$G_c = G_{c,o} \left(\frac{1}{q}\right)^{2/3} \left(\frac{1}{q_o}\right)^{1/3} \qquad 43$$

From this expression it is seen that the fracture energy for a given elastomer decreases with increasing swelling and this behaviour has been confirmed experimentally (Gent and Tobias 1982). The situation is more complex, however, for gels made with different crosslink densities. As illustrated in Fig. 8, the toughness can either increase or decrease with strand length, depending on the synthesis conditions. As illustrated in two separate studies on polyacrylamide hydrogels (Zhang et al. 2005; Tanaka et al. 2000), the toughness increases with increasing strand length when a series of gels were prepared at the same monomer concentration but with decreasing ratio of crosslinker to monomer (Tanaka et al. 2000). In contrast, a decrease in toughness with increasing strand length occurred in gels made with the same crosslinker to monomer

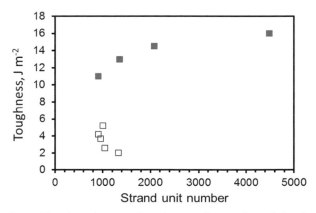

Fig. 8. Calculated strand lengths and measured toughness as for experimental data for polyacrylamide hydrogels reported by Tanaka filled squares and Zhang unfilled squares.

ratio, but with decreasing monomer concentration (Zhang et al. 2005). The latter illustrates the importance of the swelling ratio during the formation of the network (q_o) on the final network toughness.

The calculated toughness values obtained for hydrogels are small and accurately reflect the observed brittle nature of these materials. Techniques to toughen gels (for example see Naficy et al. 2011 and Zhao 2014) introduce additional mechanisms to dissipate energy during crack propagation. In 'double network' hydrogels the damage zone size is greatly increased so that many more network strands must be broken in propagating a crack. Other dissipation mechanisms involve viscoelastic effects and interactions with other phases in composite gels.

Conclusions

Hydrogels are unique and extremely useful materials by virtue of their capacity to retain significant amounts of water. Swelling by water has a profound effect on the hydrogel properties and it is important to understand these effects for proper design of hydrogel materials. Great advances have been made in the relation of basic properties of hydrogels, including mechanical properties, swelling and transport properties, by considering the topological structure of the hydrogel network and the relevant thermodynamic relations. As a result, it is possible to predict with reasonable accuracy and within certain bounds, the equilibrium swelling ratios (and the effects of external stress), the modulus, the toughness and the diffusion rates of small molecules within the hydrogels.

References

Baumberger, T., C. Caroli and D. Martina. 2006. Fracture of biopolymer gel as a viscoplastic disentanglement process. Eur. Phys. J. E 21: 81–89.

Bhowmick, A.K. 1988. Threshold fracture of elastomers. J. Macromol. Sci. C, Rev. Macromol. Chem. Phys. 28: 339–370.

Erman, B. and J.P. Flory. 1978. Theory of elasticity of polymer networks. II. The effect of geometric constraints on junctions. J. Chem. Phys. 68: 5363–5369.

Erman, B. and L. Monnerie. 1989. Theory of elasticity of amorphous networks: effect of constraints along chains. Macromolecules 22: 3342–3348.

Erman, B. and L. Monnerie. 1992. Theory of elasticity of amorphous networks: effect of constraints along chains. Macromolecules 25: 4456–4456.

Flory, P.J. 1942. Thermodynamics of high polymer solutions. J. Chem. Phys. 10: 51–61.

Flory, P.J. and J. Rehner. 1943. Statistical mechanics of cross-linked polymer networks I. Rubberlike elasticity. J. Chem. Phys. 11: 512–520.

Flory, P.J. and J. Rehner. 1944. Effect of deformation on the swelling capacity of rubber. J. Chem. Phys. 12: 412–414.

Flory, P.J. 1977. Theory of elasticity of polymer networks. The effect of local constraints on junctions. J. Chem. Phys. 66: 5720–5729.

Flory, P.J. 1979. Molecular theory of rubber elasticity. Polymer 20: 1317–1320.

Flory, P.J. and B. Erman. 1982. Theory of elasticity of polymer networks 3. Macromolecules 15: 800–806.

Fricke, H. 1924. A mathematical treatment of the electric conductivity and capacity of disperse systems I. The electric conductivity of a suspension of homogeneous spheroids. Phys. Rev. 24: 575–587.

Gaylord, R.J. and J.F. Douglas. 1987. Rubber elasticity: a scaling approach. Polym. Bull. 18: 347–354.

Gaylord, R.J. and J.F. Douglas. 1990. The localisation model of rubber elasticity. II. Polym. Bull. 23: 529–533.

Gee, G. 1946. The interaction between rubber and liquids. Some new experimental tests of a statistical thermodynamics theory of rubber–liquid systems. Trans. Faraday Soc. 42: B033–B044.

Gent, A.N. and R.H. Tobias. 1982. Threshold tear strength of elastomers. J. Polym. Sci. B 20: 2051–2058.

Gent, A.N. 1996. A new constitutive relation for rubber. Rubber Chem. Technol. 69: 59–61.

Guner, A. and M. Kara. 1998. Cloud points and θ temperature of aqueous poly(N-vinyl-2-pyrrolidone) solutions in the presence of denaturing agents. Polymer 39: 1569–1572.

Huggins, M.L. 1942. Thermodynamics properties of solutions of long-chain compounds. Ann. N. Y. Acad. Sci. 43: 1–32.

James, H.M. and E. Guth. 1943. Theory of the elastic properties of rubber. J. Chem. Phys. 11: 455–481.

Kuhn, W. 1936. Relationship between molecular size, statistical molecular shape and elastic properties of long-chain polymers. Kolloidzschr 76: 258–271.

Lake, G.J. and A.G. Thomas. 1967. The strength of highly elastic materials. Proc. Roy. Soc. London Ser. A 300: 108–119.

Mackie, J.S. and P. Meares. 1955. The diffusion of electrolytes in a cation-exchange resin membrane. I. Theoretical. Proc. R. Soc. London A 232: 498–509.

Munk, P., T.M. Aminabhavi, P. Williams, D.E. Hoffman and M. Chmelir. 1980. Some solution properties of polyacrylamide. Macromolecules 13: 871–876.

Mooney, M. 1940. A theory of large elastic deformation. J. Appl. Phys. 11: 582–592.

Naficy, S., H.R. Brown, J.M. Razal, G.M. Spinks and P.G. Whitten. 2011. Progress toward robust polymer hydrogels. Aus. J. Chem. 64: 1007–1025.

Ogden, R.W. 1972. Large deformation isotropic elasticity—On the correlation of theory and experiment for incompressible rubberlike solids. Proc. R. Soc. A 326: 565–584.

Ogston, A.G., B.N. Preston and J.D. Wells. 1973. On the transport of compact particles through solutions of chain-polymers. Pros. R. Soc. London A 333: 297–316.

Orwoll, R.A. and Y. Chong. 1999. Polyacrylamide. pp. 247. In: Mark, E.J. (ed.). Polymer Data Handbook. Oxford University Press, Oxford, U.K.

Pickup, S. and F.D. Blum. 1989. Self-diffusion of toluene in polystyrene solutions. Macromolecules 22: 3961–3968.

Rivlin, R.S. 1948. Large elastic deformations of isotropic materials. IV. Further development of the general theory. Phil. Trans. R. Soc. A 241: 379–397.

Rubinstein, M. and R.H. Colby. 2003. Polymer Physics. Oxford University Press, Oxford, U.K.

Tanaka, Y., K. Fukao and Y. Miyamoto. 2000. Fracture energy of gels. Eur. Phys. J. E. 3: 395–401.

Treloar, L.R.G. 1943. The elasticity of a network of long-chain molecules. I. Trans. Faraday Soc. 39: 36–41.

Treloar, L.R.G. 1950. The swelling of cross-linked amorphous polymers under strain. Trans. Faraday Soc. 50: 783–789.

Treloar, L.R.G. 1975. Physics of Rubber Elasticity. Oxford, U.K.

Valanis, K. and R.F. Landel. 1967. The strain-energy function of a hyperelastic material in terms of the extension ratios. J. Appl. Phys. 38: 2997.

Wall, F.T. 1942. Statistical thermodynamics of rubber. II. J. Chem. Phys. 10: 485.

Webber, R.E., C. Creton, H.R. Brown and J.P. Gong. 2007. Large strain hysteresis and Mullins effect of tough double-network hydrogels. Macromolecules 40: 2919–2927.

Xin, H., S.Z. Saricilar, H.R. Brown, P.G. Whitten and G.M. Spinks. 2013. Effect of first network topology on the toughness of double network hydrogels. Macromolecules 46: 6613–6620.

Yeoh, O.H. 1993. Some forms of the strain energy function for rubber. Rubber Chem. Technol. 66: 754–771.

Zhang, J., C.R. Daubert and E.A. Foegeding. 2005. Characterization of polyacrylamide gels as an elastic model for food gels. Rheol. Acta 44: 622–630.

Zhao, X. 2014. Multi-scale multi-mechanism design of tough hydrogels: building dissipation into stretchy networks. Soft Matter 10: 672–687.

CHAPTER 4

Mechanisms of Drug Release from Hydrogels in Medical Applications

B. McGeerver, G. Andrews and D. Jones*

Introduction

Hydrogels have proven invaluable in the field of drug delivery. Modification of the physical and chemical properties of these systems allows a network to be created in which drug molecules may be entrapped and drug release may be engineered. There are a wide range of polymers currently employed for this purpose. For example, hydrogels such as poly(2-hydroxyethylmethacrylate) (HEMA) have been used in contact lenses, catheter coatings and wound healing platforms; cellulose derivatives such as hydroxypropyl methyl cellulose (HPMC) have become one of the most popular categories of hydrophilic polymers associated with pharmaceutical systems and polyvinyl alcohol (PVA) has also been utilized in a wide range of pharmaceutical applications (Liechty et al. 2010; Hoffman 2001; Peppas et al. 2000). These polymers are capable of interacting with surrounding solvent and imbibing large quantities of water into the structure. The adaptable nature of this property creates the ideal platform for a myriad of drug loaded devices and formulations with varying release profiles (Alkayyali et al. 2012; Hoare and Kohane 2008; Vashist et al. 2014; Vasheghani-Farahani and Ganji 2009).

Hydrogels are versatile drug carriers and can be tailored for a range of applications, as previously highlighted. Drug release is dependent on the chemical nature of the platform and the network structure created. One of the most influential factors to modulate drug release from a hydrogel is the presence of cross-linking

School of Pharmacy, Queen's University, Belfast, 97 Lisburn Road, Belfast, BT9 7BL, UK.
* Corresponding author: D.Jones@qub.ac.uk

within the polymer network. Crosslinking can be categorized as physical or chemical depending on the interaction binding the polymer chains. Chemical cross-linking is defined as permanent and exists through covalent bonds; addition of a cross-linking agent is required. This form of cross-linking offers a high mechanical strength. The concentration of cross-linking can be easily adapted and is the key in modifying swelling and release of solutes from hydrogels. The density of cross-linking and distance between the cross-links directly impacts swelling capacity of the hydrogel. The mesh size of the structure created is indicative of the size of drug molecules that may be physically incorporated (Siepmann and Peppas 2011; Hoare and Kohane 2008). Notably, the cross-linking feature prevents dissolution of the polymer when exposed to solvent and enables the hydrogel to maintain the physical dimensions. Adapting the chemical properties of the cross-linker enables the production of hydrogels that offer a wide range of physical properties. For example, selecting a larger carbon chain length creates further distance between the cross-links thereby modifying swelling capacity and drug diffusion. Varying side-group moieties from the main carbon chain will also influence the fundamental characteristics, for example hydrophobic moieties may reduce swelling of the polymer or dictate the type of drug molecule incorporated. Increasing the concentration of cross-linking agent will increase the rigidity of the hydrogel structure and subsequently reducing the swelling capacity. Physical cross-linking is reversible and generally occurs through tangling of polymer chains and intermolecular ionic or hydrogen-bonding interactions (Ahmed 2015; Hoare and Kohane 2008; Berger et al. 2004). Physical cross-linking is equally valuable, for example, formulations involving HPMC-based tablets. These are created via a process of powder compaction, which consequently induces this physical cross-linking. Tablets can be moulded into specific shapes and maintain a high drug concentration whilst remaining structurally stable. Upon uptake of solvent the tablets will erode and disintegrate influencing the release of drug (Colombo et al. 1996; Gazzaniga et al. 2008).

Mathematical Modelling of Drug Release from Hydrogels

Understanding the kinetics involved in drug release from a hydrogel network can be complex, yet necessary in order to establish a relationship between drug diffusion and time. There is a range of mathematical equations in existence as a means of modelling release kinetics of drugs from respective polymeric carriers. The relevance/acceptance of the models does not suggest that these are entirely definitive of the release process and in many cases are theoretical simplifications of real systems. The accuracy of each model increases with increased model complexity. Existing models are expressed as mechanistic or empirical/semi-empirical models. The former are based on physical concepts such as diffusion, dissolution, swelling, degradation and precipitation thereby affording greater understanding of the drug release mechanism (Narasimhan 2001; Frenning et al. 2003; Frenning and Strømme 2003; Zhou and Wu 2003). The latter are considered to be descriptive and preclude many physical, chemical and biological factors affecting the release process, such as ionisation, varying temperature or pH (Singhvi and Singh 2011; Costa and Sousa Lobo 2001; Siepmann and Siepmann 2008).

In relation to the application of release kinetics in hydrogel formulations, the nature of the network structure will determine the rate-limiting step of release. Drug release from hydrogels can be classified based on the fundamental processes of diffusion, swelling or chemically induced reactions (Caló and Khutoryanskiy 2015).

Diffusion Controlled Release

Siepmann has explained that in order to rationally and correctly select the appropriate mathematical model for diffusion dominant release kinetics, the type of system, matrix or reservoir, must be identified. Furthermore, knowledge of other factors, e.g., the initial state of drug solubility within the carrier and the geometry of the drug delivery platform is required (Siepmann and Siepmann 2012). Drug loaded polymers can be designed as either reservoir (Fig. 1) or matrix (Fig. 2) systems.

The reservoir system incorporates a bank of drug surrounded by a hydrogel membrane. Drug must diffuse from the core of a supersaturated drug concentration through the hydrogel membrane; creating a concentration gradient from the formulation to surrounding media. When the membrane reaches swelling equilibrium continuous steady release rate is achieved, providing the coating remains intact. Release from the reservoir systems follow Fick's first law of diffusion as in Equation 1.

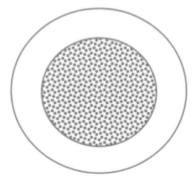

Fig. 1. Drug reservoir coated in hydrogel membrane.

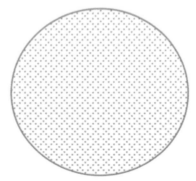

Fig. 2. Drug matrix (monolithic dispersion) in hydrogel system.

Equation 1: Fick's first law of diffusion

$$J = -D\frac{\partial c}{\partial x}$$ 1

Here, J is flux, D is the diffusion coefficient of the drug through the membrane and $\frac{\partial c}{\partial x}$ is the concentration gradient across the membrane travelling in direction x.

Diffusion from a reservoir environment has a linear relationship with time and is independent of drug concentration, therefore zero order release kinetics are achieved. Variation from this profile may be observed at the beginning of release due to a lagging effect as drug initially diffuses through the swollen membrane. Similarly this may occur towards the end of release when the core of the device is in a depleted state (Paul 2011).

Matrix or monolithic formulations are based on a homogenous dispersion of drug throughout the hydrogel as shown in Fig. 2. Diffusion from a matrix-style, swellable system occurs when the uptake of surrounding media is a rapid process, reaching equilibrium of swelling almost immediately. Dispersed drug will then diffuse through the swollen network. Fick's second law of diffusion in Equation 2 defines this mechanism of drug release and the equation must be modified relative to the geometry of the device (Ritger and Peppas 1987a).

Equation 2: Fick's second law of diffusion

$$\frac{\partial c}{\partial t} = D\frac{\partial^2 C}{\partial x^2}$$ 2

Particular experimental conditions are required for this model to apply: *sink* conditions must be maintained, diffusion from the sample must be unidirectional (drug diffusion from the sides of the sample must be negligible) and the diffusion coefficient calculated must be relative to the geometry of the sample. Ritger and Peppas simplified this model and the equation stated in Equation 3 is applicable to the diffusion process from a thin polymer slab.

Equation 3: Fick's second law of diffusion simplified by Ritger and Peppas (Ritger and Peppas 1987a)

$$\frac{M_t}{M_\infty} = 4\left(\frac{Dt}{\pi t^2}\right)^{1/2}$$ 3

This follows the assumption that drug diffusion is dependent on the square root of time multiplied by a constant: this model is applicable only to the first 60% of release (Ritger and Peppas 1987a).

Drug must diffuse through the swollen mesh network or pores depending on the structure of the hydrogel. Fickian type diffusion is defined by the diffusion coefficient (D) included in the equation and for improved accuracy and relevance of an applied mathematical model, must be calculated with relevance to one particular set of experimental conditions: meaning it is derived specifically for an individual sample (Lin and Metters 2006; Siepmann and Peppas 2011). This coefficient can be calculated by a variety of equations determined by and accounting for the nature and geometry of the polymeric meshwork structure. Equation 4 can be applied to swellable polymers where it is necessary to account for diffusion through the structure in the most swollen state. Influential properties such as polymer volume fraction and mesh size are included.

Equation 4: Prediction of drug diffusion coefficient summarized by Lin and Metters (Lin and Metters 2006)

$$\frac{D_g}{D_0} = f(r_s . v_{2.s} . \zeta)$$ 4

D_g and D_0 are the drug diffusion coefficients in the swollen hydrogel network and the pure solvent respectively, r_s is the size of the drug entrapped, $v_{2.s}$ is the polymer volume fraction in the swollen state and ζ is the mesh size of the network. The latter two components are established through calculation of network parameters of the hydrogel formulation (Ende and Peppas 1996). The size of the drug molecules involved is a necessary consideration: should this be larger than the mesh size itself, drug will remain entrapped within the structure. It is apparent through consideration of these calculations, that diffusion controlled drug release can be manipulated by the structure of the polymer network. The cross-link density will directly impact on the degree of swelling and consequently the path length for diffusion.

In relation to hydrogel formulations specifically, diffusion is not always solely dependent on time. To account for this variation Equation 5 was derived and is a highly useful tool in determining the mechanism by which release occurs from the polymer.

Equation 5: Peppas Power Law equation describing the mechanism of solute diffusion from a thin polymer slab

$$\frac{M_t}{M_\infty} = kt^n$$ 5

M_t and M_∞ are the mass of drug released at times t and infinity respectively and k is an experimentally determined parameter corresponding to a constant that incorporates structural and geometric characteristics of the system. The release exponent, n, defines this mechanism by correlating the calculated value with those in Table 1. The constants, k and n, are uniquely determined for each drug-polymer system and will vary depending on the geometry of the device (Ritger and Peppas 1987a).

Swelling Controlled Drug Release

Diffusion-controlled release from a thin device of planar geometry results in a release exponent of 0.5. Should the rate-limiting step of drug release be determined by the uptake of solvent into the formulation, release is described as Case II, with a relative diffusional exponent value of 1 (Table 1). The rate of drug release will be influenced

Table 1. Stating the diffusion exponent values describing drug release mechanisms in correlation with sample geometries.

Diffusion exponent *(n)*			
Planar	**Cylindrical**	**Spherical**	**Transport mechanism**
0.5	0.45	0.43	Fickian
0.5 < n < 1	0.45 < n < 0.89	0.43 < n < 0.85	Anomalous
1	0.89	0.85	Case II (Swelling)

by the rate of polymer relaxation occurring as solvent imbibes the system. The boundary between the polymer and solvent begins to transition from a glassy solid state, in which the drug molecules are immobile, to that of a rubbery more flexible state permitting diffusion of entrapped molecules. As relaxation occurs drug can begin to diffuse towards the external media. This process is illustrated in Fig. 3, comparing the stationary boundary present in diffusion dominant systems, with that of the moving boundary present in swellable polymers.

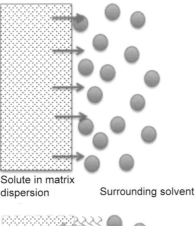

Solute diffuses outwards after swelling is maximized. The boundary of the diffusion front, where solute encounters surrounding media, remains in the same position. Solute must travel further to reach this interface as drug is depleted.

Solute in matrix dispersion   Surrounding solvent

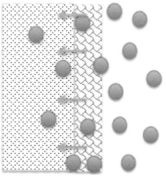

Solvent must diffuse inwards causing the polymer to swell. Solute release rate is minimal in comparison to the rate of solvent uptake. The diffusion front between formulation and media continues to move relative to time and solvent penetration continues until there is uniform swelling.

Solute in matrix dispersion   Surrounding solvent

Fig. 3. Stationary boundary in diffusion controlled swellable devices compared with the moving boundary present in swelling controlled devices (Lee 2011).

Drug release is constrained by the rate of this opposing movement at the surface of the device. Kinetics of Case II transport is defined by the constant speed at which this boundary moves, the swelling process is linear with time and therefore initially first-order release. When the swelling and drug diffusion fronts meet at a centre point, release becomes independent of time. Equation 6 below defines this mechanism (Ritger and Peppas 1987b).

Equation 6: Ritger and Peppas explanation of drug release from a thin polymer film dominated by Case-II relaxation

$$\frac{M_t}{M_\infty} = \frac{2k_o}{C_o l} t \qquad\qquad 6$$

In this equation, k_o represents a Case-II relaxation constant, l is the thickness of the film, and C_o is a constant concentration.

A *burst* release phase may be observed in swellable hydrogel formulations. This can be both advantageous and limiting depending on the desired application and release profile (Huang and Brazel 2001). It involves a large concentration of release from the surface of the device over an initial short period of time and reduces the drug concentration of the overall formulation. On formulating hydrogel based devices appropriate consideration must be made for this occurrence.

Drug release from many hydrogel formulations is influenced by both diffusion and swelling simultaneously and therefore these two processes must be fully considered. This results in non-Fickian behaviour and is classified as anomalous transport with an exponent value of $0.5 < n > 1$ for planar geometries. The driving force of the drug release process in such circumstances can be determined by calculation of the *Deborah* number derived by Brazel and Peppas, a ratio of polymer relaxation and solvent diffusion into the system as in Equation 7 (Brazel and Peppas 1999).

Equation 7: Diffusional Deborah number (Brazel and Peppas 1999)

$$D_e = \frac{\lambda}{\theta} \qquad\qquad 7$$

λ represents polymer relaxation time and θ, solvent diffusion time. Should $D_e > 1$ or <1 diffusion is Fickian, when $D_e = 1$ anomalous transport is defined. The swelling interface number (S_w) is also relevant as it relates the penetration of the surrounding solvent to that of solute diffusion and is shown in Equation 8.

Equation 8: Swelling Interface number derived by Peppas and Franson

$$Sw = \frac{v \delta r}{D} \qquad\qquad 8$$

Considering the defining exponent value associated with the mechanism of anomalous transport lies between the exponent values for Fickian diffusion and Case

II transport, Ritger and Peppas have combined the contributions from both kinetic equations to account for this as shown in Equation 9 (Ritger and Peppas 1987a).

Equation 9: Kinetics of anomalous transport comprised of both diffusion and swelling controlled drug diffusion (Ritger and Peppas 1987a)

$$\frac{M_t}{M_\infty} = k_1 t^m + k_2 t^{2m}$$

9

$k_1 t^m$ is responsible for the Fickian diffusion portion of release and $k_2 t^{2m}$ represents the polymer relaxation controlled aspect. For diffusion-controlled release from a thin, swellable polymer sample, the release exponent, in this case *m*, is equal to 0.5 therefore Equation 9 can be simplified to Equation 10.

Equation 10: Simplification of the Ritger and Peppas semi-empirical equation, by Peppas and Sahlin assuming m = 0.5 for Fickian diffusion from a thin polymer film (Peppas and Sahlin 1989)

$$\frac{M_t}{M_\infty} = k_1 \sqrt{t} + k_2 t$$

10

Figure 4 highlights the variation in release profile when the value k_2 is greater than that of k_1.

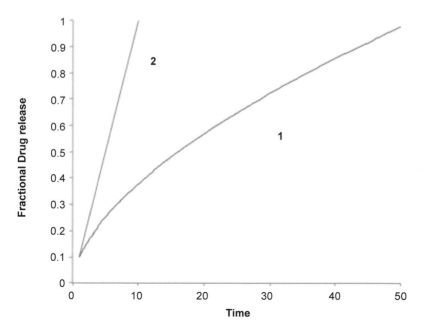

Fig. 4. Curve 1 demonstrates the release profile when $k_1 > k_2$. Curve 2 highlights the more linear relationship with time when $k_1 < k_2$. Taken from Peppas and Sahlin's, A simple equation for the description of solute release. III. Coupling of diffusion and relaxation. Int. J. Pharm. 1989 (Peppas and Sahlin 1989).

Erosion controlled release

Erosion of a hydrogel polymer can occur when there is no chemical crosslinking present or if the polymer is water-soluble in nature. Disentanglement of the polymer chains results in an increased solvent uptake and gradual disintegration of the network will occur. With respect to kinetics of controlled drug release, the rate of polymer erosion must also now be considered. Should this be the rate-limiting step of the diffusional process, drug release could be considered as erosion controlled, which in a swelling device will also result in an anomalous transport exponent. This creates an additional moving boundary whereby there is an erosion front before the swelling front as per Fig. 5.

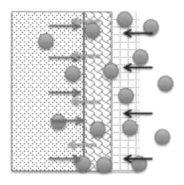

As solvent diffuses inwards the polymer structure swells. The chains being to disentangle and the structure disintegrates. There is the addition of a new boundary, the erosion front, which is moving inwards second to that of the swelling front. The diffusion front continues to move in the opposing direction.

Solute in matrix dispersion   Surrounding solvent

Fig. 5. An eroding matrix adds a third moving boundary for consideration in swelling devices (Lee 2011).

Should this erosion occur from the surface of the device, the path length for drug diffusion will gradually decrease simultaneous to decreasing drug concentration and independent of time creating zero order release kinetics. However, if erosion occurs at a slower or faster rate than drug diffusion, the release is non-zero (Sackett and Narasimhan 2011). A common example of formulations involving diffusion, swelling and erosion is release from HPMC based tablets. Many researchers have focused on mathematically predicting release from these types of devices and the extent of necessary considerations make it a complex model (Lin and Metters 2006; Wu et al. 2005; Siepmann and Peppas 2000; Göpferich 1996). The geometry of the formulation and subsequent consideration of axial and radial swelling and diffusion must be additionally considered. Upon emersion in the solvent, polymer relaxation and swelling causes expansion of the shape of the tablet. The process of chain disentanglement begins and depending on the exact polymer composition, dissolution rate of the matrix itself will vary. Peppas et al. derived a theory for modelling such kinetics, incorporating each of the mentioned phenomena (Siepmann and Peppas 2012; Siepmann et al. 1999). The rate of polymer dissolution can be accounted for in Equation 11.

Equation 11: Polymer dissolution in an eroding HPMC tablet

$$M_{pt} = M_{p0} - k_{diss} A_t t \qquad\qquad 11$$

M_{pt} and M_{p0} are the dry polymer matrix mass at time t and $t = 0$ respectively, k_{diss} is the polymer dissolution rate constant relative to the surface area of the matrix and A_t is the surface area at time t.

The diffusion and water penetration at the surface of the device are accounted for based on the theory of free volume using a Fujita type relationship displayed in Equation 12.

Equation 12: Diffusion of solute and penetration of solvent at the surface of the device relative to the free volume theory

$$D_k = D_{kcrit} \, exp \left\{ -\beta_k (1 - \frac{C_1}{C_{1crit}}) \right\} \qquad\qquad 12$$

In which, β_k is a constant, independent of concentration; D_{kcrit} represents the diffusion coefficients of water and drug at the front of polymer disentanglement. Stipulations of this theory state there must be ideal mixing between the drug, polymer and water and that the volume of the matrix is in fact additive with respect to the individual volumes (Siepmann and Peppas 2012; Narasimhan and Peppas 1996).

As with the aforementioned swellable devices, the diffusion of drug out of the matrix and diffusion of water into the system are accounted for based on Fick's second law, relative to cylindrical geometries with considerations for the radial and axial directions of diffusion as per Equation 13 (Siepmann et al. 1999; Siepmann and Peppas 2012; Narasimhan and Peppas 1996).

Equation 13: Fick's second law of diffusion relative to solute release from a device of cylindrical geometry

$$\frac{\partial C_k}{\partial t} = \frac{1}{r} \left\{ \frac{\partial}{\partial r} \left(r D_k \frac{\partial C_k}{\partial r} \right) + \frac{\partial}{\partial \theta} \left(\frac{D_k}{r} \frac{\partial C_k}{\partial \theta} \right) + \frac{\partial}{\partial z} \left(r D_k \frac{\partial C_k}{\partial z} \right) \right\} \qquad 13$$

In this equations, C_k and D_k are the concentration and diffusion co-efficient for both water (k = 1) and drug (k = 2), r represents the radial dimension of the matrix and z the axial. θ is the angle relative to the dimensions.

Alternative hydrogel delivery devices

SMART systems involve utilizing specific functionalities of the polymer backbone, creating ionisable groups or hydrogen bonds through varying pH or temperature resulting in increased or decreased polymer swelling (Colombo et al. 1996). When swelling is maximised the polymer chains expand and entrapped molecules can be released. As the surrounding environment changes, this swelling can be 'turned off' and shrinkage of the device results in a closed structure, through which drug molecules cannot diffuse. This feature can be exploited for application in targeted drug delivery. A relevant example is the delivery of drugs via injections to a site across the blood-brain barrier. Transition between gel and solution can be optimized for the process of administration with subsequent controlled release. Temperature controlled systems are generally composed of co-polymer structures. Pluronics®, which are varying ratios of poly(ethylene oxide) and poly(propylene oxide) are co-polymers defined by low critical solution temperatures (LCST). With the LCST falling close to 37°C, the formulation can undergo a phase transition at body temperature which can subsequently influence drug release as previously stated (Qiu and Park 2012; de Las Heras Alarcon et al. 2005). These SMART formulations are also of particular interest when devising pulsed release systems in an attempt to mimic natural functions of the body, such as insulin secretion or hormone dosing systems (Stubbe et al. 2004). Polymers composed of p(NIPAM) have also been researched in applications for controlled drug delivery exploiting the LCST property. The polymer chains aggregate due to hydrophobic interactions in aqueous media at low temperatures; these polymeric micelles exist in a swollen state within which the drug is entrapped (Ashraf et al. 2016; Schmaljohann 2006). At temperatures above the LCST, hydrophobic interactions cause collapse of the network and subsequent release of drug thereby rendering a responsive device (Jones et al. 2012). The thermoresponsive properties of p(NIPAM) have been confirmed in various research however specific application as a homopolymer is lacking due to the weak tensile properties of the gel (Schmaljohann 2006; Ashraf et al. 2016; Nguyen et al. 2015). Jones et al. have investigated the formation of copolymers with p(NIPAM) and additional hydrophilic and hydrophobic polymers (Jones et al. 2012). This research confirmed that while improving the tensile properties of the material, the stimuli responsive attribute desired was maintained. Application of this technology for controlled drug release purposes, as anti-infective biomaterials, was investigated and proved to be successful technology. The swelling variation is a key feature of the controlling mechanism of release in SMART formulations however other factors are suspected to be involved, all of which are not yet fully understood (Peppas 1997; Qiu and Park 2012; Zhang et al. 2002). A single kinetic model cannot be assigned to the drug delivery from this style of device given that release of this nature can result in multiple phases. Each phase can be individually modelled as previously discussed based on the relaxation, swelling, erosion and subsequent diffusion depending on the rate-limiting step in the release phase.

Chemically controlled drug release

Degradation of the polymer implies a similar outcome to erosion however it is an independent phenomena that is initiated by exploiting specifically designed aspects of the polymer structure using environmental stimuli (Lin and Metters 2006). For degradation to occur, there must be cleavage of specific bonds within the network, which result in disintegration of the structure. The cleavage can be initiated by enzyme presence or changes in swelling and is independently designed for the specific drug. Application of these hydrogels are ideal in the delivery of pro-drugs or proteins as a means of overcoming degradation prior to reaching the desired site of administration (Lin and Metters 2006). Novel formulations involving polymer-drug conjugation utilize this mechanism of action. These are distinctively different from previous formulations discussed whereby new chemical entities are formed, defined by the covalent bonding between drug and polymer (Duncan 2006). The research is based on the premise that water-soluble polymers are well established as inert within the human body; incorporating specific functionalities within the structure can render the carriers as a recognizable entity to specific target sites within the body (Kopecek 2013). Polymers that have currently been researched with this focus include N-(2-hydroxypropyl) methacrylamide, polyglutamic acid (PGA), polyethyleneglycol (PEG), polysaccharides and hydroxypropyl methacrylamide (HPMA) (Pasut and Veronese 2007; Duncan 2006; Kopecek 2013; Khandare and Minko 2006; Harris and Chess 2003). These have been utilized as co-polymer-drug conjugates incorporating low molecular weight compounds that are either conjugated directly to the polymer structure or bonded to a spacer, which is attached to the structure. The drug then assumes the form of a pro-drug in that it remains inactive while travelling through the body until reaching the site of delivery. Formulations are under clinical trial involving several anticancer drugs particularly paclitaxel, doxorubicin and camptothecin (Li and Wallace 2008; Singer 2005; Duncan 2007; Pasut and Veronese 2007). There are many associated advantages of delivering treatments using the polymeric-based carriers; improvement in solubility of hydrophobic drug molecules can ultimately increase biocompatibility and reduce side effects due to a more site specific delivery (Duncan 2006; Kopecek 2013; Surapaneni et al. 2012; Pasut and Veronese 2007; Khandare and Minko 2006; Harris and Chess 2003). In addition, these carriers have proven to overcome multi-drug resistance by operating in opposite gradients from treatment of the independent drug. Research has investigated carriers composed of two polymers conjugated with two individual drugs but also a single polymer conjugating with one or two drugs, depending on the treatment or targeted delivery required (Kopecek 2013). Other applications of these systems have been researched for treatment of musculoskeletal conditions and inflammatory or infectious diseases. The macromolecular structures involved in the formulations inhibits administration via the traditional oral route due to poor bioavailability therefore parental administration is utilized (Duncan 2006). Combining the processes of polymer-drug conjugation and triggered release, the theory has been applied in relation to coatings of biomedical devices. McCoy et al. investigated release of the known antimicrobially active agent naladixic acid by conjugation with various esters for co-polymerization with the hydrophilic monomer HEMA, utilizing an environmental trigger to stimulate release and treat infection. The elevation in pH in the presence of urease releasing bacteria induced cleavage of the ester from the polymeric network with subsequent release of the naladixic acid (McCoy et al. 2016). In using water-soluble polymers as a carrier device, the previously discussed phenomena apply with regards to swelling and/or erosion of the device itself. Currently, modelling release kinetics of the mentioned formulations has not been defined. The nature of the formulations discussed demonstrates unique tailoring. Cleavage of the drug from the network structure would be the expected rate-limiting factor given the specific delivery of these applications. Specific bonding between drugs and polymers or spacers results in subsequent triggered release and can be associated with intracellular mechanisms or enzymatic cleavage: a universal model predicting release kinetics is not possible (Lin and Metters 2006).

Concluding Remark

To conclude, this chapter has highlighted that several parameters may be considered in determining the kinetics involved in hydrogel based drug delivery formulations. Many of factors that contribute to the development of a potential drug-carrier device can be exploited in an attempt to augment the release profile achieved. These attributing factors are tailored for specific medical indications. It has been shown that the theoretical methods used to describe drug release are in fact models and should be treated as generalizations or over simplifications of real phenomena. It is implausible to assume that every variable impacting upon the release profile has been accounted for. This is of particular relevance within the hydrogel domain due to the anomalous mechanism of drug release often associated with these materials.

References

Ahmed, E.M. 2015. Hydrogel: preparation, characterization, and applications: a review. J. Adv. Res. 6(2): 105–121.

Alkayyali, L.B., O.A. Abu-Diak, G.P. Andrews and D.S. Jones. 2012. Hydrogels as drug-delivery platforms: physicochemical barriers and solutions. Ther. Deliv. 3(6): 775–86.

Ashraf, S., H.K. Park, H. Park and S.H. Lee. 2016. Snapshot of phase transition in thermoresponsive hydrogel PNIPAM: role in drug delivery and tissue engineering. Macromol. Res. 24(4): 297–304.

Berger, J., M. Reist, J.M. Mayer, O. Felt and R. Gurny. 2004. Structure and interactions in chitosan hydrogels formed by complexation or aggregation for biomedical applications. Eur. J. Pharm. Biopharm. 57(1): 35–52.

Brazel, C.S. and N.A. Peppas. 1999. Dimensionless analysis of swelling of hydrophilic glassy polymers with subsequent drug release from relaxing structures. Biomat. 20(8): 721–732.

Caló, E. and V.V. Khutoryanskiy. 2015. Biomedical applications of hydrogels: a review of patents and commercial products. Eur. Poly. J. 65: 252–267.

Colombo, P., R. Bettini, P. Santi and N.A. Peppas. 1996. Analysis of the swelling and release mechanisms from drug delivery systems with emphasis on drug solubility and water transport. J. Control. Release. 39(2-3): 231–237.

de Las Heras Alarcon, C., S. Pennadam and C. Alexander. 2005. Stimuli responsive polymers for biomedical applications. Chem. Soc. Rev. 34(3): 276–285.

Duncan, R. 2006. Polymer conjugates as anticancer nanomedicines. Nat. Rev. Cancer. 6(9): 688–701.

Duncan, R. 2007. Designing polymer conjugates as lysosomotropic nanomedicines. Biochem. Soc. Trans. 35(Pt 1): 56–60.

Ende, M.T.A. and N.A. Peppas. 1996. Transport of ionizable drugs and proteins in crosslinked poly (acrylic acid) and poly (acrylic acid-co-2-hydroxyethyl methacrylate) hydrogels. J. Control. Release. 59: 673–685.

Frenning, G. and M. Strømme. 2003. Drug release modeled by dissolution, diffusion, and immobilization. Int. J. Pharm. 250(1): 137–45.

Frenning, G., A. Tunón and G. Alderborn. 2003. Modelling of drug release from coated granular pellets. J. Control. Release. 92(1-2): 113–23.

Gazzaniga, A., L. Palugan, A. Foppoli and M.E. Sangali. 2008. Oral pulsatile delivery systems based on swellable hydrophilic polymers. Eur. J. Pharm. Biopharm. 68(1): 11–8.

Göpferich, A. 1996. Mechanisms of polymer degradation and erosion. Biomate. 17(2): 103–114.

Harris, J.M. and R.B. Chess. 2003. Effect of pegylation on pharmaceuticals. Nat. Rev. Drug Discovery. 2(3): 214–221.

Hoare, T.R. and D.S. Kohane. 2008. Hydrogels in drug delivery: progress and challenges. Poly. 49(8): 1993–2007.

Hoffman, A.S. 2001. Hydrogels for biomedical applications. Annals of the New York Academy of Sciences. 944: 62–73.

Huang, X. and C.S. Brazel. 2001. On the importance and mechanisms of burst release in matrix-controlled drug delivery systems. J. Control. Release. 73(2-3): 121–136.

Jones, D.S., G.P. Andrews, D.L. Caldwell, C. Lorimer, S.P. Gorman and C.P. McCoy. 2012. Novel semi-interpenetrating hydrogel networks with enhanced mechanical properties and thermoresponsive engineered drug delivery, designed as bioactive endotracheal tube biomaterials. Eur. J. Pharm. Biopharm. 82(3): 563–571.

Khandare, J. and T. Minko. 2006. Polymer-drug conjugates: progress in polymeric prodrugs. Prog. Poly Sci. 31(4): 359–397.

Kopecek, J. 2013. Polymer-drug conjugates: origins, progress to date and future directions. Adv. Drug. Deliv. Rev. 65(1): 49–59.

Lee, P.I. 2011. Modeling of drug release from matrix systems involving moving boundaries: approximate analytical solutions. Int. J. Pharm. 418(1): 18–27.

Li, C. and S. Wallace. 2008. Polymer-drug conjugates: recent development in clinical oncology. Adv. Drug. Deliv. Rev. 60(8): 886–898.

Liechty, W.B., D.R. Kryscio, B.V. Slaughter and N.A. Peppas. 2010. Polymers for drug delivery systems. Annu. Rev. Chem. Biomol. Eng. 1(1): 149–173.

Lin, C.C. and A.T. Metters. 2006. Hydrogels in controlled release formulations: network design and mathematical modeling. Adv. Drug. Deliv. Rev. 58(12-13): 1379–1408.

McCoy, C.P., N.J. Irwin, C. Brady, D.S. Jones, L. Carson, G.P. Andrews et al. 2016. An infection-responsive approach to reduce bacterial adhesion in urinary biomaterials. Mol. Pharmaceutics. 13(8): 2817–2822.

Narasimhan, B. 2001. Mathematical models describing polymer dissolution: consequences for drug delivery. Adv. Drug. Deliv. Rev. 48(2-3): 195–210.

Narasimhan, B. and N.A. Peppas. 1996. Disentanglement and reptation during dissolution of rubbery polymers. J. Poly Sci. Part B. 34(5): 947–961.

Nguyen, H.H., B. Payré, J. Fitremann, N. Lauth-de Viguerie and J. Marty. 2015. Thermoresponsive properties of PNIPAM-based hydrogels: effect of molecular architecture and embedded gold nanoparticles. Langmuir. 31(16): 4761–4768.

Pasut, G. and F.M. Veronese. 2007. Polymer-drug conjugation, recent achievements and general strategies. Prog. Poly Sci. 32(8-9): 933–961.

Paul, D.R. 2011. Elaborations on the Higuchi model for drug delivery. Int. J. Pharm. 418(1): 13–7.

Peppas, N.A. and J.J. Sahlin. 1989. A simple equation for the description of solute release. III. Coupling of diffusion and relaxation. Int. J. Pharm. 57(2): 169–172.

Peppas, N.A. 1997. Hydrogels and drug delivery. Curr. Opin. Colloid. Interface Sci. 2(5): 531–537.

Peppas, N.A., P. Bures, W. Leobandung and H. Ichikawa. 2000. Hydrogels in pharmaceutical formulations. Eur. J. Pharm. Biopha. 50(1): 27–46.

Qiu, Y. and K. Park. 2012. Environment-sensitive hydrogels for drug delivery. Adv. Drug Deliv. Rev. 64(SUPPL.): 49–60.

Ritger, P.L. and N.A. Peppas. 1987a. A simple equation for description of solute release I. Fickian and non-fickian release from non-swellable devices in the form of slabs, spheres, cylinders or discs. J. Control. Release. 5(1): 23–36.

Ritger, P.L. and N.A. Peppas. 1987b. A simple equation for description of solute release II. Fickian and anomalous release from swellable devices. J. Control. Release. 5(1): 37–42.

Sackett, C.K. and B. Narasimhan. 2011. Mathematical modeling of polymer erosion: consequences for drug delivery. Int. J. Pharm. 418(1): 104–114.

Schmaljohann, D. 2006. Thermo- and pH-responsive polymers in drug delivery. Adv. Drug Deliv. Rev. 58(15): 1655–1670.

Siepmann, J., H. Kranz, R. Bodmeier and N.A. Peppas. 1999. HPMC-matrices for controlled drug delivery: a new model combining diffusion, swelling, and dissolution mechanisms and predicting the release kinetics. Pharm. Res. 16(11): 1748–1756.

Siepmann, J. and N.A. Peppas. 2000. Hydrophilic matrices for controlled drug delivery: an improved mathematical model to predict the resulting drug release kinetics (the & quot; sequential layer & quot; model). Pharm. Res. 17(10): 1290–8.

Siepmann, J. and F. Siepmann. 2008. Mathematical modeling of drug delivery. Int. J. Pharm. 364: 328–343.

Siepmann, J. and N.A. Peppas. 2011. Higuchi equation: derivation, applications, use and misuse. Int. J. Pharm. 418(1): 6–12.

Siepmann, J. and F. Siepmann. 2012. Modeling of diffusion controlled drug delivery. J. Control. Release. 161(2): 351–362.

Siepmann, J. and N.A. Peppas. 2012. Modeling of drug release from delivery systems based on hydroxypropyl methylcellulose (HPMC). Adv. Drug Deliv. Rev. 64(SUPPL.): 163–174.

Singer, J.W. 2005. Paclitaxel poliglumex (XYOTAX???, CT-2103): a macromolecular taxane. J. Control. Release. 109(1-3): 120–126.

Singhvi, G. and M. Singh. 2011. Review: *in vitro* drug release characterization models. Int. J. Pharm. Stud. Res. II(I): 77–84.

Stubbe, B.G., S.C. De Smedt and J. Demeester. 2004. Programmed polymeric devices for pulsed drug delivery. Pharm. Res. 21(10): 1732–1740.

Surapaneni, M.S., S.K. Das and N.G. Das. 2012. Designing paclitaxel drug delivery systems aimed at improved patient outcomes: current status and challenges. ISRN Pharmacol. 2012: 623139.

Vasheghani-Farahani, E. and F. Ganji. 2009. Hydrogels in controlled drug delivery systems. Iranian. Poly J. 18(1): 63–88.

Vashist, A., A. Vashist, Y.K. Gupta and S. Ahmad. 2014. Recent advances in hydrogel based drug delivery systems for the human body. J. Mater. Chem. B. 2(2): 147–166.

Wu, N., L.S. Wang, D.C. Tan, S.M. Moochhala and Y.Y. Yang. 2005. Mathematical modeling and *in vitro* study of controlled drug release via a highly swellable and dissoluble polymer matrix: polyethylene oxide with high molecular weights. J. Control. Release. 102(3): 569–581.

Zhang, X.Z., R.X. Zhuo, J.Z. Cui and J.T. Zhang. 2002. A novel thermo-responsive drug delivery system with positive controlled release. Int. J. Pharm. 235(1-2): 43–50.

Zhou, Y. and X.Y. Wu. 2003. Modeling and analysis of dispersed-drug release into a finite medium from sphere ensembles with a boundary layer. J. Control. Release. 90(1): 23–36.

CHAPTER 5

Hydrogel Coatings for Medical Device Applications

Nicola J. Irwin,* Colin P. McCoy and *Johann L. Trotter*

Introduction

Upon implantation of a medical device into the body, initial interactions with the surrounding tissue are governed by properties of the device surface, such as hydrophilicity, surface energy, roughness and conductivity (Goodman et al. 2013). Facile manipulation of these surface properties to enhance the success of device integration within the body is now possible via the application of hydrogel coatings. The exact range of desired properties is dependent on the intended application and site of device implantation, however requisite properties common to all medical device coatings include biocompatibility, ease of application, flexibility, stability for the intended duration of use, adherence to the substrate, and durability to withstand mechanical trauma and shear forces encountered during implantation and *in vivo* (Lawrence and Turner 2005). In this chapter, osseointegration, haemocompatibility and lubricity, which are of key importance for bone-contacting, blood-contacting and urinary devices respectively, will be considered in turn (Kulkarni et al. 2014).

Hydrogel-coated devices have been used clinically for over two decades (Metha et al. 2015). These polymers constitute attractive materials for medical device coatings on the basis of their characteristic biocompatibility, resistance to non-specific macromolecular adhesion and similar degree of flexibility to body tissue (Yu et al. 2008). In addition, the swelling capacity of hydrogels facilitates the entrapment and subsequent release of therapeutically-relevant doses of active agents, including antibiotics, silver ions, growth factors and antimicrobial peptides (Mattioli-Belmonte

School of Pharmacy, Queen's University Belfast, 97 Lisburn Road, Belfast BT9 7BL, Northern Ireland, UK.
* Corresponding author: n.irwin@qub.ac.uk

et al. 2014; Cleophas et al. 2014). Localised release of therapeutic agents from 'active' coatings offers several advantages over systemic administration of drugs, such as reduced risk of toxicity and side effects resulting from the use of lower doses and improved site-specific targeting (Goodman et al. 2013). Additional design criteria for bioactive-releasing coatings include the ability to efficiently load and modulate the release of required doses of active agents, whilst retaining therapeutic activity (Goodman et al. 2013).

Anti-Biofouling Coatings

Biofouling is a biological process initiated with the deposition of host proteins to the device surface, which subsequently induces the adhesion of complement-related proteins and triggers an inflammatory response. Further cellular recruitment, with subsequent adhesion, is triggered by monocytes and macrophages, often resulting in failure of the medical device. The improved performance of hydrogel-coated glucose biosensors *in vivo,* in association with the observed reduction in the foreign body reaction at the tissue-device interface, has previously been attributed to the ability of hydrogel coatings to resist protein adsorption in physiological solution (Yu et al. 2008). In addition to long-term biocompatibility and durability, biosensor coatings must possess sufficient porosity for reliable and rapid analyte measurements *in vivo.* Following subcutaneous implantation in rats, hydroxyethyl methacrylate-2,3-dihydroxypropyl methacrylate-based hydrogel-coated glucose sensors maintained their function for at least three weeks, and histological examination after four weeks *in vivo* revealed the presence of thinner fibrous capsules around the hydrogel-coated sensors (50–100 μm) than around their uncoated counterparts (100–500 μm). Porosity and durability of the copolymer coatings were optimised by the addition of *N*-vinyl-2-pyrrolidinone and ethylene glycol dimethacrylate respectively (Yu et al. 2008).

Surfaces of implanted medical devices also constitute attractive niches for microorganism colonization. The preference of planktonic bacteria to grow on surfaces was first reported in 1943 (ZoBell 1943) and the inherent susceptibility of implanted devices to bacterial adherence is now widely recognized. Infection can originate from numerous sources: perioperative contamination of implant surfaces resulting from inadequate sterilization prior to, and aseptic technique during, insertion of medical devices; bacterial haematogenous spreading from distant sites in the body; direct seeding from adjacent tissues harbouring infectious microorganisms; or, in the immediate post-operative period in hospital (Subbiahdoss et al. 2010; Subbiahdoss et al. 2009). Indeed, the presence of a foreign implant material has a profound influence on host defence mechanisms, increasing the risk of infection more than 100,000-fold (Zimmerli et al. 1982; Zimmerli 2014) and permitting transient bacteraemias of less than 100 colony forming units to establish successful surface colonization (Elek and Conen 1957; Zimmerli and Sendi 2011; Hickok and Shapiro 2012). Furthermore, biomaterial-associated infections remain the most common cause of failure of many indwelling medical devices (Muszanska et al. 2012; Campoccia et al. 2006) and account for over half of the annual two million nosocomial infections in Europe (Chopra et al. 2008). Device-associated infections are estimated to extend hospital stays by an average of two to three days, increase hospital expenditure by approximately $1 billion in the US (Behlau and Gilmore 2008), cause approximately 100,000 deaths per annum in US hospitals and an annual 40,000 deaths in European hospitals and, furthermore, have unquantifiable effects on patient morbidity (Francolini and Donelli 2010).

Biomaterial-associated infections are characterized by their recalcitrance to conventional treatments due to the nature of bacterial growth within highly regulated sessile microbial communities encased in self-produced amorphous matrix substances, known as biofilms (Donlan and Costerton 2002) (Fig. 1). Implant removal and revision surgeries are often required, causing additional expense for the healthcare provider, and increased patient morbidity and potential mortality (McCann et al. 2008).

The device surface itself often lends to an increased susceptibility to microbial colonization as a consequence of factors such as surface energy, hydrophilicity, roughness and chemistry. Modification of these properties to render surfaces less attractive for bacterial adherence therefore constitutes a rational method to prevent infection, and can be achieved through coating with hydrogels such as polyethylene oxide or polyethylene glycol (Kaper et al. 2003; Kingshott et al. 2003). The antimicrobial efficacy of these 'passive' coatings is, however, limited and dependent on the bacterial challenge. Alternatively, drug-eluting device coatings, developed to combat infection through the localized release of bioactive agents and the subsequent generation of high concentrations of drug directly at the biomaterial-tissue interface, thus mitigating concerns over systemic toxicity (Campoccia et al. 2006), have become one of the most widely researched strategies to prevent device-associated infection (Zilberman and Elsner 2008). Antibiotic use is associated with issues such as the possible emergence of super-infections, promotion of bacterial resistance, and changes in the local microbiological flora (Goodman et al. 2013), therefore the employment of non-antibiotic agents is preferred. Release kinetics must be carefully controlled to achieve therapeutically-active concentrations of drug when required and prevent premature exhaustion of the active agent (Goodman et al. 2013).

Up to 25% of bloodstream infections reported in intensive care units are a consequence of bacterial adherence to central venous catheters, thus highlighting the

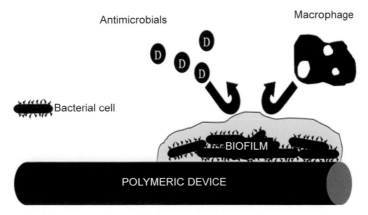

Fig. 1. Biofilm-associated bacterial resistance to the innate immune system and administered antimicrobials.

need for effective infection prevention strategies, especially in critically ill patients (Brun-Buisson et al. 2004). Hydrogel coatings impregnated with antiseptics are currently one of the most widely researched measures to reduce line infections and sepsis (Fischer et al. 2015), and the utilization of silver-hydrogel-coated central venous catheters dates back to 1998 (Gatter et al. 1998). The potential toxicity of silver to healthy human cells, however, limits use of this agent in medical device coatings (Beer et al. 2012).

In addition, orthopaedic reconstructive and fixation procedures in the US are associated with an average infection rate of 5%, representing an approximate 100,000 cases per annum, therefore making infection one of the most common complications associated with bone implants (Moriarty et al. 2010; Goodman et al. 2013). Sequelae include delayed bone healing and implant loosening, which often necessitate debridement, surgical removal and replacement of the device with complex antibiotic therapy to eradicate the infection (Moriarty et al. 2010). The significant financial burden of these infections, and the associated patient morbidity and mortality, has driven research into preventative strategies. The potential to reduce infection rates by coating orthopaedic prostheses with antibacterial-loaded resorbable hydrogel copolymers, for example comprising hyaluronic acid and biodegradable polyesters such as polylactic acid, has received limited attention (Giamonna et al. 2010).

Negatively charged layer-by-layer hydrogel thin-film coatings with pH-triggered hydrophobicity and bactericidal activity have recently been reported as a promising antibiotic-free strategy towards the prevention of biofilm growth on implanted medical device surfaces (Lu et al. 2015). Acidification of the surrounding media due to bacterial proliferation induces hydrophilic-to-hydrophobic transitions of the immobilized poly(2-alkylacrylic acid) polymers, for example polymethacrylic acid, poly(2-ethylacrylic acid), poly(2-n-propylacrylic acid) and poly(2-n-butylacrylic acid), and dehydration of the coating, which becomes selectively toxic to bacterial cells but remains cytocompatible with human osteoblasts. Furthermore, antimicrobial peptides such as inverso-CysHHC10 and cateslytin (CTL) have been incorporated into hydrogels to form thin coatings. These coatings have demonstrated retention of antimicrobial activity and stability under physiological conditions (Cleophas et al. 2014). One representative system employs multi-layered films of CTL-functionalized hyaluronic acid and chitosan. Release of the antimicrobial peptide, and subsequent antimicrobial activity, is triggered via enzymatic degradation of the film in the presence of the enzyme hyaluronidase, which is released by pathogens such as *Staphylococcus aureus* and *Candida albicans* at the onset of infection (Cado et al. 2013).

Coatings to Promote Osseointegration

The incidence of musculoskeletal diseases, including osteoporosis and bone fractures, is rising steadily as a direct consequence of the ageing population, thereby leading to an increased need for orthopaedic surgeries such as spinal reconstruction, fracture fixation and joint arthroplasties (Zimmerli 2014). Of relevance here is the doubling in the number of hip replacements performed in the US between 1990 to 2007, and the approximate five-fold increase in the number of knee replacements recorded over the same time period, resulting in the performance of an estimated 200,000 and 550,000 hip and knee procedures in 2007 respectively (Zimmerli 2014; Del Pozo et al. 2009).

Until recently, the focus of orthopaedic implants was largely mechanical, with the biological outcomes of device implantation regarded as a secondary consequence of stable integration with the host bone tissue (Goodman et al. 2013). The importance of cellular interactions at the tissue-device interface in determining the ultimate success of implant integration has, however, now been recognised. Device failure with consequent implant rejection can be a result of the foreign body reaction, bacterial infection, or micromovements of the implant itself (Kulkarni et al. 2014). This often leads to difficult revision surgeries, which extend patient recovery times and increase hospital costs (Peivandi et al. 2013). Modulation of the biological milieu surrounding the implant site to facilitate osseointegration, prevent adverse tissue reactions and implant rejection, and ultimately improve clinical outcomes is now possible with the advent of biological coatings (Goodman et al. 2013).

Much interest has been generated in the use of the osteoconductive mineral hydroxyapatite for enhancing osseointegration of bone implants. Coatings of hydroxyapatite are, however, difficult to apply. Currently used processes, including sputter techniques and plasma spraying, are limited by the suboptimal robustness and consequent failure of the coating to withstand mechanical wear and the restrictions surrounding implant geometry. Mineralization of gelatin methacrylate hydrogel coatings on titanium surfaces with hydroxyapatite by a facile biomimetic method, involving pre-functionalization of the metallic surfaces with an organic matrix embedded with bioactive nucleating agents to induce formation of the calcium phosphate crystals, has recently been proposed as a promising surface optimization technique. The resulting stable macroporous surfaces are expected to promote osseointegration and host acceptance of titanium-based implants, however further *in vitro* and *in vivo* studies are required (Tan et al. 2013).

In addition to enhancing osseointegration through biofunctionalization with hydroxyapatite, hydrogel coatings also provide a mechanism to achieve localized, site-specific delivery of therapeutic agents to promote osseointegration and/or prevent infection (Fig. 2). Much research has previously been focussed on prolonging the duration of antimicrobial release from active coatings to prevent biofilm formation, however it is now widely recognised that the "race for the surface" is contested within the first four hours (Costerton 2005). In line with this, a resorbable hydrogel coating, termed the Disposable Antibacterial Coating, has now been developed, which demonstrates complete antimicrobial release within 96 hours and can also withstand the widely reported issue of orthopaedic coating detachment during press-fit insertion (Drago et al. 2014).

The range of delivered agents has recently been extended to include bioactive agents such as DNA and growth factors to further augment new bone formation, particularly in challenging environments such as cases of previous infection or extensive trauma of the host tissue (Goodman et al. 2013). For example, polyethylene oxide-based prepolymers (NCO-sP(EO-stat-PO)) with surface-bound growth factors to optimize bone integration have been developed into hydrogel coatings which display promising osseointegrative properties, biocompatibility and preservation of growth

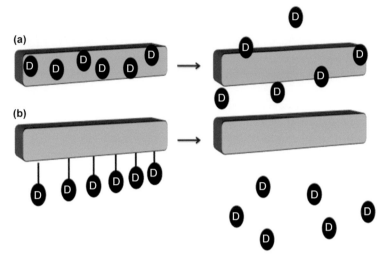

Fig. 2. Release from drug-loaded hydrogel coatings: (a) Physical loading of drug within the hydrogel matrix and (b) drug attachment via labile spacer groups.

factor functionality (Neuerburg et al. 2013). Bisphosphonate-modified hyaluronan hydrogels have also been synthesized as vehicles to adsorb and subsequently release proteins, such as the osteogenic bone morphogenetic protein-2, when in contact with bodily fluids, thereby enhancing osseointegration (Berts et al. 2014).

In another study, multifunctional copolymeric hydrogel coatings of poly-2-hydroxyethyl methacrylate-2-methacryloyloxyethyl phosphate were electrosynthesized on titanium substrates and loaded with recombinant human vascular endothelial growth factor (rhVEGF) in an attempt to enhance bone regeneration by promoting deposition of hydroxyapatite-like calcium phosphate and formation of blood vessels. The ability of the coating to promote calcification in an *in vitro* model with simulated body fluid was attributed to the presence of negatively-charged phosphate groups. Sustained release of the entrapped rhVEGF is expected to enhance angiogenesis and thus stimulate proliferation of bone cells *in vivo*, however this remains to be tested in culture systems (De Giglio et al. 2010).

Athrombogenic Coatings

Haemocompatibility of blood-contacting medical devices, for example central venous catheters, heart valves, stents and vascular grafts, is of paramount importance. Following introduction of a foreign device into the circulation, plasma proteins, such as fibrinogen, rapidly adsorb to the surface triggering the clotting cascade, a pathway of interconnected reactions which ultimately lead to the generation of thrombi and formation of a crosslinked fibrin mesh (Jaffer et al. 2015; Kulkarni et al. 2014). Thrombi formation on the implant surface is a common cause of device failure and, moreover, escape of the clot to the patient's circulation can have potentially life-threatening consequences (Fig. 3). Modification of the surface of blood-contacting

Protein deposition

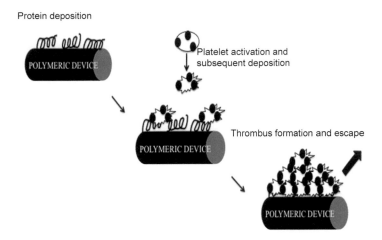

Platelet activation and subsequent deposition

Thrombus formation and escape

Fig. 3. Overview of the clotting cascade.

medical devices by the application of hydrogel coatings designed to inhibit adsorption of biomacromolecules, in particular proteins, is therefore a rationale strategy to prevent thrombus formation.

Poly(vinyl pyrrolidone) (PVP) has gained importance as a hydrophilic medical device coating material due to its biocompatibility (Leone et al. 2011), resistance to hydrolysis (Butruk-Raszeja et al. 2015), non-antigenicity and non-toxicity (Biazar et al. 2012). Of key importance to blood-contacting devices is the haemocompatibility of PVP, which was reportedly used as a human plasma substitute during World War II (Seldon 1954) and is now widely employed as a hydrogel coating to increase biocompatibility of devices such as intravascular catheters (Francois et al. 1996). Reductions in surface-adsorbed platelets (Butruk-Raszeja et al. 2015), albumin, fibrinogen (Butruk-Raszeja et al. 2015) and fibronectin (Francois et al. 1996) have all been demonstrated on PVP-coated surfaces.

A novel two-phase free radical-based grafting-crosslinking method has recently been reported for the formation of highly biocompatible, athrombogenic hydrogel coatings on polyurethane surfaces. In addition to the controllable density and equilibrium water content of the applied hydrogel layer, this two-phase application process, involving initial substrate immersion in an organic solution containing cumene hydroperoxide, the free radical generator species, and ethylene glycol dimethacrylate, the grafting and cross-linking agent, followed by immersion in an aqueous solution of PVP and iron (II) chloride ($FeCl_2$), ensures high grafting efficiency and leads to the formation of a durable, covalently-anchored coating. The presence of the hydrated PVP coating resulted in a 50% reduction in adhesion of fibrinogen after a one hr incubation period in platelet-poor plasma and significantly reduced the aggregation of platelets in whole human blood under dynamic conditions simulating arterial flow, with the percentage of remaining platelets in the blood samples approximating 35% and 80% after incubation of unmodified and PVP-coated polyurethane materials respectively (Butruk-Raszeja et al. 2015).

Lubricious Coatings

Low friction surfaces serve a dual role in improving ease of use and preventing tissue damage when devices such as guidewires and urinary catheters are manoeuvred through tortuous pathways and bodily cavities. The lubricity, or slipperiness, and roughness of such material surfaces are therefore of utmost importance (Jones et al. 2004; Cox 1987). It is widely reported that as the roughness of the coated surface decreases, the lubricity increases, leading to a corresponding increase in the ease of device insertion (Jones et al. 2004).

Initially employed on Cook arterial introducer sheaths (Cook Medical, Bloomington, IN, USA) to reduce the coefficient of friction between the device surface and blood vessel walls, hydrophilic coatings are now found on an extensive range of neurointerventional and cardiovascular devices, such as peripherally-inserted central catheters, arterial lines and infusion microcatheters (Mehta et al. 2010; Metha et al. 2015). The advent of these hydrogel-coated devices has enabled the utilization of less invasive surgical procedures with corresponding reductions in the incidence of arterial spasms and degree of patient discomfort, as highlighted in multiple studies, and ultimately leading to enhanced patient outcomes (Rathore et al. 2010).

While hydrophilic-coated devices have revolutionized endovascular surgery, their use is not without risk. Dissociation of polymer coating particulates from the device surface *in vivo* during catheter implantation or manipulation can lead to widespread embolization within the vasculature of the heart, lung, brain and/or lower extremities, with associated clinical sequelae including ischaemia, gangrene, stroke and death (Mehta et al. 2010; Metha et al. 2015). First described in 2010, the prevalence rate of this potentially fatal phenomenon, known as hydrophilic polymer embolism (HPE), has recently been estimated as 13% and is predicted to rise in line with the growing number of hydrophilic-coated catheters and delivery devices employed in vascular interventional procedures (Mehta et al. 2010; Metha et al. 2015).

Hydrogel coatings have played a major role in the evolvement of intermittent catheters from painful-to-use devices into much more acceptable and patient-friendly urine drainage instruments. Low friction urinary catheter coatings have, to-date, been largely based on poly(vinylpyrrolidone) (PVP), which has demonstrated efficacy in increasing wettability and improving frictional properties of the catheter surface, thereby reducing damage to the urethra, especially upon device implantation (Nurdin et al. 1996). Coatings are activated to a lubricious state by soaking in water or saline solution, or by bursting a hydration compartment within the packaging prior to insertion of the catheter (Sutherland et al. 1996). In one comparative study, SpeediCath® (a catheter with a ready-to-use hydrophilic coating) demonstrated a significantly lower mean withdrawal force of friction than the uncoated, gel-lubricated counterpart. However, an alternative hydrophilic-coated catheter (LoFric®) showed a significantly higher mean withdrawal force of friction than both the gel-lubricated and SpeediCath® hydrophilic-coated catheters. In this study, urine dipstick analysis was carried out to further ascertain the effect of these catheters on urethral trauma. Significantly less haematuria was observed in the urine collected after use of the hydrophilic-coated catheters in comparison to the urine collected after use of the gel-lubricated catheter. Finally, upon questioning the patients undergoing catheterization, 93% of participants preferred the hydrophilic-coated catheters (Stensballe et al. 2005). The relatively rapid dry out and ready detachment of most currently-available hydrophilic coatings from the device surface means that, in practice, the surface is often in a dried out or uncoated state during removal of the device, causing much pain and damage to the urethra from the resulting frictional forces (Stensballe et al. 2005).

Multifunctional Coatings

Optimal performance of many medical devices requires a combination of the previously described surface properties. For example, surfaces of blood-contacting medical devices should ideally resist bacterial adhesion, but not at the expense of their inherent haemocompatibility. Multilayer hydrogel coatings exhibiting a desirable combination of antibacterial and athrombogenic properties have recently been developed from silver nanoparticle-containing poly(ethylene glycol) (PEG)-heparin hydrogel films. An outer silver-free hydrogel coating on the silver-loaded PEG-heparin hydrogel layer performs the dual role of shielding mammalian cells from the silver nanoparticles, while also serving as a diffusion barrier for prolonged bioactive release (Fischer et al. 2015).

Orthopaedic devices, in particular, have a dual requirement to integrate within the bone while also remaining resistant to bacterial colonization. This balance can be challenging to achieve on the basis of the similar mechanisms of cellular surface adhesion between host tissue cells and infecting bacterial cells. Surface modifications which reduce bacterial adherence are therefore often detrimental to the process of host tissue integration, and vice versa (Goodman et al. 2013). For example, the addition of antibacterial agents to the biomaterial can have undesirable effects on host tissue cells, while also compromising the mechanical performance of the device itself. Chitosan, however, is a biocompatible polysaccharide with antibacterial activity deriving from the presence of a cationic amino group which targets bacterial cell membranes. Materials based on this biocompatible polysaccharide have, in addition, demonstrated the ability to enhance host cell adhesion and proliferation (Gaharwar et al. 2010). Of relevance here is the synthesis of chitosan-gentamycin sulfate hydrogels as candidate orthopaedic coatings which both reduce infection and improve osteogenic activity. These materials successfully inhibited biofilm formation while also stimulating the adhesion, proliferation and differentiation of MC3T3-E1 osteoblast cells during an *in vitro* study (Meng et al. 2014).

The development of dual lubricious and bacterial-repelling urinary catheter surfaces represents a promising strategy to both improve patient comfort and prevent unwanted complications, namely urinary infections and associated cases of catheter encrustation and blockage. With up to 80% of all nosocomial urinary infections resulting from the implantation of indwelling urinary catheters (Nicolle 2010), and treatment complicated by the nature of bacterial growth within highly regulated biofilm communities (Tambyah and Oon 2012), there is an urgent need for effective solutions to prevent catheter-associated urinary tract infections.

Future Developments

Significant improvements in device performance have undoubtedly been realized with the advent of hydrogel coatings. Benefits include enhanced biocompatibility, lubricity, athrombogenicity and infection resistance, all of which should consequentially improve patient outcomes, decrease morbidity and prevent premature mortality. Hydrogel coatings are, however, typically characterized by poor abrasion resistance, thus limiting potential applications. Future research should focus on improving coating durability to withstand mechanical wear throughout the duration of implantation, in addition to the initial and often highly abrasive implantation process (Goodman et al. 2013). Furthermore, the development of durable, biocompatible and infection-resistant coatings is regarded as a matter of urgency to combat the increasing incidence of device-associated infections.

Hydrogel coatings have made the targeted site-specific delivery of bioactive agents a real possibility, with potential benefits including reduced systemic toxicity of therapeutic agents and antimicrobial resistance problems, improved compliance and, ultimately, enhanced therapeutic outcomes. An expanding range of incorporated bioactive agents, in combination with advances in nanotechnology, could enable the controlled delivery of chemotherapeutic agents from coated peripherally inserted central catheters (Mehta et al. 2010). In consideration of these potential capabilities, the ever-evolving nanotechnologies and implantable 'smart' devices will continue to be coated with hydrogels (Metha et al. 2015).

Future development of bioactive hydrogel coatings will be focussed on delivering agents in tune with *in vivo* requirements, with the aim of mimicking the natural biological milieu and initiating multiple cellular cascades in a controlled fashion. Bone healing, for example, requires the sequential delivery of multiple growth factors to stimulate angiogenesis and bone formation respectively (Goodman et al. 2013). Initial success has been achieved with the use of polyelectrolyte multilayer coatings. Recombinant human vascular endothelial growth factor (rhVEGF) and recombinant human bone morphogenetic proteins (rh-BMP) were incorporated into these multilayer coatings and eluted over eight days and two weeks respectively, demonstrating the potential to fine tune biological drug delivery *in vivo* (Shah et al. 2011). Sequential, tailored delivery of BMP-2 and BMP-7 has been achieved in another study where in growth factor-loaded nanocapsules of poly(lactic-*co*-glycolic acid) and poly(3-hydroxybutyrate-*co*-3-hydroxyvalerate) were incorporated into fiber scaffolds of chitosan and chitosan-polyethylene oxide (Yilgor et al. 2009).

With regards to blood-contacting devices, despite lifelong administration of complex anticoagulation therapy to patients, thrombosis remains the most common cause of device failure. For example, thromboembolic complications of mechanical heart valves are reported at a rate of up to 6.4% per patient year (Jaffer et al. 2015; Bluestein et al. 2013). Novel strategies to eliminate the risk of medical device-induced thrombosis are therefore urgently needed. This goal will only be realised through further understanding of the pathogenesis of thrombus formation at the interface between the blood-contacting device surface and the circulatory system, in combination with advancements in materials science (Jaffer et al. 2015). Hydrogel-coated surfaces which inhibit protein adhesion are promising, however human studies to test their efficacy on more advanced mechanical circulatory support devices, such as ventricular assist devices, are needed (Jaffer et al. 2015). Furthermore, systematic studies of the pathological sequelae of HPE, novel diagnostic tests and further histopathological investigations of autopsy tissue are required to increase understanding of the aetiology of this vascular embolization process and subsequently facilitate the development of effective preventative measures (Metha et al. 2015; Sanon et al. 2014).

In conclusion, the application of hydrogels as medical device coatings offers a promising strategy to address these problems, and may ultimately lead to the development of infection-resistant devices which can be inserted with ease, integrate successfully within the body and, finally, can be removed after the required duration of implantation with no associated tissue damage—the so-called 'ideal' device.

References

Beer, C., R. Foldbjerg, Y. Hayashi, D.S. Sutherland and H. Autrup. 2012. Toxicity of silver nanoparticles-nanoparticle or silver ion? Toxicol. Lett. 208: 286–292.

Behlau, I. and M.S. Gilmore. 2008. Microbial biofilms in ophthalmology and infectious disease. Archiv. Ophthalmol. 126: 1572–1581.

Berts, I., D. Ossipov, G. Fagneto, A. Frisk and A.R. Rennie. 2014. Polymeric smart coating strategy of titanium implants. Adv. Eng. Mat. 16: 1–11.

Biazar, E., Z. Roveimiab, G. Shahhosseini, M. Khataminezhad, M. Zafari and A. Majdi. 2012. Biocompatibility evaluation of a new hydrogel dressing based on polyvinylpyrrolidone/polyethylene glycol. J. Biomed. Biotechnol. 2012: 343989.

Bluestein, D., S. Einav and M.J. Slepian. 2013. Device thrombogenicity emulation: a novel methodology for optimizing the thromboresistance of cardiovascular devices. J. Biomech. 46: 338–344.

Brun-Buisson, C., F. Doyon, J.P. Sollet, J.F. Cochard, Y. Cohen and G. Nitenberg. 2004. Prevention of intravascular catheter-related infection with newer chlorhexidine-silver sulfadiazine-coated catheters: a randomized controlled trial. Intensive Care Med. 30: 837–43.

Butruk-Raszeja, B.A., I. Lojszczyk, T. Ciach, M. Koscielniak-Ziemniak, K. Janiczak, R. Kustosz et al. 2015. Athrombogenic hydrogel coatings for medical devices—Examination of biological properties. Colloids Surf. B Biointerfaces. 130: 192–198.

Cado, G., R. Aslam, L. Seon, T. Garnier, R. Fabre, A. Parat et al. 2013. Self-defensive biomaterial coating against bacteria and yeasts: polysaccharide multilayer film with embedded antimicrobial peptide. Adv. Funct. Mater. 23: 4801–4809.

Campoccia, D., L. Montanaro and C.R. Arciola. 2006. The significance of infection related to orthopedic devices and issues of antibiotic resistance. Biomaterials. 27: 2331–2339.

Chopra, I., C. Schofield, M. Everett, A. O'Neill, K. Miller, M. Wilcox et al. 2008. Treatment of health-care-associated infections caused by Gram-negative bacteria: a consensus statement. Lancet Infect. Dis. 8: 133–139.

Cleophas, T.C., J. Sjollema, H.J. Busscher, W. Kruijtzer and R.M.J. Liskamp. 2014. Characterization and activity of an immobilized antimicrobial peptide containing bactericidal PEG-hydrogel. Biomacromolecules. 15: 3390–3395.

Costerton, J.W. 2005. Biofilm theory can guide the treatment of device-related orthopaedic infections. Clin. Orthop. and Relat. Res. 437: 7–11.

Cox, A.J. 1987. Effect of a hydrogel coating on the surface topography of latex-based urinary catheters: an SEM study. Biomaterials. 8: 500–502.

De Giglio, E., S. Cometa, M.A. Ricci, A. Zizzi, D. Cafagna, S. Manzotti et al. 2010. Development and characterization of rhVEGF-loaded poly(HEMA-MOEP) coatings electrosynthesized on titanium to enhance bone mineralization and angiogenesis. Acta Biomater. 6: 282–290.

Del Pozo, J. and R. Patel. 2009. Infection associated with prosthetic joints. N. Engl. J. Med. 361: 787–794.

Donlan, R.M. and J.W. Costerton. 2002. Biofilms: survival mechanisms of clinically relevant microorganisms. Clin. Microbiol. 15: 167–193.

Drago, L., W. Boot, K. Dimas, K. Malizos, G.M. Hansch, J. Stuyck et al. 2014. Does implant coating with antibacterial-loaded hydrogel reduce bacterial colonization and biofilm formation *in vitro*? Clin. Orthop. Rel. Res. 472: 1–13.

Elek, S.D. and P.E. Conen. 1957. The virulence of staphylococcus pyogenes for man; a study of the problems of wound infection. Brit. J. Exper. Pathol. 38: 573–586.

Fischer, M., M. Vahdatzadeh, R. Konradi, J. Friedrichs, M.F. Maitz, U. Freudenberg et al. 2015. Multilayer hydrogel coatings to combine hemocompatibility and antimicrobial activity. Biomaterials. 56: 198–205.

Francois, P., P. Vaudaux, N. Nurdin, H.J. Mathieu, P. Descouts and D.P. Lew. 1996. Physical and biological effects of a surface coating procedure on polyurethane catheters. Biomaterials. 17: 667–676.

Francolini, I. and G. Donelli. 2010. Prevention and control of biofilm based-medical device related infections. FEMS Immunol. Med. Microbiol. 59: 227–238.

Gaharwar, A.K., P.J. Schexnailder, Q. Jin, C.J. Wu and G. Schmidt. 2010. Addition of chitosan to silicate cross-linked PEO for tuning osteoblast cell adhesion and mineralization. ACS Appl. Mater. Interfaces. 2: 3119–3127.

Gatter, N., W. Kohnen and B. Jansen. 1998. *In vitro* efficacy of a hydrophilic central venous catheter loaded with silver to prevent microbial colonization. Zentralbl. Bakteriol. 287: 157–169.

Giamonna, G., G. Pitarresi, F. Palumbo, C.L. Romano, E. Meani and E. Cremascoli. 2010. Antibacterial Hydrogel and Use Thereof in Orthopedics. US Patent # 20110280921.

Goodman, S.B., Z. Yao, M. Keeney and F. Yang. 2013. The future of biologic coatings for orthopaedic implants. Biomaterials. 34: 3174–3183.

Hickok, N.J. and I.M. Shapiro. 2012. Immobilized antibiotics to prevent orthopaedic implant infections. Adv. Drug Deliv. Rev. 64: 1165–1176.

Jaffer, I.H., J.C. Fredenburgh, J. Hirsh and J.I. Weitz. 2015. Medical device-induced thrombosis: what causes it and how can we prevent it? J. Thromb. Haemost. 13: S72–S81.

Jones, D.S., C.P. Garvin and S.P. Gorman. 2004. Relationship between biomedical catheter surface properties and lubricity as determined using textural analysis and multiple regression analysis. Biomaterials. 25: 1421–1428.

Kaper, H.J., H.J. Busscher and W. Norde. 2003. Characterization of poly(ethylene oxide) brushes on glass surfaces and adhesion of Staphylococcus epidermidis. J. Biomater. Sci. Polym. Ed. 14: 313–324.

Kingshott, P., J. Wei, D. Bagge-Ravn, N. Gadegaard and L. Gram. 2003. Covalent attachment of poly(ethylene glycol) to surfaces, critical for reducing bacterial adhesion. Langmuir. 19: 6912–6921.

Kulkarni, M., A. Mazare, P. Schmuki and A. Iglic. 2014. Biomaterial surface modification of titanium and titanium alloys for medical applications. pp. 111–136. *In*: Seifalian, A., A. de Mel, and D.M. Kalaskar (eds.). Nanomedicine. One Central Press, Manchester, UK.

Lawrence, E.L. and I.G. Turner. 2005. Materials for urinary catheters: a review of their history and development in the UK. Med. Eng. Phys. 27: 443–453.

Leone, G., M. Consumi, G. Greco, C. Bonechi, S. Lamponi, C. Rossi et al. 2011. A PVA/PVP hydrogel for human lens substitution: synthesis, rheological characterization, and *in vitro* biocompatibility. J. Biomed. Mater. Res. Part B Appl. Biomater. 97: 278–288.

Lu, Y., Y. Wu, J. Liang, M.R. Libera and S.A. Sukhishvili. 2015. Self-defensive antibacterial layer-by-layer hydrogel coatings with pH-triggered hydrophobicity. Biomaterials. 45: 64–71.

McCann, M.T., B.F. Gilmore and S.P. Gorman. 2008. Staphylococcus epidermidis device-related infections: pathogenesis and clinical management. J. Pharm. Pharmacol. 60: 1551–1571.

Mehta, R.I., O.E. Solis, R. Jahan, N. Salamon, J.M. Tobis, W.H. Yong et al. 2010. Hydrophilic polymer emboli: an under-recognized iatrogenic cause of ischemia and infarct. Mod. Pathol. 23: 921–930.

Meng, G., J. He, Y. Wu, F. Wu and Z. Gu. 2014. Antibiotic-loaded chitosan hydrogel with superior dual functions: Antibacterial efficacy and osteoblastic cell responses. ACS Appl. Mater. Interfaces. 6: 10005–10013.

Metha, R.I., J.M. Choi, A. Mukherjee and R.J. Castellani. 2015. Hydrophilic polymer embolism and associated vasculopathy of the lung: prevalence in a retrospective autopsy study. Hum. Pathol. 46: 191–201.

Moriarty, T.F., U. Schlegel, S. Perren and R.G. Richards. 2010. Infection in fracture fixation: Can we influence infection rates through implant design? J. Mater. Sci. Mater. Med. 21: 1031–1035.

Muszanska, A.K., M. Reza Nejadnik, Y. Chen, E.R. van den Heuvel, H.J. Busscher, H.C. van der Mei et al. 2012. Bacterial adhesion forces with substratum surfaces and the susceptibility of biofilms to antibiotics. Antimicrob. Agents Chemother. 56: 4961–4964.

Neuerburg, C., S. Recknagel, J. Fiedler, J. Groll, M. Moeller, K. Bruellhoff et al. 2013. Ultrathin sP(EO-stat-PO) hydrogel coatings are biocompatible and preserve functionality of surface bound growth factors *in vivo*. J. Mater. Sci. Mater. Med. 24: 2417–2427.

Nicolle, L.E. 2010. Catheter-acquired urinary tract infection: the once and future guidelines. Infect. Control Hosp. Epidemiol. 31: 327–329.

Nurdin, N., E. Weilandt, M. Textor, M. Taborelli, N.D. Spencer and P. Descouts. 1996. Reduced frictional resistance of polyurethane catheter by means of a surface coating procedure. J. Appl. Polym. Sci. 61: 1939–1948.

Peivandi, M.T., M.R. Yusof-Sani and H. Amel-Farzad. 2013. Exploring the reasons for orthopedic implant failure in traumatic fractures of the lower limb. Arch. Iran. Med. 16: 478–482.

Rathore, S., R.H. Stables, M. Pauriah, A. Hakeem, J.D. Mills, N.D. Palmer et al. 2010. Impact of length and hydrophilic coating of the introducer sheath on radial artery spasm during transradial coronary intervention: a randomized study. JACC. Cardiovasc. Interv. 3: 475–483.

Sanon, S., J.J. Maleszewski and C.S. Rihal. 2014. Hydrophilic polymer embolism induced acute transcatheter aortic valve thrombosis: a novel complication. Catheter. Cardiovasc. Interv. 83: 1152–1155.

Seldon, T.H. 1954. Plasma expanders. Anesth. Analg. 33: 346–348.

Shah, N.J., M.L. Macdonald, Y.M. Beben, R.F. Padera, R.E. Samuel and P.T. Hammond. 2011. Tunable dual growth factor delivery from polyelectrolyte multilayer films. Biomaterials. 32: 6183–6193.

Stensballe, J., D. Looms, P.N. Nielsen and M. Tvede. 2005. Hydrophilic-coated catheters for intermittent catheterisation reduce urethral micro trauma: a prospective, randomised, participant-blinded, crossover study of three different types of catheters. Eur. Urol. 48: 978–983.

Subbiahdoss, G., R. Kuijer, D.W. Grijpma, H.C. van der Mei and H.J. Busscher. 2009. Microbial biofilm growth vs. tissue integration: "the race for the surface" experimentally studied. Acta biomaterialia. 5: 1399–404.

Subbiahdoss, G., R. Kuijer, H.J. Busscher and H.C. van der Mei. 2010. Mammalian cell growth versus biofilm formation on biomaterial surfaces in an *in vitro* post-operative contamination model. Microbiology. 156: 3073–3078.

Sutherland, R.S., B.A. Kogan, L.S. Baskin and R.A. Mevorach. 1996. Clean intermittent catheterization in boys using the LoFric catheter. J. Urol. 156: 2041–2043.

Tambyah, P.A. and J. Oon. 2012. Catheter-associated urinary tract infection. Curr. Opin. Infect. Dis. 25: 365–370.

Tan, G., L. Zhou, C. Ning, Y. Tan, G. Ni, J. Liao et al. 2013. Biomimetically-mineralized composite coatings on titanium functionalized with gelatin methacrylate hydrogels. Appl. Surf. Sci. 279: 293–299.

Yilgor, P., K. Tuzlakoglu, R.L. Reis, N. Hasirci and V. Hasirci. 2009. Incorporation of a sequential BMP-2/BMP-7 delivery system into chitosan-based scaffolds for bone tissue engineering. Biomaterials. 30: 3551–3559.

Yu, B., C. Wang, Y.M. Ju, L. West, J. Harmon, Y. Moussy et al. 2008. Use of hydrogel coating to improve the performance of implanted glucose sensors. Biosens. Bioelectron. 23: 1278–1284.

Zilberman, M. and J.J. Elsner. 2008. Antibiotic-eluting medical devices for various applications. J. Control. Rel. 130: 202–215.

Zimmerli, W., F.A. Waldvogel, P. Vaudaux and U.E. Nydegger. 1982. Pathogenesis of foreign body infection: description and characteristics of an animal model. J. Infect. Dis. 146: 487–497.

Zimmerli, W. and P. Sendi. 2011. Pathogenesis of implant-associated infection: The role of the host. Sem. Immunopathol. 33: 295–306.

Zimmerli, W. 2014. Clinical presentation and treatment of orthopaedic implant-associated infection. J. Intern. Med. 276: 111–119.

ZoBell, C.E. 1943. The effect of solid surfaces upon bacterial activity. J. Bacteriol. 46: 39–56.

CHAPTER 6

Hydrogels for Bone Regeneration

An Overview

Sreekanth Pentlavalli,[1] *Helen O. McCarthy*[1] *and*
Nicholas J. Dunne[1,2,]*

Introduction

Bone is a unique type of connective tissue, which is both strong and light. In order for its supportive and protective function, bone acts as a reservoir for inorganic ions; it plays an important role in the homeostasis of calcium in the body. The extracellular matrix (ECM) of this tissue comprises of a non-mineralized phase (osteoid), containing type I collagen and glycosaminoglycans (GAGs), and a mineralized phase, comprising calcium phosphate salts (Marks Jr. and Odgren 2002). During embryonic development, bone formation is achieved via direct or indirect ossification. Flat bones of the skull, e.g., the mandible, maxilla, and clavicles are formed via intramembranous ossification, during which mesenchymal stem cells (MSCs) differentiate directly into osteogenic cells function (Marks Jr. and Odgren 2002; Wozney 2002). In contrast, long bones and other load-bearing bones form via endochondral ossification, during which MSCs first differentiate into cartilage that is subsequently replaced by weak woven bone with randomly organised collagen fibres. Woven bone is gradually replaced by mature and rigid lamellar bone, consisting of highly organised concentric layers of inorganic and organic ECM (Marks Jr. and Odgren 2002).

[1] School of Pharmacy, Queen's University, Belfast, United Kingdom.
[2] School of Mechanical and Manufacturing Engineering, Dublin City University, Dublin, Ireland.
* Corresponding author: nicholas.dunne@dcu.ie

In adults, bone continues to undergo constant remodelling in response to mechanical load, changes in local calcium levels, and a wide range of paracrine and endocrine factors. This dynamic process regulates the balance between bone formation and resorption, which occurs in both compact and trabecular bone, and is governed by bone-producing cells (osteoblasts) and bone-resorbing cells (osteoclasts). The remodelling starts by osteoblasts triggering osteoclasts to break down bone matrix. The activated osteoclasts form a ruffled border in the area of bone resorption and release organic acids and lysosomal enzymes to break down the inorganic and organic bone components, respectively. As a result of this process, calcium is released into the bloodstream. Over time, osteoblasts replace osteoclasts and begin to lay down new lamellar bone on top of the old bone (Marks Jr. and Odgren 2002; Raggatt and Partridge 2010).

Most bones in the body are comprised of two morphologically and functionally different forms of bone. The outer layer consists of compact bone, also referred to as cortical bone. Compact bone is made up of densely packed collagen fibrils, which form concentric rings (lamellae). The lamellae are organised in perpendicular frames giving compact bone its rigid properties suitable for mechanical support. The inner layer is composed of a loosely organised and porous trabecular bone, also known as cancellous or spongy bone. Trabecular bone, which surrounds the bone marrow, has a more metabolic function (Marks Jr. and Odgren 2002). Cartilage is a connective tissue, which does not have any neural, lymphatic or vascular supply. The cells embedded in the dense ECM of the cartilage are called chondrocytes (Temenoff et al. 2000). The ECM of cartilage is made up of proteoglycans and collagen, which is responsible for the mechanical strength and architecture of the tissue (Ringe et al. 2002). Cartilage is predominantly present in between the joints of the long bone. As a result, they are subjected to continuous wear and tear, thereby leading to its degeneration. Cartilage can be damaged even due to trauma like sport injuries or accidents (Mano and Reis 2007; Hunziker 2002). For the cartilage to regenerate efficiently it is important to mimic its ECM. Hence the main focus for tissue engineering is the regeneration of the ECM. Since hydrogels resembles the aqueous rich environment of a cartilage tissue, they are considered suitable for cartilage tissue engineering (Lee et al. 2001; Li et al. 2009).

Bone defects can occur due to trauma, surgical excisions, congenital anomalies and degenerative disorders. More than 500,000 bone graft procedures are performed every year to address bone fractures and other orthopaedic-related injuries resulting from a variety of surgical, degenerative and traumatic causes (Greenwald et al. 2001; Laurencin et al. 2006). Injuries to the oral and maxillofacial complex are particularly challenging to repair as morphologically complex structures are damaged. The current treatment options such as autologous or allograft bone inadequately address the functional and aesthetic reconstruction of craniofacial bone due to limited supply, lack of contouring, donor-site morbidity, and other associated surgical complications (Kim et al. 2009; Schwartz et al. 2009; Sen et al. 2007). This chapter will focus on the use of hydrogels for bone regeneration. Briefly discuss about various types of hydrogel synthesis and parameters to be considered for designing of hydrogel for bone regeneration.

Human Bones

Functions of bone

Bones are responsible for ensuring structural support within the body and give protection for vital organs (Amini et al. 2012). In addition to this bone provide an environment for marrow, which is where blood cells are produced, and act as a storage location for minerals (Amini et al. 2012).

Structure and composition of bone

The loading situations acting on the skeleton influence the growth of the most macroscopically diverse bone structures *in vivo*, creating carefully tailored shapes, mechanical properties and spatial distributions (Stevens 2008). There are 206 different bones that make up the human skeletal structure (Stevens 2008). These include long bones that are found in the limbs, short bones in the wrist and ankles, flat bones in the sternum and skull and irregular bones in the vertebra (Stevens 2008). An average bone is usually enveloped in a dense layer of vascular connective tissue known as periosteum; joints are exempt (Donald 2014). This is followed by a dense and tough outer layer, of cortical (compact) bone, and beneath this is a spongy layer called trabecular (Cancellous) bone which is lighter, slightly flexible with enclosed spaces containing blood and marrow (Donald 2014). The bone is further built up of collagen and non-collagenous proteins, inorganic mineral salts and bone forming and reabsorbing cells (Amini et al. 2012). The bone forming cells are called osteoblasts and osteocytes and the bone reabsorbing cells are named osteoclasts (Amini et al. 2012). In mature bones, trabeculae are organized in orderly patterns that allow for continuous units of bone tissue aligned parallel with lines of compressive and tensile forces (Donald 2014). Hence trabeculae create a series of complex cross-branched interior struts arranged so that maximal rigidity is gained with as minimal material as needed (Donald 2014).

Bone regeneration process

It is also important to understand bone regeneration process. This will happen in two stages; the initial stage is known as formation of woven bone where collagen formed randomly with weak mechanical strength. During the second stage, collagen aligns as sheets (lamellae), which provides appropriate mechanical strength known as lamellar bone. Almost all bones in a healthy adult are lamellar bone in nature (Amini et al. 2012).

Bone healing

Bone repair restores damaged tissue to its previous physical and mechanical state. Bone healing occurs in three distinct but overlapping stages: (1) early inflammatory stage; (2) repair stage and (3) remodeling stage (Kalfas 2001). During the early inflammatory stage a hematoma develops within the fracture site. Inflammatory cells and fibroblasts enter the fracture site and initiate the formation of granulation tissue, ingrowth of vascular tissue and migration of MSCs (Kalfas 2001). Fibroblasts then begin to lay down a stoma that helps support vascular ingrowth. As vascular ingrowth progresses, a collagen matrix is laid down while osteoid is secreted and then mineralized. This results in the formation of a soft callus around the fracture-undergoing repair. After a period, the callus turns into bony tissue forming a bridge of woven bone between the broken fragments. However, if proper immobilization is not applied the callus will not ossify and unstable fibrous unions will occur (Kalfas 2001). The remodeling stage is complete when the healing bone is restored to its original shape, structure and mechanical strength. This process can occur over months or years depending on the age of the patient and is accomplished by mechanical stresses acting on the bone.

Function of bone cells in healing

Bone, unlike most organs and tissues, has a natural tendency to regenerate and heal. According to the Diamond concept there are four conditions required for successful healing in fractures (Verdonk et al. 2015). The four conditions refer to the presence of an appropriate mechanical environment and osteoconductivity (scaffolds) and encouraging osteoconductivity with growth factors and cell to induce effective osteogenesis (Verdonk et al. 2015). This concept is dependent on each of the bone cells fulfilling their respective roles in the healing process (Table 1).

Table 1. Types of bone cells and function in healing (Amini et al. 2012).

Cell Type	Function
Osteoblasts	Cells that are derived from MSCs and are responsible for bone matrix (osteoid) synthesis and its subsequent mineralization.
Osteocytes	These cells are osteoblasts that become integrated within the newly formed osteoid, which eventually becomes calcified bone. They are ideally situated so they can respond to changes in physical forces that are subjected on the bone and to transduce information to cells on the bone surface guiding them to sites that require resorption or formation responses.
Osteoclasts	Osteoclasts function in the reabsorption of mineralized tissue and are found attached to the bone surface at sites of active bone resorption. Their characteristic feature is a ruffled edge where active resorption takes place with the secretion of bone-resorbing enzymes, which digest the bone matrix.

Common Bone Diseases and Available Solutions

Bone defects can occur due to trauma, surgical excisions, congenital anomalies and degenerative disorders.

Union and non-union fractures

Unfortunately, the expected union of the bone as a result of this normal bone healing process does not always occur. Union of a bone is a process influenced by various factors, which can be delayed or even inhibited in 5–10% of all fractures resulting in major implications for the individual and increased economic costs to society

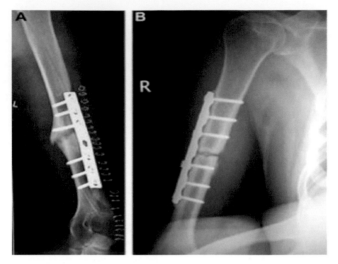

Fig. 1. Illustrations of (A) Hypertrophic; (B) Atrophic.

(Tosounidisa et al. 2009). There are two main types of non-union fractures: (1) hypertrophic and (2) atropic (Fig. 1) that are routinely classified according to their radiological appearance and lack of evidence of progression in fracture healing six months post-injury (Verdonk et al. 2015).

This complication may result from inadequate fixation (too rigid or too loose) in long bone fractures or may be attributed to other general risk factors, e.g., age, gender, history of osteoporosis, smoking, diabetes, cachexia, infection and the limited impacted of some medications such as non-steroidal anti-inflammatory drugs (NSAIDs) and steroids.

Bone diseases

There are many diseases that can affect the structure and composition of bone a few of which include: bone cancer, osteogenesis imperfecta, Rickets and osteoporosis (MedlinePlus 2016). All these diseases result in a reduction in bone density that makes the bone weaker and brittle (MedlinePlus 2016). Osteoporosis is becoming more common as the age expectation of the populace increases and with it an increase in treatment has occurred and lead to the advancements of these treatments.

Autografts

This method is currently the most favoured for treatment as it has the best clinical outcome due to the fact that the autologous bone integrates reliably with the host bone and lacks immune and disease related complications associated with allografts (Stevens 2008). This method is used to promote bone repair after severe non-union fractures, spinal fusions, joint revisions and to fill bone defects left by the removal of tumors and involves the harvesting of bone from a non-load-bearing site in the patient and transplanting it into the defective site (Stevens 2008). The drawback of this method of treatment is that it is restricted by the supply and morbidity of the donor sites related to harvesting bone tissue (Stevens 2008).

Allografts

Allografts are an alternative but less favoured method of treatment for the promotion of bone repair. The donor bone for this treatment is harvested from another patient and requires the recipient to take daily immunosuppressive drugs (Basha et al. 2015). The challenges with this treatment are: limited amount of availability, risk of disease transmission and infection (Basha et al. 2015).

Biomaterials for bone repair

Biomaterials were traditionally defined as inert and would not interact with the hosts biological chemistry; wood is one such material that was once used to replace lost tissue after a trauma (e.g., Prosthetics) (Lee and Mooney 2011). However, as research into synthetic materials has progressed it has led to a new definition of what is currently accepted as a biomaterial.

Biomaterials are defined *"as material intended to interface with the biological systems to evaluate, treat, augment or replace any tissue, organ or function of the body"* (Lee et al. 2011).

It is proposed that advancements in science, engineering and technology enable the limitations of the previous two treatments to be overcome by the use of a biomaterial substitute (Basha et al. 2015). The materials that are used for bone treatment must be osteoconductive (promote bone growth and encourage ingrowth of surrounding bone) and be able to integrate into surrounding bone (Kalfas 2001). Previous biomaterials can be categorized into four generations (Table 2) (Basha et al. 2015).

While the first-generation materials had excellent mechanical properties, they were not bioresorbable or bioactive and had to be surgically replaced as they have a limited lifetime. The scaffolds developed by the second generation of materials proved to be too brittle for load bearing conditions and the polymeric scaffolds also lacked bioactivity and adequate mechanical strength. By combining scaffolds with other materials third generation biomaterials were developed. The third-generation classification of biomaterials that benefit from combined the strength, stiffness and osteoconductivity of ceramic scaffolds with the flexibility, toughness and resorbability of the polymer scaffolds. Further advances incorporated osteogenic cells and growth

Table 2. The Four Generations of Biomaterials.

Generation	Biomaterials
First generation	Metal and alloy bone grafts
Second generation	Bioactive ceramic and bioresorbable polymer scaffolds
Third generation	Composite scaffolds
Fourth generation	Polymer-ceramic composite scaffolds with an incorporation of osteogenic cells

factors or bone morphogenetic proteins (BMPs) together or individually to create polymer-ceramic composite scaffolds. This illustrates that scientists have shifted from bioinert to more bioactive materials that integrate with biological molecules or cells and help with the regeneration of tissue (Stevens 2008). The ideal premise of biomaterials is that they should be able to be reabsorbed and replaced over time by the body's own regenerated biological tissue (Stevens 2008). For these reasons, Hydrogels have become of increasing interest in this sector of research.

Current Strategies and Materials

Modern medicines provide several options for patients with severe bone loss, of which autologous bone grafting is considered to be the gold standard. In general, during this treatment, bone from the iliac crest of the patient's own pelvis is transplanted to the site of the defect. Despite the prevalence of this technique it has severe drawbacks, such as donor site morbidity, additional pain and risk of infection. Furthermore, the autologous grafts can often be insufficient due to the limited supply of suitable donor tissue from one individual, anatomical and structural problems and high resorption levels. Another opinion is surgical transplantation of bone tissue from other donors (allografts). However, this requires the patients to be treated with immunosuppressive drugs during the remainder of their lives. Treatment with allografts also introduces the risk of disease transmission (Saito et al. 2003; Gautschi et al. 2007).

The aforementioned limitations of the existing treatments motivated the search for alternative materials, which would enhance bone formation via one or several of the three basic mechanisms: Osteoconduction, osteoinduction and osteogenesis. During osteoconduction bone formation is triggered from existing bone by the introduction of a scaffold with a three-dimensional structure similar to that of bone tissue. Osteoinduction implies that endogenous or transplanted osteoprogenitor cells in response to biomolecules, e.g., growth factors, form new bone. Osteogenesis can be initiated by manipulating the natural process of bone remodelling, e.g., by inhibiting bone resorption (Athanasiou et al. 2000).

Bone morphogenetic proteins

Bone morphogenetic proteins (BMPs) were discovered in 1965 by an orthopaedic surgeon, Dr. Marshall R. Urist, who showed that extracts of demineralised bone could induce ectopic bone and cartilage formation when it was implanted in non-skeletal tissue in rats (Urist 1965; Urist and Strates 1971). This discovery commenced a new research era, the main goal of which was to identify, purify and employ new growth factors to regenerate damaged or missing tissue. Some of the most frequently used growth factors in modern regenerative medicine are listed below.

Due to short biological half-life of these proteins, many carrier systems have been developed for sustained and local delivery with a common goal to retain its bioactivity at the site implantation long enough for the cells to migrate in and initiate differentiation into osteoblasts (Seeherman et al. 2002; Bessa et al. 2008). Some of the major materials and carriers used are listed below.

Table 3. Growth factors and its function (Chen et al. 2003).

Growth Factor	Abbreviation	Physiological Function
Basic fibroblast growth factor	bFGF/FGF-2	Proliferation of fibroblasts and initiation of angiogenesis
Bone morphogenetic protein	BMP-2 BMP-7	Differentiation and migration of bone-forming cells
Epidermal growth factors	EGF	Proliferation of epithelial, mesenchymal, and fibroblast cells
Platelet-derived growth factor	PDGF-AA PDGF-AB PDGF-BB	Proliferation and chemoattractant agent for smooth muscle cells; extra cellular matrix synthesis and deposition
Transforming growth factors-α	TGF-α	Migration and proliferation of keratinocytes; extra cellular matrix synthesis and deposition
Transforming growth factors-β	TGF-β	Proliferation and differentiation of bone-forming cells; chemoattractant for fibroblasts
Vascular endothelial growth factor	VEGF	Migration, proliferation, and survival of endothelial cells

Table 4. Cargos for BMP-2 delivery.

Materials	Examples
Ceramics	Hydroxyapatite Bioglass Tri-calcium phosphate (TCP)
Natural biopolymers	Collagen Fibrin Gelatin Alginate Chitosan Hyaluronan
Synthetic polymers	Poly(lactic acid) (PLA) Poly(glycolic acid) (PGA) Poly(lactic-co-glycolic acid) (PLGA) PLA-hyaluronan
Composites	Chitosan-gelatin Poly(caprolactone) (PCL)-collagen–TCP

Hydrogels

There have been many graft substitutes such as decellularized bone matrix, bioglass, calcium phosphate cements, calcium sulfate, hydroxyapatite powder, blocks and shapes (Bohner 2010). However, these materials are difficult to deliver into deeper and more complex shaped skeletal tissues (Kretlow et al. 2009). Injectable ceramic cements tend to become brittle thereby leading to improper repair. Furthermore, scaffolds leave some voids in the defect area, which results in impaired bone healing and regeneration. While considering these limitations, injectable hydrogel systems have an upper hand. Injectable hydrogels can adapt well into the margins of the defect, can be placed with minimal invasiveness into deep defect sites. Thus, injectable hydrogels can greatly reduce the surgical time, scar formation, post-operative pain and recovery time (Zhao et al. 2010). Hydrogels, which can adapt well to the defect margins, will provide better opportunities for cell recruitment and neovascularization from the adjacent healthy tissues. Furthermore, most of the hydrogels can mimic the native ECM, thus providing a favorable environment for the cells to proliferate and differentiate (Tibbitt et al. 2009). By incorporating different osteoinductive components (Gkioni et al. 2010; Eglin et al. 2006), growth factors (Tabata et al. 1998; Yamamoto et al. 2000), drugs like antibiotics (Niranjan et al. 2013), etc., one can further improve outcome of the treatment.

Hydrogels consists of three-dimensional crosslinked hydrophilic polymeric networks that absorb and retain large amounts of water or biological fluids (Kopecek 2007). Hydrogels have several unique characteristic features, which include resemblance of tissue, ECM, supports cell proliferation and migration, controlled release of growth factors, minimal mechanical irritation to surrounding tissue and nutrient diffusion that supports the viability and proliferation of cells (Uludag et al. 2000; Slaughter et al. 2009; Tan et al. 2010). These properties allow their usage in tissue engineering and regenerative medicine (TERM) as carriers for growth factors (Cai et al. 2005), cells (Gerecht et al. 2007), drugs (Tiller 2003) and genes (Li et al. 2003). TERM is an interdisciplinary field which aims in supporting, rejuvenating and/ or replacing the partially functioning or the damaged tissues, caused either by acute trauma, surgical removal, congenital diseases or chronic problems (Furth et al. 2007).

Conventional methods for tissue regeneration, like preformed hydrogels or scaffolds, face the problem of surgical implantation, increasing the risk of infections and improper adaptation to the defect site, which could lead to scaffold failure. By overcoming these problems, injectable hydrogels are gaining importance in the field of TERM as they can reach the defects in very deep tissues, with minimum invasiveness and provide better defect margin adaptation. This would result in reduce risk of infection, less scarring and less pain (Patenaude et al. 2014). Overall it reflects the importance of injectable hydrogels in tissue engineering area compared with traditional scaffolds. In this chapter, recent developments in several injectable hydrogels for bone regeneration are highlighted.

Based on their origins two kinds of biodegradable polymers are used for preparation of injectable hydrogels: Naturally derived and synthetic polymers. In comparison with synthetic polymers, most but not all naturally derived polymers are expected to have better interaction with cells along with increased cell proliferation and differentiation (Stevens et al. 2005). On the other hand, synthetic polymers possess tuneable mechanical properties and degradation profile (Drury et al. 2003). Mutually exclusive advantages of these polymers have motivated the researchers to investigate combinational systems of synthetic and naturally derived polymers, thereby improving the properties injectable hydrogels (Sionkowska 2011). Injectable hydrogels are prepared using various physical and chemical crosslinking methods.

Hydrogel Synthesis Methods

Chemical crosslinked hydrogels

Chemical crosslinked hydrogels represents a hydrogel class that can change from a liquid state to a gel state by forming new covalent bonds in a polymer network through chemical reactions. These types of hydrogels have typically been used for implantable applications. These types of hydrogels have also been used as injectable devices by forming *in-situ* forming hydrogels. Chemical crosslinked reactions take place by various mechanisms, such as redox reactions, photo-polymerization; click chemistry, Michael reaction, Schiff's base reaction, enzymatic reactions or disulfide-forming reactions. Irrespective of the type of reaction, new covalent bonds formed from these reactions to construct a polymeric three-dimensional network structure in which water can be entrapped and therapeutic agent or living cells can be encapsulated. Each type of reaction involves different synthesis protocol and produces different properties of hydrogels. In this section, some of the main strategies for fabricating injectable chemically cross-linked hydrogels will be addressed.

Photo-crosslinking

Photo-crosslinking usually taken place in the presence of electromagnetic radiation in the visible and UV region. Photo-initiators are interacting with light to generate free radicals, which reacts with photo-curable polymers to initiate crosslinking reaction to form hydrogels (Fig. 2). Broadly, photo-initiation is classified based on the polymerization reaction, which includes radical photo-polymerization by photo-cleavage, radical photo-polymerization by hydrogen abstraction and cationic polymerization. Because of toxicity issues, cationic photo-initiators are generally avoided, as they tend to generate protonic acids (Peiffer et al. 1997; Decker 1987). Photo-crosslinking is a three step-process comprising of initiation, propagation and termination. During the initiation step, the illumination causes the excitation of photo-

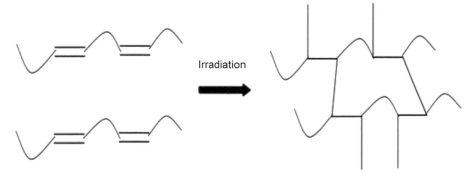

Fig. 2. Schematic representation of photo-crosslinking of vinyl groups.

initiators and results in free radical. Then they react with photo curable macromers giving rise to reactive species that could take part in propagation. Stepwise growth by crosslinking happens during propagation. The termination step is characterized by the end of the crosslinking in the 3D-polymeric network (Ifkovits et al. 2007).

Photo-polymerization has been a crosslinking technique with several advantages, including low energy and rapid reactions under mild conditions. Photo-polymerisable hydrogels have been exploited for a decade in biomedical and pharmaceutical applications, mostly in tissue engineering (Nguyen et al. 2002; Ifkovits and Burdick 2007). Photo-crosslinked systems can be formulated from aqueous solutions of polymers/monomers containing photo-sensitive molecules and a catalyst upon exposure to an external irradiation source such as ultraviolet (UV) or visible light, thus forming free radicals and catalysing the polymerization. Polymers used for these reactions usually have unsaturated groups for example methacrylate or acrylate groups, which undergoes rapid polymerization in the presence of light irradiation. This approach allows for the spatial control of the cross-linked network. Moreover, the gelation rate can also be controlled timely; resulting in the formation of patterned structured hydrogels for specific applications. Alsberg et al. 2001 introduced a biodegradable photo-crosslinked hydrogel based on heparin/alginate for affinity-based growth factors delivery (Jeon et al. 2011). Different growth factors such as FGF-2, VEGF, TGF-b1 and BMP-2 were successfully released over three weeks in a sustained manner, which was attributed to the strong affinity interaction between heparin and the growth factor. Subsequently released BMP-2 and VEGF were examined for their period of bioactivity, i.e., 2 and 3 weeks, respectively.

Click chemistry

Generally, the term "click" chemistry is being defined by Sharpless and coworkers as certain reaction types that have high efficiency, excellent specificity, bioorthogonality and mild reaction conditions (Kold et al. 2001). Click chemistry has played a significant role in polymer synthesis and bio-conjugation as a flexible and efficient method-to connect functionalized molecules. Click chemistry has been a great interest in the fabrication of hydrogels, nanogels and microgels as an emerging platform for tissue engineering and drug delivery. Typically, a wide and diverse range of reactions, including Cu(I) catalyzed alkyne-azide cycloaddition (CuAAc) reactions, catalyst-free alkyne-azide coupling reactions, Diels-Alder cycloaddition, Radical-mediated thiol-Michael reactions and Schiff's base reactions, could be considered to be 'click' chemistry (Fig. 3).

Thiol-based Michael reactions

Michael reaction refers to the nucleophilic addition of a nucleophile to a α, β-unsaturated carbonyl compound. Particularly, nucleophile components are thiol- and amine-bearing molecules, whereas unsaturated carbonyl components are commonly associated with acrylate, methacrylate and vinyl sulfone groups (Fig. 4). The advantages of Michael reactions are: mild conditions required, controllable reaction rate, high chemical yield

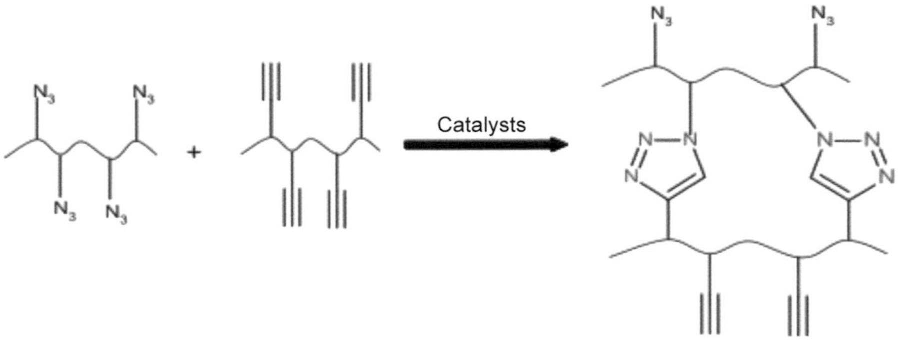

Fig. 3. Schematic representation of alkyne-azide clicks reaction.

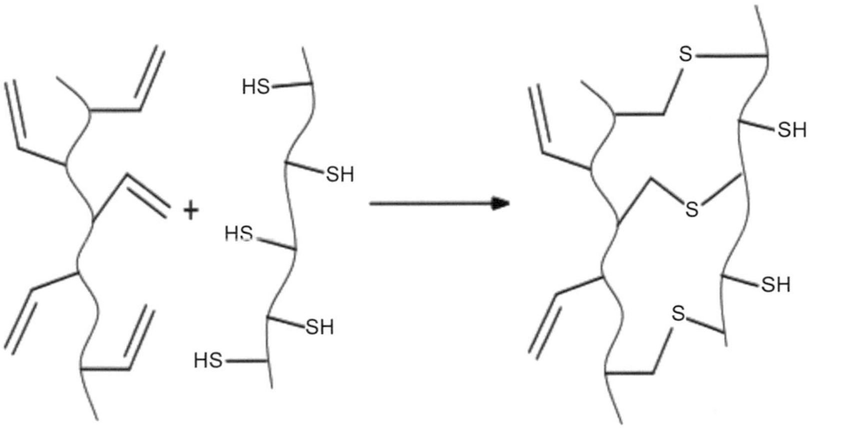

Fig. 4. Schematic representation of Michael addition of vinyl and thiol groups.

and relatively inertness to biomolecules. Michael reactions between thiol and vinyl groups have been extensively investigated to construct injectable *in situ* cross-linked hydrogels for therapeutic applications.

Schiff's base reactions

Schiff base crosslinked injectable gels are prepared by utilising the reaction between nucleophilic amines or hydrazides and electrophilic carbon atoms of aldehydes or ketones. Schiff's base reactions can occur without any chemicals or catalysts under physiological conditions (Fig. 5). The main parameters such as gelation time and strength of the hydrogel depend on the number of amines and aldehydes groups. Changing the pH of the reaction mixture can control these reactions. One must be careful while choosing the ratios of aldehyde and amines. If any unreacted aldehyde may react with amine groups of bioactive molecules, which may lead for toxicity.

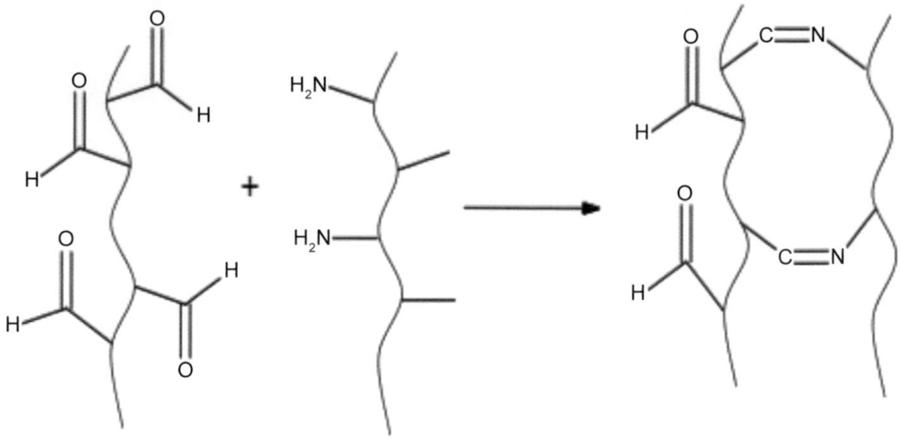

Fig. 5. Schematic representation of Schiff's base reaction.

Physically crosslinked hydrogels

Physical crosslinking hydrogels have different mechanism then chemically crosslinked hydrogels. By changing the intermolecular forces such as hydrogen bonding, hydrophobic interaction, electrostatic, ionic force, intermolecular assemblies such as guest-host inclusion, stereo-complexation and complementary binding. These changes can be induced by external stimuli such as heat, pH, temperature, light and electrical field (Qui et al. 1998). The advantages of these types of gels are to avoid toxic crosslinkers and catalysts to formulate injectable hydrogels. Also, one can design hydrogels with different mechanical strength, gelation time and rate of degradation.

Thermoresponsive hydrogels

In early generation physical crosslinked hydrogels, thermoresponsive hydrogels plays an important role. Temperature can induce a change in the solubility of a whole polymer network, thereby causing the sol-gel phase transition. The temperature at which phase transition occurs is called lower critical solution temperature (LCST) (Skrabania et al. 2007). This property is used to prepare *in situ* hydrogels, where polymer solution exists in liquid state below LCST and forms a solid gel at above LCST. Most of these gels are designed in such a way that the LCST is around or near body temperature (37°C). Some of the most widely used non-biodegradable thermoresponsive gels synthesised using N-isopropylacrylamide (NIPAAm), Pluronics and various PEG-based polymers. Pluronics is a triblock copolymer composed of PEO and PPO (PEO-PPO-PEO), which exhibit sol-gel transition at physiological temperatures (Fig. 6). The composite consists of chondrocytes suspended in Pluronics resulted in a bone-cartilage interface for mandibular condylar reconstruction (Weng et al. 2001). The main advantages of Pluronics are mild gelation, good biocompatibility, increase the stability of encapsulated proteins, however, the low mechanical integrity, non-degradability, high permeability limits its biomedical application (Liu et al. 2007). Thermosensitive chitosan-Pluronic

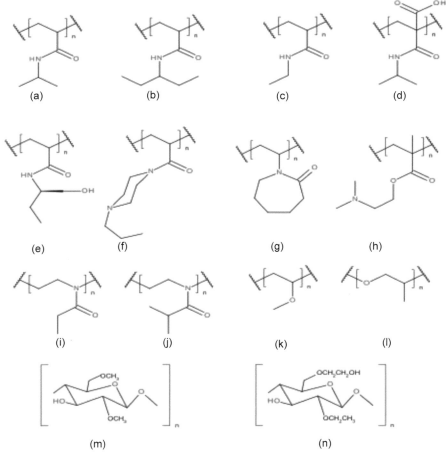

Fig. 6. Commonly used thermoresponsive polymers chemical structures: (a) poly (N-isopropylacrylamide); (b) poly (N,N-diethylacrylamide); (c) poly (N-ethylacrylamide); (d) poly (2-carboxyisopropylamide); (e) poly (N-(L)-(1-hydroxymethyl)) propylmethacrylamide; (f) poly (N-acryloyl-N'-propilpiperazine); (g) poly (N-vinylcaprolactam); (h) poly (2-domethylamino)ethyl methacrylate; (i) poly (2-ethyl-2-oxazoline); (j) poly (2-isopropyl-2-oxazoline); (k) poly (vinyl methyl ether); (l) poly (propylene oxide); (m) methylcellulose; (n) ethyl(hydroxyethyl)cellulose.

hydrogel has proven itself to be a successful injectable delivery carrier for cartilage regeneration (Park et al. 2009). Composite thermosensitive hydrogel using Pluronic derivatives and crosslinked hyaluronic acid loaded with TGF-β1 have been shown to increase benefits in the induction of chondrogenic differentiation of human adipose-derived stem cells in a full-thickness defect of rabbit knee articular cartilage mode (Jung et al. 2010).

pH-sensitive hydrogels

pH is a notable environmental parameter that can be used for stimuli-sensitive system because each site in the human body possesses a different pH value. A well-designed

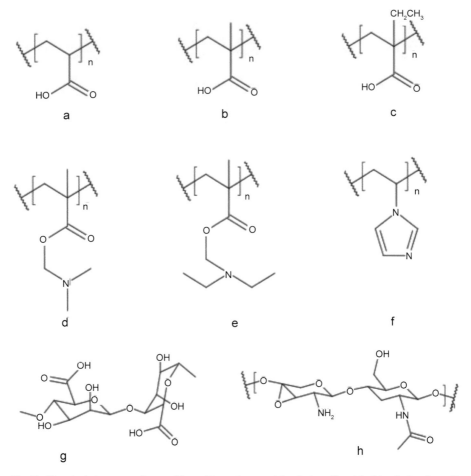

Fig. 7. Chemical structures of some pH-sensitive polymers: (a) poly (acrylic acid); (b) poly (methacrylic acid); (c) poly (2-ethyl acrylic acid); (d) poly (N,N-dimethyl aminoethyl methacrylate); (e) poly (N,N-diethyl aminoethyl methacrylate); (f) poly (vinyl imidazole); (g) alginate; (h) chitosan.

pH-sensitive system can be applied to the delivery of bioactive agents to any site in the body. pH-triggered phase transition between soluble-insoluble mainly occurs via the protonation-deprotonation of ionosable groups around the *pKa* value. pH-sensitive polymers are usually weak polyelectrolytes based on either acidic moieties such as carboxylic acid, sulfonamide or basic tertiary-amine groups that ionise at high or low pH, respectively (Fig. 7).

Ionic crosslinking

Ionic crosslinking is one of the methods used to crosslink ionisable polymers using di- and/or tri-valent cations (Fig. 8). Commonly used polymers are alginate and pectin, where divalent metal ions such as Ca^{2+} are used to cross-link anionic chains of polycarboxylates (Atala et al. 1993; Munarin et al. 2011). The polymeric solution

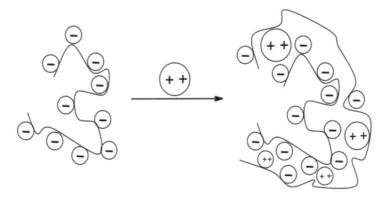

Fig. 8. Schematic representation of ionic interaction.

Table 5. Various hydrogel materials, crosslinking initiators and mechanism.

Material	Gel Precursor	Crosslink Mechanism
Pluronics	Macromer(s): PEO-PPO-PEO Initiator: temperature (37°C)	Physical (Ruel-Gariepy et al. 2004)
Chitosan-Pluronics	Macromer(s): Chitosan and pluronics Initiator: temperature (37°C)	Physical (Weng et al. 2001)
Chitosan-AHP	Macromer(s): Chitosan and AHP Initiator: temperature (37°C)	Physical (Nair et al. 2007)
Chitosan-Glycerol Phosphate	Macromer(s): Chitosan and glycerol phosphate Initiator: temperature (37°C)	Physical (Ahmadi et al. 2008)
PPF-Co-Ethylene Glycol	Macromer(s): hydrophobic PPF and hydrophilic PEG Initiator: light	Chemical (Fisher et al. 2004)
Hyaluronic Acid	Macromer(s): tyramine substituted hyaluronic acid Initiator: HRP enzyme	Physical (Darr et al. 2009)
SMO-PCLA-PEG-PCLA-SMO copolymer hydrogel	Macromer(s): pH-sensitive SMOs and thermo-sensitive PCLA-PEG-PCLA Initiator: temperature (37°C) and pH (7.4)	Physical (Shim et al. 2006)
Oxidised Alginate, Gelatin and Biphasic Calcium Phosphate	Macromer(s): oxidized alginate, gelatin and biphasic calcium phosphate	Chemical (Nguyen and Lee 2012)

and ionic solution of calcium chloride or aqueous slurry of calcium salts such as calcium sulfate, calcium carbonate was injected using dual syringe. The gels were formed instantaneously upon reacting with Ca^{2+} ions. Gelation time depends on the temperature and concentration of calcium ions.

The main drawbacks of alginate hydrogels are very poor bioresorption and rate of degradation. This gel does not undergo hydrolytic cleavage or enzymatic degradation under physiological conditions. However, partial oxidation of alginate using sodium periodate shows faster degradation rate, as it is susceptible to hydrolysis. Oxidized alginate hydrogels showed faster degradation there by enhancing new bone formation, when compared to unoxidized alginate hydrogel (Kong et al. 2004).

Consideration of Hydrogel Design for Bone Applications

In TERM applications, it is essential to mimic the ECM for regenerating the damaged tissue. As hydrogels are capable of forming three-dimensional network with high porosity and absorbs considerable amount of water, they serve as a delivery vehicle for tissue engineering. It is important to understand the properties of natural tissue while designing the hydrogels as every tissue in our body has specific properties. The following key parameters need to be considered while designing injectable hydrogels.

Stiffness and strength

The stiffness and strength of the hydrogels varies based on the application and mimic the native tissue. Usually the strength of the hydrogels is measured in terms of elastic modulus and yield stress. For example, the hydrogels should have considerable strength for bone applications where as for skin this requirement is less demanding. The cellular processes such as adhesion and differentiation (Cukierman et al. 2011), motility (Lo et al. 2000) and phagocytosis (Beningo and Wang 2002) are depending on stiffness of the gel. The stiffness of the hydrogels depends on various parameters such as polymer concentration (West et al. 2007), preparation method (Drury et al. 2003) and degree of crosslinking (Nicodemus et al. 2008; Dadsetan et al. 2007). Shear thinning is a property shown by certain class of hydrogels where they start flow when external shear is applied. In the absence of shear, hydrogels behave like a solid and retain their original shape. Many researchers are developing this type of gels for ease of handling and minimal invasiveness to use in tissue regeneration (Van Vlierberghe et al. 2011).

Porosity/permeability

Another important parameter to be considered in tissue regeneration is porosity of the hydrogel, which helps cell migration and nutrient supply. These interconnected porous networks create a platform for faster cell growth and proliferation (Kretlow et al. 2007; Hunt et al. 2010). The pore size plays important role in controlled release of drugs and growth factors. The appropriate pore size is however still a topic of debate. Some studies shown that smaller pore size hydrogels are better since natural tissues are in nanometer scale. However, some researchers have demonstrated that better cell proliferation and matrix content production when hydrogels have large interconnected pores (Griffon et al. 2006). Brauker et al. showed the importance of pore size for cell growth. The average pore size (0.8–8 um) enhanced the cell growth in the gels (Brauker et al. 1995). It is important to design a hydrogel with appropriate pore size and strength for controlled delivery of drugs or growth factors. At the same time size of the molecules should be smaller than size of the pores to enable free movement inside the pores and controlled release. Such release also depends on the pore size, pore volume fraction, the interconnectivity of pores, crosslinking density and interaction between the polymer and macromolecules (Hoffman 2002). The best way to tailor the hydrogel porosity is by varying concentration of crosslinker. The concentration of crosslinker is indirectly proportional to the size of the gels. When pores are small, the gels might be stiffer and low swelling.

Various techniques such as solvent casting/particle leaching, gas foaming and freeze-drying have been developed to include micro or macro pores in the hydrogel. In solvent casting/particle leaching, polymer homogenous solution is mixed with porogens and solidified. In an appropriate solvent, the solid mass is immersed to dissolve porogens to create porous network (Ford et al. 2006). Alginate hydrogels are formulated by bubbling CO_2 gas into the hydrogel to create porous network. The average pore size created using this method is approximately 23–250 um (Partap et al. 2006). The most common technique used to create porous network is freeze-drying. The polymeric solution is rapidly frozen and lyophilized to form pores hydrogels.

Hydrophilicity and charge

Highly hydrophilic hydrogels contain large amounts of water, which helps cells to grow and proliferate efficiently. Also, these hydrophilic hydrogels degrade and release entrapped cells, drugs or growth factors (Kwon et al. 2000). For using synthetic polymers as scaffolds, charged gels show better cell proliferation than uncharged gels. It is also noteworthy that cells prefer positively charged scaffold surface for attachment due to electrostatic interactions (Schneider et al. 2004).

Biocompatibility

Biocompatibility is a key parameter one can consider when designing a biomaterial or a hydrogel. Any biomaterial, which helps for cell growth without causing any toxicity or immunological response, called as biocompatible material. Since these materials have constant interactions with surrounding tissues, it is important that they should not trigger the immune system. While comparing synthetic polymers with natural polymers, all natural polymers have monomeric units similar to native ECM that are more biocompatible than synthetic polymers (Lee and Mooney 2001).

Biodegradability

Biodegradation is another important parameter to be considered while designing any hydrogel. The degradation of material over a period must be equal to or comparable to rate of tissue regeneration. In some cases, a slow rate of degradation restricts the native tissue regeneration (Nguyen et al. 2002). Hence the ideal property of hydrogel should be gradual degradation that helps native tissue growth. However, in certain applications such as cartilage or cornea tissue regeneration fast degradation is not required. In such applications, partial degraded material integrates with native tissue to provide support and helps to regenerate effectively. Biodegradation is a process where the three-dimensional network cleaves either by enzymatic degradation or hydrolysis. The materials that have these properties must be included while designing any biodegradable hydrogel. At the same time one should consider while choosing monomer/polymer that the nature of degraded products should not be toxic. The preferred degraded products must show the properties of natural occurring products in the body such as lactic acid, colic acid, succinic acid and glucose. The main advantage of biodegradation is to release encapsulated drugs, growth factors and cells in a controlled manner from hydrogel, which helps the tissue regeneration. Based on nature of application one can tailor the degradation rate of the hydrogel by choosing appropriate polymers.

Hydrogel Applications

Cartilage

Cartilage is an important structural component of the body. It is a firm tissue but is softer and much more flexible than bone. Cartilage is made up of specialized cells called chondrocytes. These cells produce large amounts of ECM composed of collagen fibers, proteoglycan and elastin fibers. As cartilage does not have any blood vessels to supply nutrients to cells, they grow very slowly compare to other tissues. So it vital to design any biomaterial for cartilage repair should mimic ECM. Since hydrogels resemble aqueous rich environment of a cartilage tissue, they are considered suitable for cartilage tissue engineering.

Various hydrogels have been developed for cartilage repair. Natural polymers like alginate and fibrin hydrogels have been used to encapsulate cells for cartilage regeneration (Cao et al. 1998; Sims et al. 1998). Collagen gels, encapsulated with chondrocytes showed glycosaminoglycan content along with higher expression of Type II collagen and aggrecan (Taguchi et al. 2005). Chitosan based hydrogels were used to encapsulate chondrocytes. Chitosan-hydroxyapatite based hydrogel, formed by Schiff-base reaction encapsulated with bovine articular chondrocytes showed good cell attachment and proliferation as well as good mechanical stability (Hong et al. 2007). Park et al. developed hydrogel from methacrylated glycol chitosan (MeGC) and HA (Park et al. 2013). Injectable hydrogel was prepared from gelatin-hydroxy phenylpropionic acid (Gtn-HPA) conjugate, in which the HPA was enzymatically crosslinked using hydrogen peroxide and HRP. Chondrocytes encapsulated in Gtn-HPA hydrogels with medium stiffness (G' = 1000 Pa) showed higher levels of sGAG (Sulfated Glycosaminoglycan) production, higher collagen I & II gene expression, better ectopic cartilage formation and better integration with the surrounding cartilage *in vivo* (Wang et al. 2014). Photo-polymerized PEG based hydrogels encapsulated with chondrocytes (Elisseeff et al. 2000) and bone marrow-derived MSCs (Williams et al. 2003) were developed injected subcutaneously and photo-polymerized trans dermally in animal models. These gels showed good dynamic stiffness and equilibrium moduli, which increased with time. Histological studies showed tissue structure similar to the native neocartilage. Numerous other PEG based hydrogels were developed that showed good cartilage regeneration potential (Bryant et al. 2001; Fisher et al. 2004; Buxton et al. 2007).

Hydrogels have also been encapsulated with growth factors like transforming growth factor-beta (TGF-β), insulin-like growth factor-1 (IGF-1), BMP-2, commonly found in the ECM of the cartilage. These encapsulated growth factors are expected to provide a more conductive environment for the cells to grow within the hydrogel scaffold. To improve mechanical properties of hydrogel Gelatin was photo crosslinked with methacrylic acid. These gels when incorporated with TGF-β1, showed good chondrocyte growth and proliferation along with maintenance of chondrocytic phenotype and ECM secretion (Hu et al. 2009). Kim et al. developed an oligo poly(ethylene glycol) fumarate (OPF) hydrogel and encapsulated with gelatin microparticles loaded human recombinant IGF-1 and TGF-β3 (Kim et al. 2013). Though such a dual growth factor delivery system was expected to increase the osteochondral defect healing, single delivery of IGF-1 showed better results. Holland et al. also showed similar results (Holland et al. 2007). Furthermore, IGF-1 along with BMP-2 when encapsulated in OPF hydrogel showed a synergistic effect on the two growth factors and enhance the bone growth and repair in rabbit medial femoral condyle osteochondral defect (Lu et al. 2014). Thus it can be said that only certain combinations of growth factors interact positively with each other and show better results. Hence, optimum combinations of growth factors should be kept in mind while designing the hydrogel for enhanced tissue engineering.

Bone

Alginate hydrogels along with poly(aldehyde guluronate) (PAG) have been encapsulated with rat calvarial osteoblasts and implanted ectopically in mice. Bone tissue formation was observed at the end of nine weeks (Lee et al. 2001). RGD peptide modified alginate injectable hydrogel have also been developed to improve cell interactions and showed significant bone formation *in vivo* studies in mice (Alsberg et al. 2001). Photo-crosslinked hydrogel have been prepared with tunable biodegradation properties (Jeon et al. 2009). The use of platelet rich plasma, which is rich in growth factors, in an injectable form along with MSCs, has also been used to improve osteogenesis (Yamada et al. 2004). Kim et al. encapsulated MSCs and BMP-2 in sulfamethazine oligomers (SMOs) to both ends of a thermo-sensitive poly(ε-caprolactone-co-lactide)-poly(ethylene glycol)-(ε-caprolactone-co-lactide) (PCLA-PEG-PCLA). This injectable gel was both pH and thermoresponsive and showed mineralised tissue formation ectopically in mice (Kim et al. 2008). Similarly Kim et al. synthesised injectable acrylated HA gel-using tetrathiolated PEG as a crosslinker. This delivery system was used to deliver MSCs and BMP-2. The *in vivo* studies in rat calvarial defects showed that MSCs could differentiate into osteoblasts and endothelial cells due to the microenvironment of the site (Kim et al. 2007). Burdick et al. developed injectable RGD modified PEG hydrogel by photo-crosslinking method to encapsulate osteoblasts (Burdick et al. 2002). It was demonstrated that with RGD conjugation a large number of cells could be encapsulated and good cell attachment and spreading could be achieved within the photo cross-linked hydrogel. Chitosan has been synthesized into an *in situ* gelling system by the addition of ammonium hydrogel phosphate. By varying the phosphate salt concentration, a gelation time at 37°C could be achieved within

5 min (Nair et al. 2007). Injectable Chitin-PCL-nanohydroxyapatite microgels have been prepared through simple regeneration chemistry without crosslinkers. This microgel system demonstrated an early osteodifferentiation and mineralisation *in vitro* (Kumar et al. 2015). The use of growth factors such as VEGF, TGF-β (Park et al. 2007), FGF (Dyondi et al. 2013) were loaded in the gels and showed significantly improve in the neovascularisation and bone formation. For example, silk hydrogel was used for the delivery of VEGF and BMP-2 into maxillary sinus floor. This system demonstrated the potential of using such a delivery system for deeper and irregular bony defect regeneration (Zhang et al. 2011). Chitosan-alginate injectable hydrogels have also been used successfully to deliver BMP-2 along with MSCs for bone regeneration (Park et al. 2005).

Challenges and Future Directions

Currently the TERM field is growing and focusing on novel delivery systems. The key to success is designing the construct or scaffold based on specific application. For example, when one desires to engineer bone or cartilage, load bearing capacity of new tissue plays an important role. Also, delivery of bioactive molecules to the target and rate of delivery will play important role in regeneration. Hydrogels have many different functions in the field of TERM. They are applied as space filling agents, as delivery vehicles for bioactive molecules and 3D structures that organize cells and present stimuli to direct the formation of a desired tissue. Many hydrogels (natural, synthetic or combination of both) have been developed and patented with different properties to address bone regeneration but only handful are commercially available. Most of them fulfill one or two requirements (e.g., biocompatibility, controlled delivery) without considering other design parameters (e.g., degradation profile, mechanical properties and method of delivery). Many studies so far have shown promising results at the pre-clinical phase. However, unable to overcome controlled release of growth factors and/or cells, batch-to-batch variation of natural polymers, production of growth factors for human use have hindered clinical translation. As our understanding of biological process of tissue regeneration expands, this information must be incorporated into the design of new hydrogel where target oriented delivery system with appropriate bio-chemical properties. It is vital to understand the interactions occurring at the cell surface and material interface to develop clinical applications. By using different synthetic methods, many new hydrogel systems are already underway. For example, controlled degradation of hydrogels, cell adhesion ligands have been attached to these material and growth factors have been incorporated into them to specifically regulate cell fate. Also, different synthetic protocols enhance the material biocompatibility as well as mechanical properties. Similarly, these methods have been developed to control porosity, improve diffusion and gently incorporate cells into the scaffold. These advances have the potential to improve materials properties and support the development of more natural and functional tissue. It is noteworthy to mention briefly about new type of hydrogels such as three dimensional printed hydrogels, memory shaped hydrogels and the advent four dimensional/active printed materials that could change their shape and under various stimuli. With further research in this field, hydrogels for bone regeneration will have better patient compliance.

References

Ahmadi, R. and J.D. de Bruijn. 2008. Biocompatibility and gelation of chitosan-glycerol phosphate hydrogels. J. Biomed. Mater. Res. A. 86: 824–832.

Alsberg, E., K. Anderson, A. Albeiruti, R. Franceschi and D. Mooney. 2001. Cell-interactive alginate hydrogels for bone tissue engineering. J. Dent. Res. 80: 2025–2029.

Amini, A.R., C.T. Laurencin and S.P. Nukavarapu. 2012. Bone tissue engineering: Recent advances and challenges. Crit. Rev. Biomed. Eng. 40: 363–408.

Arun Kumar, R., A. Sivashanmugam, S. Deepthi, S. Iseki, K.P. Chennazhi, S.V. Nair et al. 2015. Injectable chitin–poly(e-caprolactone)/nanohydroxyapatite composite microgels prepared by simple regeneration technique for bone tissue engineering. ACS Appl. Mater. Interfaces. 7: 9399–9409.

Atala, A., L.G. Cima, W. Kim, K.T. Paige, J.P. Vacanti and A.B. Retik. 1993. J. Urol. 150: 745–747.

Athanasiou, K.A., C.F. Zhu, D.R. Lanctot, C.M. Agrawal and X. Wang. 2000. Fundamentals of biomechanics in tissue engineering of bone. Tissue Engineering 6: 361–381.

Basha, R.Y., T.S. Sampath Kumar and M. Doble. 2015. Design of biocomposite materials for bone tissue regeneration. Materials Science and Engineering: C. 57: 452–463.

Beningo, K.A. and Y.L. Wang. 2002. Fc-receptor-mediated phagocytosis is regulated by mechanical properties of the target. J. Cell. Sci. 115: 849–856.

Bessa, P.C., M. Casal and R.L. Reis. 2008. Bone morphogenetic proteins in tissue engineering: the road from laboratory to clinic, part II (BMP delivery). Journal of Tissue Engineering and Regenerative Medicine. 2: 81–96.

Bohner, M. 2010. Resorbable biomaterials as bone graft substitutes. Mater. Today. 13: 24–30.

Brauker, J.H., V.E. Carr-Brendel, L.A. Martinson, J. Crudele, W.D. Johnston and R.C. Johnson. 1995. Neovascularization of synthetic membranes directed by membrane microarchitecture. J. Biomed. Mater. Res. 29: 1517–1524.

Bryant, S.J. and K.S. Anseth. 2001. The effects of scaffold thickness on tissue engineered cartilage in photocrosslinked poly(ethylene oxide) hydrogels. Biomaterials. 22: 619–626.

Burdick, J.A. and K.S. Anseth. 2002. Photoencapsulation of osteoblasts in injectable RGD-modified PEG hydrogels for bone tissue engineering. Biomaterials. 23: 4315–4323.

Buxton, A.N., J. Zhu, R. Marchant, J.L. West, J.U. Yoo and B. Johnstone. 2007. Design and characterization of poly(ethylene glycol) photopolymerizable semiinterpenetrating networks for chondrogenesis of human mesenchymal stem cells. Tissue Eng. 13: 2549–2560.

Cai, S., Y. Liu, X. Zheng Shu and G.D. Prestwich. 2005. Injectable glycosaminoglycan hydrogels for controlled release of human basic fibroblast growth factor. Biomaterials. 26: 6054–6067.

Cao, Y., A. Rodriguez, M. Vacanti, C. Ibarra, C. Arevalo and C.A. Vacanti. 1998. Comparative study of the use of poly(glycolic acid), calcium alginate and pluronics in the engineering of autologous porcine cartilage. J. Biomater. Sci. Polym. Ed. 9: 475–487.

Chen, R.R. and D.J. Mooney. 2003. Polymeric growth factor delivery strategies for tissue engineering. Pharmaceutical Research. 208: 1103–1112.

Cukierman, E., R. Pankov, D.R. Stevens and K.M. Yamada. 2011. Taking cell-matrix adhesions to the third dimension. Science. 294: 1708–1712.

Dadsetan, M., J.P. Szatkowski, M.J. Yaszemski and L. Lu. 2007. Characterization of photo-cross-linked oligo [poly(ethylene glycol) fumarate] hydrogels for cartilage tissue engineering. Biomacromolecules. 8: 1702–1709.

Darr, A. and A. Calabro. 2009. Synthesis and characterization of tyramine-based hyaluronan hydrogels. J. Mater. Sci. Mater. Med. 20: 33–44.

Decker, C. 1987. UV-curing chemistry: past, present and future. J. Coat. Technol. 59: 97–106.

Donald, G. 2014. Bone Anatomy. http://www.britannica.com/science/bone-anatomy (Accessed: 12th April 2016).

Drury, J.L. and D.J. Mooney. 2003. Hydrogels for tissue engineering: scaffold design variables and applications. Biomaterials. 24: 4337–4351.

Dyondi, D., T.J. Webster and R. Banerjee. 2013. A nanoparticulate injectable hydrogel as a tissue-engineering scaffold for multiple growth factor delivery for bone regeneration. Int. J. Nanomed. 8: 47–59.

Eglin, D., S. Maalheem, J. Livage and T. Coradin. 2006. *In vitro* apatite forming ability of type I collagen hydrogels containing bioactive glass and silica sol-gel particles. J. Mater. Sci. Mater. Med. 17: 161–167.

Elisseeff, J., W. McIntosh, K. Anseth, S. Riley, P. Ragan and R. Langer. 2000. Photoencapsulation of chondrocytes in poly(ethylene oxide)-based semi-interpenetrating networks. J. Biomed. Mater. Res. 51: 164–171.

Fisher, J.P., S. Jo, A.G. Mikos and A.H. Reddi. 2004. Thermoreversible hydrogel scaffolds for articular cartilage engineering. J. Biomed. Mater. Res. A. 71: 268–74.

Ford, M.C., J.P. Bertram, S.R. Hynes, M. Michaud, Q. Li, M. Young et al. 2006. A macroporous hydrogel for the coculture of neural progenitor and endothelial cells to form functional vascular networks *in vivo*. Proc. Natl. Acad. Sci. 103: 2512–2517.

Furth, M.E., A. Atala and M.E. van Dyke. 2007. Smart biomaterials design for tissue engineering and regenerative medicine. Biomaterials. 28: 5068–5073.

Gautschi, O.P., S.P. Frey and R. Zellweger. 2007. Bone morphogenetic proteins in clinical applications. ANZ Journal of Surgery. 77: 626–631.

Gerecht, S., J.A. Burdick, L.S. Ferreira, S.A. Townsend, R. Langer and G. Vunjak-Novakovic. 2007. Hyaluronic acid hydrogel for controlled self-renewal and differentiation of human embryonic stem cells. Proc. Natl. Acad. Sci. 104: 11298–11303.

Gkioni, K., S.C. Leeuwenburgh, T.E. Douglas, A.G. Mikos and J.A. Jansen. 2010. Mineralization of hydrogels for bone regeneration. Tissue Eng. B. 16: 577–585.

Greenwald, A., S. Boden, V. Goldberg, Y. Khan, C. Laurencin and R. Rosier. 2001. Bone graft substitutes: facts, fictions & applications. American Academy of Orthopaedic Surgeons. San Francisco, CA. 1–6.

Griffon, D.J., M.R. Sedighi, D.V. Schaeffer, J.A. Eurell and A.L. Johnson. 2006. Chitosan scaffolds: interconnective pore size and cartilage engineering. Acta Biomater. 2: 313–320.

Hoffman, A.S. 2002. Hydrogels for biomedical applications. Adv. Drug Deliv. Rev. 54: 3–12.

Holland, T., E. Bodde, V. Cuijpers, L. Baggett, Y. Tabata, A. Mikos et al. 2007. Degradable hydrogel scaffolds for *in vivo* delivery of single and dual growth factors in cartilage repair. Osteoarthr. Cartil. 15: 187–197.

Hong, Y., H. Song, Y. Gong, Z. Mao, C. Gao and J. Shen. 2007. Covalently crosslinked chitosan hydrogel: properties of *in vitro* degradation and chondrocyte encapsulation. Acta Biomater. 3: 23–31.

Hu, X., L. Ma, C. Wang and C. Gao. 2009. Gelatin hydrogel prepared by photo-initiated polymerization and loaded with TGF-b1 for cartilage tissue engineering. Macromol. Biosci. 9: 1194–1201.

Hunt, N.C. and L.M. Grover. 2010. Cell encapsulation using biopolymer gels for regenerative medicine. Biotechnol. Lett. 32: 733–742.

Hunziker, E. 2002. Articular cartilage repair: basic science and clinical progress. A review of the current status and prospects. Osteoarthr. Cartil. 10: 432–463.

Ifkovits, J.L. and J.A. Burdick. 2007. Photopolymerizable and degradable biomaterials for tissue engineering applications. Tissue Eng. 13: 2369–85.

Jeon, O., K.H. Bouhadir, J.M. Mansour and E. Alsberg. 2009. Photocrosslinked alginate hydrogels with tunable biodegradation rates and mechanical properties. Biomaterials. 30: 2724–2734.

Jeon, O., C. Powell, L.D. Solorio M.D. Krebs and E. Alsberg. 2011. Affinity based growth factor delivery using biodegradable, photocrosslinked heparin-alginate hydrogels. J. Controlled Release. 154: 258–66.

Jung, H.H., K. Park and D.K. Han. 2010. Preparation of TGF-beta 1-conjugated biodegradable pluronic F127 hydrogel and its application with adipose-derived stem cells. J. Control Release. 147: 84–91.

Kalfas, I.H. 2001. Principles of bone healing. Neurosurg. Focus. 10: E1.

Kim, D.H., R. Rhim, L. Li, J. Martha, B.H. Swaim, R.J. Banco et al. 2009. Prospective study of iliac crest bone graft harvest site pain and morbidity. Spine J. 9: 886–892.

Kim, H.K., W.S. Shim, S.E. Kim, K.H. Lee, E. Kang, J.H. Kim et al. 2008. Injectable *in situ*-forming pH/ thermo-sensitive hydrogel for bone tissue engineering. Tissue Eng. A. 15: 923–933.

Kim, J., I.S. Kim, T.H. Cho, K.B. Lee, S.J. Hwang, G. Tae et al. 2007. Bone regeneration using hyaluronic acid-based hydrogel with bone morphogenic protein-2 and human mesenchymal stem cells. Biomaterials. 28: 1830–1837.

Kim, K., J. Lam, S. Lu, P.P. Spicer, A. Lueckgen, Y. Tabata et al. 2013. Osteochondral tissue regeneration using a bilayered composite hydrogel with modulating dual growth factor release kinetics in a rabbit model. J. Control. Release. 168: 166–178.

Kold, H.C., M.G. Finn and K.B. Sharpless. 2001. Click chemistry: diverse chemical function from a few good reactions. Angew. Chem. Int. Ed. 40: 2004–2021.

Kong, H., D. Kaigler, K. Kim and D.J. Mooney. 2004. Controlling rigidity and degradation of alginate hydrogels via molecular weight distribution. Biomacromolecules. 5: 1720–1727.

Kopecek, J. 2007. Hydrogel biomaterials: a smart future? Biomaterials. 28: 5185–5192.

Kretlow, J.D., L. Klouda and A.G. Mikos. 2007. Injectable matrices and scaffolds for drug delivery in tissue engineering. Adv. Drug Deliv. Rev. 59: 263–273.

Kretlow, J.D., S. Young, L. Klouda, M. Wong and A.G. Mikos. 2009. Injectable biomaterials for regenerating complex craniofacial tissues. Adv. Mater. 21: 3368–3393.

Kwon, O.H., A. Kikuchi, M. Yamato, Y. Sakurai and T. Okano. 2000. Rapid cell sheet detachment from poly(N-isopropylacrylamide)-grafted porous cell culture membranes. J. Biomed. Mater. Res. 50: 82–89.

Laurencin, C., Y. Khan, M. Kofron, A. El-Amin, E. Botchwey, X. Yu et al. 2006. Tissue engineering bone and ligament: a 15-year perspective. Clin. Orthop. Relat. Res. 447: 221–236.

Lee, K.Y. and D.J. Mooney. 2001. Hydrogels for tissue engineering. Chem. Rev. 101: 1869–1880.

Lee, K.Y. and D.J. Mooney. 2011. Alginate: properties and biomedical applications. Progress in Polymer Science. 37: 106–126.

Lee, Y., E. Alsberg and D.J. Mooney. 2001. Degradable and injectable poly(aldehyde guluronate) hydrogels for bone tissue engineering. J. Biomed. Mater. Res. 56: 228–233.

Li, H., Q. Zheng, Y. Xiao, J. Feng, Z. Shi and Z. Pan. 2009. Rat cartilage repair using nanophase PLGA/HA composite and mesenchymal stem cells. J. Bioact. Compat. Polym. 24: 83–99.

Li, Z., W. Ning, J. Wang, A. Choi, P.Y. Lee, P. Tyagi et al. 2003. Controlled gene delivery system based on thermosensitive biodegradable hydrogel. Pharm. Res. 20: 884–888.

Liu, Y., W.L. Lu, J.C. Wang, H. Zhang, X.Q. Wang and T.Y. Zhou. 2007. Controlled delivery of recombinant hirudin based on thermo-sensitive Pluronics F127 hydrogel for subcutaneous administration: *in vitro* and *in vivo* characterization. J. Control. Release. 117: 387–395.

Lo, C.M., H.B. Wang, M. Dembo and Y.I. Wang. 2000. Cell movement is guided by the rigidity of the substrate. Biophys. J. 79: 144–152.

Lu, S., J. Lam, J.E. Trachtenberg, E.J. Lee, H. Seyednejad, J.J. van den Beucken et al. 2014. Dual growth factor delivery from bilayered, biodegradable hydrogel composites for spatially guided osteochondral tissue repair. Biomaterials. 35: 8829–8839.

Mano, J. and R. Reis. 2007. Osteochondral defects: present situation and tissue engineering approaches. J. Tissue Eng. Regen. Med. 1: 261–273.

Marks, Jr., S.C. and P.R. Odgren. 2002. Structure and development of the skeleton in Principles of Bone Biology. 2nd ed., Bilezikian, J.P., Raisz, L.G., and Rodan, G.A., Eds., Academic Press, San Diego: 3–15.

Munarin, F., S.G. Guerreiro, M.A. Grellier, M.C. Tanzi, M.A. Barbosa, P. Petrini et al. 2011. Pectin-based injectable biomaterials for bone tissue engineering. Biomacromolecules. 12: 568–577.

Nair, L.S., T. Starnes, J.W. Ko and C.T. Laurencin. 2007. Development of injectable thermogelling chitosan-inorganic phosphate solutions for biomedical applications. Biomacromolecules. 8: 3779–85.

Nguyen, K.T. and J.L. West. 2002. Photopolymerizable hydrogels for tissue engineering applications. Biomaterials. 23: 4307–14.

Nguyen, T.P. and B.T. Lee. 2012. Fabrication of oxidized alginate-gelatin-BCP hydrogels and evaluation of the microstructure, material properties and biocompatibility for bone tissue regeneration. J. Biomater. Appl. 27: 311–321.

Nicodemus, G.D. and S.J. Bryant. 2008. Cell encapsulation in biodegradable hydrogels for tissue engineering applications. Tissue Eng. B. 14: 149–165.

Niranjan, R., C. Koushik, S. Saravanan, A. Moorthi, M. Vairamani and N. Selvamurugan. 2013. A novel injectable temperature-sensitive zinc doped chitosan/bglycerophosphate hydrogel for bone tissue engineering. Int. J. Biol. Macromol. 54: 24–29.

Park, D.J., B.H. Choi, S.J. Zhu, J.Y. Huh, B.Y. Kim and S.H. Lee. 2005. Injectable bone using chitosan-alginate gel/mesenchymal stem cells/BMP-2 composites. J. Cranio Maxill. Surg. 33: 50–54.

Park, H., J.S. Temenoff, Y. Tabata, A.I. Caplan and A.G. Mikos. 2007. Injectable biodegradable hydrogel composites for rabbit marrow mesenchymal stem cell and growth factor delivery for cartilage tissue engineering. Biomaterials. 28: 3217–3227.

Park, H., B. Choi, J. Hu and M. Lee. 2013. Injectable chitosan hyaluronic acid hydrogels for cartilage tissue engineering. Acta Biomater. 9: 4779–4786.

Park, K.M., S.Y. Lee, Y.K. Joung, J.S. Na, M.C. Lee and K.D. Park. 2009. Thermosensitive chitosan-Pluronic hydrogel as an injectable cell delivery carrier for cartilage regeneration. Acta Biomater. 5: 1956–1965.

Partap, S., I. Rehman, J.R. Jones and J.A. Darr. 2006. Supercritical carbon dioxide in water emulsion-templated synthesis of porous calcium alginate hydrogels. Adv. Mater. 18: 501–504.

Patenaude, M., N. Smeets and T. Hoare. 2014. Designing injectable, covalently cross-linked hydrogels for biomedical applications. Macromol. Rapid Commun. 35: 598–617.

Peiffer, R., A. Scranton and A. Bowman. 1997. Photopolymerization: fundamentals and applications. ACS Symposium Series.

Qui, Y. and K. Park. 1998. Environment-sensitive hydrogels for drug delivery. Adv. Drug. Delive. Rev. 31: 197–221.

Raggatt, L.J. and N.C. Partridge. 2010. Cellular and molecular mechanisms of bone remodeling. Journal of Biological Chemistry. 285: 25103–25108.

Ringe, J., C. Kaps, G.R. Burmester and M. Sittinger. 2002. Stem cells for regenerative medicine: advances in the engineering of tissues and organs. Naturwissenschaften. 89: 338–351.

Ruel-Gariepy, E. and J.C. Leroux. 2004. *In situ*-forming hydrogels—review of temperature-sensitive systems. Eur. J. Pharm. Biopharm. 58: 409–26.

Saito, N. and K. Takaoka. 2003. New synthetic biodegradable polymers as BMP carriers for bone tissue engineering. Biomaterials. 24: 2287–2293.

Salgado, A.J., O.P. Coutinho and R.L. Reis. 2004. Bone tissue engineering: state of the art and future trends. Macromol. Biosci. 4: 743–765.

Schneider, G.B., A. English, M. Abraham, R. Zaharias, C. Stanford and J. Keller. 2004. The effect of hydrogel charge density on cell attachment. Biomaterials. 25: 3023–3028.

Schwartz, C.E., J.F. Martha, P. Kowalski, D.A. Wang, R. Bode, L. Li et al. 2009. Prospective evaluation of chronic pain associated with posterior autologous iliac crest bone graft harvest and its effect on postoperative outcome. Health Qual. Life Outcomes. 7: 49–52.

Seeherman, H., J. Wozney and R. Li. 2002. Bone morphogenetic protein delivery systems. Spine. 27: S16–S23.

Sen, M.K. and T. Miclau. 2007. Autologous iliac crest bone graft: should it still be the gold standard for treating nonunions? Injury. 38: S75–S80.

Shim, W.S., J.H. Kim, H. Park, K. Kim, I. Chan Kwon and D.S. Lee. 2006. Biodegradability and biocompatibility of a pH- and thermo-sensitive hydrogel formed from a sulfonamide-modified poly(epsilon-caprolactone-*c*o-lactide)-poly(ethylene glycol)-poly(epsiloncaprolactone-*co*-lactide) block copolymer. Biomaterials. 27: 5178–85.

Sims, D.C., P.E. Butler, Y. Cao, R. Casanova, M.A. Randolph, A. Black et al. 1998. Tissue engineered neocartilage using plasma derived polymer substrates and chondrocytes, Plast. Reconstr. Surg. 101: 1580–1585.

Sionkowska, A. 2011. Current research on the blends of natural and synthetic polymers as new biomaterials: review. Prog. Polym. Sci. 36: 1254–1276.

Skrabania, K., J. Kristen, A. Laschewsky, O. Akdemir, A. Hoth and J.F. Lutz. 2007. Design, synthesis and aqueous aggregation behavior of nonionic single and multiple thermoresponsive polymers. Langmuir. 23: 84–93.

Slaughter, B.V., S.S. Khurshid, O.Z. Fisher, A. Khademhosseini and N.A. Peppas. 2009. Hydrogels in regenerative medicine. Adv. Mater. 21: 3307–3329.

Stevens, M.M. and J.H. George. 2005. Exploring and engineering the cell surface interface. Science. 310: 1135–1138.

Stevens, M.M. 2008. Biomaterials for bone tissue engineering. Materials Today. 11: 18–24.

Tabata, Y., K. Yamada, S. Miyamoto, I. Nagata, H. Kikuchi, I. Aoyama et al. 1998. Bone regeneration by basic fibroblast growth factor complexed with biodegradable hydrogels. Biomaterials. 19: 807–815.

Taguchi, T., L. Xu, H. Kobayashi, A. Taniguchi, K. Kataoka and J. Tanaka. 2005. Encapsulation of chondrocytes in injectable alkali-treated collagen gels prepared using poly(ethylene glycol)-based 4-armed star polymer. Biomaterials. 26: 1247–1252.

Tan, H. and K.G. Marra. 2010. Injectable, biodegradable hydrogels for tissue engineering applications. Materials. 3: 1746–1767.

Temenoff, J.S. and A.G. Mikos. 2000. Tissue engineering for regeneration of articular cartilage. Biomaterials. 21: 431–440.

Tibbitt, M.W. and K.S. Anseth. 2009. Hydrogels as extracellular matrix mimics for 3D cell culture. Biotechnol. Bioeng. 103: 655–663.

Tiller, J.C. 2003. Increasing the local concentration of drugs by hydrogel formation. Angew. Chem. Int. Ed. 42: 3072–3075.

Tosounidisa, T., G. Kontakisa, V. Nikolaoub and A.P.P.V. Giannoudisb. 2009. Fracture healing and bone repair: an update. Trauma. 11: 145–156.

U.S. National Library of Medicine. 2016. Bone Diseases. Available at: https://www.nlm.nih.gov/medlineplus/bonediseases.html (Accessed: 7 March 2016).

U.S. National Library of Medicine. 2016. Bone Diseases. http://www.nlm.nih.gov/medlineplus/bonediseases.html (Accessed: 4th April 2016).

Uludag, H., P. De Vos and P.A. Tresco. 2000. Technology of mammalian cell encapsulation. Adv. Drug Deliv. Rev. 42: 29–64.

Urist, M.R. 1965. Bone: formation by autoinduction. Science. 150: 893–899.

Urist, M.R. and B.S. Strates. 1971. Bone morphogenetic protein. Journal of Dental Research. 50: 1392–1406.

Van Vlierberghe, S., P. Dubruel and E. Schacht. 2011. Biopolymer-based hydrogels as scaffolds for tissue engineering applications: a review. Biomacromolecules. 12: 1387–1408.

Verdonk, R., Y. Goubau, F.K. Almqvist and P. Verdonk. 2015. Biological methods to enhance bone healing and fracture repair. Arthoscopic and Related Surgery. 31: 715–718.

Wang, L.S., C. Du, W.S. Toh, A.C.A. Wan, S.J. Gao and M. Kurisawa. 2014. Modulation of chondrocyte functions and stiffness-dependent cartilage repair using an injectable enzymatically crosslinked hydrogel with tunable mechanical properties. Biomaterials. 35: 2207–2217.

Weng, Y., Y. Cao, C.A. Silva, M.P. Vacanti and C.A. Vacanti. 2001. Tissue-engineered composites of bone and cartilage for mandible condylar reconstruction. J. Oral Maxillofac. Surg. 59: 185–190.

West, E.R., M. Xu, T.K. Woodruff and L.D. Shea. 2007. Physical properties of alginate hydrogels and their effects on *in vitro* follicle development. Biomaterials. 28: 4439–4448.

Williams, C.G., T.K. Kim, A. Taboas, A. Malik, P. Manson and J. Elisseeff. 2003. *In vitro* chondrogenesis of bone marrow-derived mesenchymal stem cells in a photopolymerizing hydrogel. Tissue Eng. 9: 679–688.

Wozney, J.M. 2002. Overview of bone morphogenetic proteins. Spine. 27: S2–S8.

Yamada, Y., M. Ueda, T. Naiki, M. Takahashi, K.I. Hata and T. Nagasaka. 2004. Autogenous injectable bone for regeneration with mesenchymal stem cells and platelet-rich plasma: tissue-engineered bone regeneration. Tissue Eng. 10: 955–964.

Yamamoto, M., Y. Tabata, L. Hong, S. Miyamoto, N. Hashimoto and Y. Ikada. 2000. Bone regeneration by transforming growth factor b1 released from a biodegradable hydrogel. J. Control. Release. 64: 133–142.

Zhang, W., X. Wang, S. Wang, J. Zhao, L. Xu, C. Zhu et al. 2011. The use of injectable sonication-induced silk hydrogel for VEGF and BMP-2 delivery for elevation of the maxillary sinus floor. Biomaterials. 32: 9415–9424.

Zhao, L., M.D. Weir and H.H. Xu. 2010. An injectable calcium phosphate-alginate hydrogel-umbilical cord mesenchymal stem cell paste for bone tissue engineering. Biomaterials. 31: 6502–6510.

CHAPTER 7

Hydrogels in Wound Management

Enrica Caló,[1] *Lucy Ballamy*[2] and
Vitaliy V. Khutoryanskiy[1,*]

Introduction

One of the most prevalent applications of hydrogels is wound management. Thanks to their high water content and unique physical properties, hydrogels could potentially resemble biological tissues including human skin (Peppas et al. 2000; Gupta et al. 2010; Caló and Khutoryanskiy 2015; Jones et al. 2006). There is active interest in the development of new and advanced hydrogel-based products from both an academic and industrial perspective. In fact, hydrogels exhibit many characteristics of the 'ideal' wound dressing. These include: the capability of maintaining a moist environment at the wound site allowing gas exchange (moisture vapour transmission), biocompatibility, fast absorption of wound exudate, protection of newly formed or delicate skin and easy and relatively painless dressing removal (Thomas 1990; Gupta et al. 2010; Vowden and Vowden 2014; Boateng and Catanzano 2015). In this chapter we will provide the reader with an overview of the most recent hydrogel materials designed for wound management.

Skin Anatomy

The skin is considered to be the largest organ in the human body. It is responsible for protecting the body from external agents, thermoregulation and balance of water loss (Nicol 2005). Three different layers can be differentiated within the skin structure

[1] University of Reading, Reading, Berkshire, RG6 6AD, United Kingdom.
[2] ConvaTec Ltd., First Avenue-Deeside Industrial Park, Flintshire CH5 2NU, Wales, United Kingdom.
* Corresponding author: v.khutoryanskiy@reading.ac.uk

(Fig. 1): epidermis, dermis and subcutis (or hypodermis). The epidermis is composed of 80% keratinocytes that differentiate and migrate towards the surface (this process is called keratinization), resulting in the formation of four different 'strata' (inwards from the outer skin layer): corneum, granulosum, spinosum and basale (Keng and Lau 2015; Nicol 2005). The stratum corneum (10–20 μm thick) has a peculiar organization in which corneocytes (representing the physical barrier) are arranged in the well-known 'bricks in mortar' system within the lipid matrix; the lipid matrix is composed of ceramides, free-fatty acid and cholesterol (Michaels et al. 1975; Menon et al. 2012; van Smeden et al. 2014). This layer is always damaged when a wound occurs. It also represents one of the major obstacles within topical drug delivery (Williams 2003).

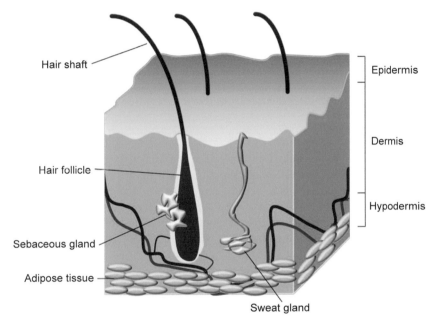

Fig. 1. Schematical representation of human skin structure.

Classification of Wounds

A wound is defined as a disruption of skin integrity, which can be a symptom of a pre-existing pathological condition or caused by mechanical, thermal or chemical damage (Thomas 1990). Wounds can be classified into two main types, depending on the healing time and response to treatments: acute or chronic (Harper et al. 2014). The correct diagnosis of each wound (by identifying the causes and types of tissue present) can greatly influence the choice of treatment and the healing outcome (Trudie 2015).

Acute wounds

Acute or 'superficial' wounds usually heal within a period of three weeks and involve only the epidermis and dermis (they are then called 'superficial') or they can expand into the subcutaneous layer ('full-thickness'). Abrasions, surgical wounds, burns and lacerations are considered acute wounds (Dreifke et al. 2015). Burns can be further classified into: first-degree (resulting from exposure to moderate intensity heat and involving primarily only the epidermis), second-degree (involving a large part of the dermis as well) and third-degree or full-thickness burns (the skin is completely damaged) (Thomas 1990).

Chronic wounds

Chronic wounds take a minimum of eight weeks and sometimes even up to many years, in some cases, to heal or respond to therapy. They can seriously affect the quality of life of the patient causing mobility limitations and sometimes depression. These type of wounds are often caused by vascular, haemostaseological or metabolic disorders, as well as inflammatory skin diseases, cancer or infections (Erfurt-Berge and Renner 2015). Hospitalization is often required with consequent high costs for the healthcare system. For example, approximately 2% of health budgets are used for chronic wound therapies and care (Harding et al. 2002; Schreml et al. 2010).

The Healing Process

Wound healing can be described as a cascade of four different events: haemostasis, inflammation, proliferation and maturation. Through this dynamic phenomenon, which requires the contribution of several molecules, cells and growth factors, the equilibrium is re-established in the body and the wound closes (Hanna and Giacopelli 1997; Gurtner et al. 2008). Considering the complexity of the healing cascade it is very impressive to observe how often everything proceeds without any problems (Harper et al. 2014). In the case of chronic wounds, the process is delayed by complications such as a secondary infection, and it can take much longer for the wound to heal (Timmons 2006). For instance, when there has been considerable tissue loss, wound closure is not immediately possible because the edges are too distant or for the presence of sepsis, in which case the microbial load must be managed so that the wound can heal without trapping bacteria inside the body. This represents the so-called closure by secondary intention, which is different from wound closure by primary intention which results from suturing wounds that involve minimal tissue loss, such as surgical incisions (Harper et al. 2014).

Haemostasis

During haemostasis, uncontrolled blood loss is prevented and vascular integrity is restored. After tissue damage, the formation of a localized thrombus is promoted: subendothelial collagen and von Willebrand factor (vWF) are exposed on the lower face of the endothelium, stimulating platelet adhesion. Plasminogen activator inhibitor is produced, allowing fibrin generation through the proteolytic cleavage of fibrinogen by thrombin. Cross-linked fibrin then binds to platelets leading to the formation of a clot, which is visible to the naked eye (Austin 2013; Baum and Arpey 2006). The fibrin and platelets are the main components of the clot matrix formed, which represents an indispensable scaffold for all the cells that are recruited to the wound during the first steps of the healing process (Gurtner et al. 2008; Baum and Arpey 2006).

Inflammation

In order for the healing process to take place the fibrin clot is destroyed (through a process called fibrinolysis), facilitating cell migration to the wound site. Fluid movement to the wound is promoted through local vasodilation triggered by growth factors released from platelets, and enhancement in the permeability of capillaries in the area (Baranoski and Ayello 2004). The complement system (which involves a variety of different plasma proteins) is then activated: this complicated enzyme-triggered cascade is responsible for opsonization, phagocytosis and ultimately, the destruction of bacterial cells (Charles et al. 2001). Chemotactic substances (such as chemotaxin) are released attracting polymorphonuclear (PMN) neutrophils and monocytes, which will differentiate into macrophages (Mulder et al. 2002). Neutrophils produce important inflammatory factors such as interleukin-1 (IL-1) and tumor necrosis factor alpha (TNF-α), and proteases which are able to break down damaged extracellular matrix (ECM) components. Macrophages play many roles, including phagocytizing bacteria, as well as producing collagenases, elastase, other growth factors and many types of cytokines. Evident symptoms of inflammation are: erythema, swelling and an increase of the temperature in the injured area (Granick and Teot 2012).

Proliferation

This phase is characterized by two events that are crucial for the progress of healing: angiogenesis, which is defined as the process of formation of new blood vessels or repairing of pre-exiting ones allowing blood supply to the site of injury, and the production of new ECM (Flanagan 2013; Tonnesen et al. 2000). Formation of capillary buds from vascular endothelial cells is promoted by angiogenesis factors, such as vascular endothelial growth factor (VEGF) and fibroblast growth factor-2 (FGF-2). Fibroblasts migrate to the wound in response to the transforming growth factor-β (TGF-β) which is released from macrophages, proliferate and start the production of collagen fibres and other connective tissue proteins. As a result, so-called 'granulation tissue' is formed: newly formed blood vessels within the ECM appear red and granular (Huether and McCance 2013). Myofibroblasts (differentiated fibroblasts, similar to smooth muscle cells due to the presence of parallel fibres in their cytoplasm) present in the granulation tissue are responsible for wound contraction, which usually starts 6 to 7 days post-injury (Hinz et al. 2007; Huether and McCance 2013). The choice of the initial dressing in this phase is crucial and it has to consider that any mechanical stress could lead to renewed bleeding, special care has to be taken to manage the wound and encourage the best healing outcome (Davey and Ince 1999).

Maturation

The maturation phase usually starts 20 days after the injury in acute wounds and it can last from six to 18 months, depending on several factors, such as skin type, age and genetic predisposition of the subject (McCulloch and Kloth 2010; Davey and Ince 1999). The aim of this phase is for the injured skin to regain its strength and elasticity. This delicate process is controlled by metalloproteinases (MMPs), which are responsible for matrix tissue degradation, and their inhibitors (Hess 2008). Approximately 50% of the tensile strength is already regained by the wound two weeks after re-epithelization. However after having some types of wounds, especially chronic wounds, the repaired tissue may not recover completely (Davey and Ince 1999).

Classification of Wound Dressings

The choice of the appropriate dressing is very important and it has to be made in accordance with the overall wound management plan specific to each individual. This process is of course directly determined by the diagnosis of the wound, which is related to a great extent to the aspect and state of the wound bed (colour and tissue types present) (Vowden and Vowden 2014). Wound dressings can be generally classified into: dry and moist products. Dry dressings, such as gauzes, are usually easily available, very cheap, indicated for low-exuding wounds and they can strongly adhere to the newly formed tissue causing painful removal (Jones et al. 2006). Moist dressings include different types of materials: transparent films, hydrocolloids, alginates, foams and hydrogels. Transparent film dressings (such as Tegaderm® by 3M Health Care) are made from polyurethane or co-polyester and are flexible with an adhesive backing but are incapable of absorbing wound fluids, therefore they should be used on dry non-infected wounds only (Sood et al. 2014). Hydrocolloids (such as DuoDERM® by ConvaTec) are usually composed of two layers: the inner adhesive layer in contact with the wound containing pectin, gelatin and/or sodium carboxymethylcellulose, and the outer polyurethane layer impermeable to water. They conform to the wound surface absorbing slight to moderate amounts of exudate and they do not require frequent changes (they can be kept in place for a maximum of seven days) (Hanna and Giacopelli 1997). Alginates (such as Kaltostat® by ConvaTec) are derived from the calcium and sodium salts of alginic acid formed in *Phaeophyceae*, brown seaweed. They are made up of repeating units of mannuronic and guluronic acid and the ratio between the two units greatly influences their absorptive capacity and their tensile strength. They are suitable for medium to highly exuding wounds (Jones et al. 2006). In the presence of high exudate, foam dressings (such as Allevyn® by Smith and Nephew) can be used as well, because they can absorb a large amount of wound fluid within their porous structure, the limitations being that the dressing must be changed frequently so that pooling and spread of wound fluid does not cause breakdown of the surrounding skin (maceration). They are commonly represented by polyurethane or silicon foams (Murphy and Evans 2012). Dressings containing Hydrofiber® technology (such as AQUACEL® by ConvaTec) are made up of sodium carboxymethyl cellulose fibres. The fibres form a gel on contact with wound fluid which conforms well to the wound bed. Dressings containing Hydrofiber® technology are suitable for low to medium exudate levels and due to their gel-like nature can be easily removed from the wound bed without damaging new cells. Hydrogel dressings (which will be explored further in the next section) can be made of natural or synthetic cross-linked polymeric networks able to absorb large amounts of biological fluids. Their so-called 'moisture donor effect' promotes collagenase production accelerating autolytic debridement of necrotic wounds (Stashak et al. 2004).

Hydrogel-based Products for Wound Care

Although hydrogels are now recognized as an alternative to more conventional wound care products, they are not routinely employed and there are few products currently available on the market. The high production and final costs may prevent the industry from manufacturing these materials on a large scale and healthcare professionals from extensively using them on patients (Caló and Khutoryanskiy 2015; Sood et al. 2014). Hydrogel-based products for wound care are usually designed as flat transparent sheets, which are very useful for instance in the treatment of pressure wounds, or as amorphous gels, which can be applied to wounds at difficult anatomical locations such as cavity wounds (acting as fillers) (Figs. 2 and 3) (Jones and Vaughan 2005). However, independently from the shape or design, all hydrogel products must exhibit specific characteristics, such as very high absorption capacity, moisture donation capability, transparency, good mechanical properties and biocompatibility in order to have the best performance (Holbock and Yeao 2011).

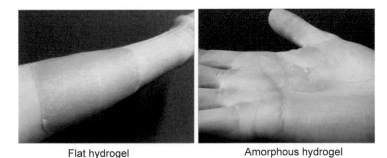

Flat hydrogel   Amorphous hydrogel

Fig. 2. Flat and amorphous hydrogel products for wound care.

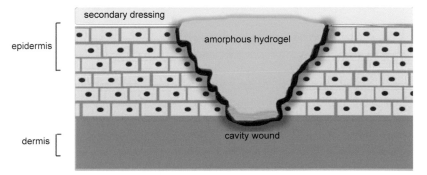

Fig. 3. Amorphous hydrogel acting as filler for cavity wound.

Commercially available hydrogels

The wound management industry has experienced a period of incredible development in the last five decades, continuously designing more advanced technologies and products (Schreml et al. 2010). Since Winter (1962) established that a moist environment effectively helps and accelerates wound healing, moist wound dressings, such as hydrogels, started gaining popularity over gauze and dry materials (Jones 2005; Jones and Vaughan 2005; Jones et al. 2006). Whilst bearing in mind that the 'perfect' dressing for every type of wound and every stage of healing would be very difficult to create, efforts have been made to manufacture new products with specific features (such as particular designs for an easier application or active ingredients added) and keeping the final prices as low as possible (Jones et al. 2006; Leaper 2006). We will mention a few in order to give the reader an idea of the range of hydrogel-based products for wound care now available on the market.

Granugel® (ConvaTec) is an amorphous clear hydrogel containing pectin, carboxymethyl cellulose and propylene glycol. It is indicated for the management of partial and full-thickness wound (such as leg and pressure ulcers) (Williams 1996). Intrasite® Gel (Smith and Nephew) is made from modified carboxymethyl cellulose and propylene glycol and it is used for surgical wounds, venous ulcers, diabetic foot and pressure ulcers. It is relatively simple to apply thanks to an applicator (Applipak system) and is available in different sizes (Williams 1994; Vernon 2000; Eaglstein 2001). Purilon® Gel (Coloplast) also has an applicator, and it is composed of sodium carboxymethyl cellulose, calcium alginate and water. It is usually used in conjunction with a secondary dressing, on dry and necrotic wounds (Caló and Khutoryanskiy 2015). Aquaform™ (Aspen Medical), more specifically its newer version, contains glycerol, starch copolymer, methylparaben and imidazolidyl urea (as preservatives) and purified water. It can be used on flat and cavity wounds with low or no exudate (Timmons et al. 2008). Aquaflo® (Covidien) is a flat hydrogel dressing and is produced from polyethylene glycol and propylene glycol. It has a unique disc shape and is transparent to aid monitoring of the wound. First Water Ltd., which was recently acquired by Scapa Group plc, manufactures Woundtab®, a flat hydrogel containing carboxymethylcellulose, sulphonated copolymer, glycerol and water indicated for chronic wounds (Caló and Khutoryanskiy 2015). Another well-known hydrogel composition is a Kikgel™ developed by Rosiak et al., which is made from the combination of a natural polymer (such as agar) and a synthetic one (such as polyvinyl pyrrolidone) crosslinked by gamma radiation (Rosiak 1995; Dabbagh et al. 2010), this dressing is intended for chronic ulcers and burns. Nu-Gel® (Systagenix) is a hydrogel dressing made of polyvinyl pyrrolidone and water, indicated for dry, partial and full-thickness wounds (Ovington 2007; Eaglstein 2001).

Hydrogel wound care products now often contain active ingredients such as antimicrobial agents in order to prevent bacteria colonization of the wound and infections that would delay healing (Leaper 2006). For instance, colloidal or ionic silver has been proposed in several wound care products as an efficient antimicrobial to be used against pathogens such as *Pseudomonas aeruginosa* and *Staphylococcus aureus* (Foster 1996; Seth et al. 2012). Silvasorb® (Medline) is a polyacrylate gel produced using the MicroLattice™ technology, containing ionic silver. It is suitable for chronic deep wounds with moderate drainage and can be changed every 3 (amorphous form) to 7 days (gel sheets) (Hess 2008; Ovington 2007). Povidone-iodine loaded hydrogel dressings became very popular as well, such as Vigilon™ (Bard, distributed by Seton Healthcare Group plc), and are claimed to inhibit bacteria growth and proliferation at the wound site (Mertz et al. 1986).

Future hydrogel technologies

Academia is the cradle of new ideas and exciting findings par excellence, which has always inspired industry. Many research projects for the development of advanced wound care technologies have been successful resulting from productive collaborations between academia and industry, and have led to significant progress in the field (Salcido 1999). From simple dressings, hydrogels become systems for the delivery of agents that can accelerate the healing process and actually make a big difference to the condition of patients. Gong et al. (Gong et al. 2013) proposed a thermosensitive *in situ* forming hydrogel containing curcumin-loaded micelles, which reported very good *in vitro* wound healing activity. The composite made of poly(ethylene glycol)- poly(ε-caprolactone)-poly(ethylene glycol) (PEG-PCL-PEG), would gel at body temperature adhering to the tissue and offering a sustained release of curcumin over a period of 14 days. Curcumin (extracted from the rhizome of *Curcuma longa*) has been used as a traditional medicine in Southeast Asia for its anti-oxidant, anti-bacterial and anti-inflammatory activities. However, it has poor solubility in water and oral bioavailability, problems that have been bypassed using this system (Gong et al. 2013). Miguel et al. (Miguel et al. 2014) presented an *in situ* thermoresponsive and antimicrobial chitosan-agarose hydrogel that accelerates skin regeneration. *In vitro* (using human dermal fibroblasts), and *in vivo* (using Wistar rats) testing reported, shows that this material is able to allow cell migration and proliferation, and to enhance autolytic debridement, promoting re-epithelization. Patients with burns can present particularly unpleasant scarring and may benefit from formulations such as this (Miguel et al. 2014). Burns can also have prolonged recovery (up to 10 weeks) especially when the dermis is compromised (full and partial-thickness burns).

Loo et al. (Loo et al. 2014) designed a very interesting hydrogel, formed from ultrashort peptides (motif composed of three to seven aliphatic amino acids) in a nanofibrous network, that can be used as a primary dressing for these types of burn injuries. These peptides undergo self-assembly in aqueous conditions and can retain up to 99.9% of water, as the peptides convert into hydrogels, they are able to keep the wound hydrated and can be removed easily. The resemblance of the network formed with the ECM facilitates cell adhesion and tissue regeneration, resulting in a faster healing when compared with the standard dressing (Loo et al. 2014). Reyes-Ortega et al. (Reyes-Ortega et al. 2015) loaded a gelatin/hyaluronic acid hydrogel with proadrenomedullin N-terminal 20 peptide (PAMP). This peptide naturally occurs in the skin and it is known for its proangiogenic, anti-inflammatory and antibacterial activities. The system presented in this work is composed of two different sections, both bio-functionalized. The external layer is made of polyurethane and loaded with bioresorbable nanoparticles containing bemiparin (low molecular weight form of heparin able to complex with growth factors such as FGF and VEGF enhancing their activity). The internal layer is represented by the biodegradable hydrogel releasing PAMP to the wound. This dressing has been proposed for the compromised wounds, such as diabetic ulcers, or in the presence of problematic epidermal regeneration, as in the elderly (Reyes-Ortega et al. 2015). One of the most popular strategies to speed up healing is indeed the delivery of peptides, polysaccharides and other molecules that naturally take part in this process. For instance, hyaluronic acid (HA), present in the aforementioned work as well, has been extensively explored for the role that it plays in the early stages, promoting keratinocytes proliferation and migration. Catanzano et al. (Catanzano et al. 2015) developed a hydrogel dressing made of alginate (ALG) and HA by internal gelation, the technique that involves the slow release of calcium ions which can form complexes with ALG leading to the formation of an ionically cross-linked homogenous network without the addition of any toxic cross-linking agents. Here, the presence of HA was shown to significantly reduce the time to wound closure as demonstrated by the *in vivo* excision wound model carried out on rats (Catanzano et al. 2015). Researchers are also considering natural molecules extractable from different sources such as bacteria and insects. A good example is the work presented by Shi et al. (Shi et al. 2015) that combined poly(γ-glutamic acid) (γ-PGA, polyamino acid secreted by some *Bacilli*) and silk sericin (SS, protein obtained from silkworm *Bombyx mori*) to produce an antibacterial hydrogel dressing (Shi et al. 2015). Chitosan-based hydrogel products have been widely investigated because of chitosan's intrinsic activity against bacteria and fungi, and of course due to the biocompatibility of this polymer, but no products are known to have been commercialized yet (Paul and Sharma 2004).

When the wound is microscopic in size or affects particularly delicate organs of the body such as the eyes, treatment can be very challenging. Tsai et al. (Tsai et al. 2016) proposed a thermosensitive chitosan/gelatine/glycerophosphate hydrogel for the delivery of ferulic acid (FA) to corneal burns that may be caused by chemicals or ultraviolet-B light exposure. In this condition, an abnormal production of reactive oxygen species (ROS) is often observed, and it can be very hard for the endogenous anti-oxidant system to manage this high level. FA is a polyphenol, natural anti-oxidant compound that can prevent ROS damages. However, it has low bioavailability and residence time when administered topically in the eye. Its inclusion in the hydrogel system presented by Tsai et al. allows its successful sustained release to the cornea with very interesting clinically relevant results *in vitro* and *in vivo* (Tsai et al. 2016).

Conclusions

Hydrogels represent an excellent choice of treatment for many types of wounds, which can be difficult to manage with traditional dry dressings. However, patients would benefit from more advanced, efficient, cost-effective hydrogel products in order to significantly enhance healing time and quality. For these reasons, it is important that industry and academia continue to join their efforts and expertise. In future, it is hoped that specific novel computer technologies and equipment will enable the development of improved wound management techniques. For instance, new wound image evaluation systems such as the one proposed by Veredas et al. (Veredas et al. 2015) could give healthcare professionals a great help establishing the correct diagnosis in the shortest possible time (Veredas et al. 2015; Engel et al. 2011). The healthcare system, which annually sustains huge costs for the treatment of chronic wounds (of non-hospitalized and hospitalized patients), would greatly benefit, from innovative low-cost hydrogel-based wound care solutions for routine use (Ramos et al. 2015; Sen et al. 2009).

Acknowledgement

The authors would like to thank the University of Reading and ConvaTec Ltd. for funding Enrica Caló's PhD project. The authors confirm that there is no conflict of interest.
®/TM all trademarks are the property of their respective owners.

References

Austin, S.K. 2013. Haemostasis. Medicine (Baltimore). 41: 208–211.
Baranoski, S. and E.A. Ayello. 2004. Wound Care Essentials: Practice Principles. Lippincott Williams & Wilkins, Philadelphia, USA.
Baum, C.L. and C.J. Arpey. 2006. Normal cutaneous wound healing: Clinical correlation with cellular and molecular events. Dermatologic Surg. 31: 674–686.
Boateng, J. and O. Catanzano. 2015. Advanced therapeutic dressings for effective wound healing—A review. J. Pharm. Sci. 104: 1–28.
Caló, E. and V.V. Khutoryanskiy. 2015. Biomedical applications of hydrogels: a review of patents and commercial products. Eur. Polym. J. 65: 252–267.
Catanzano, O., V. D'Esposito, S. Acierno, M.R. Ambrosio, C. Caro, C. De Avagliano et al. 2015. Alginate-hyaluronan composite hydrogels accelerate wound healing process. Carbohydr. Polym. 131: 407–414.
Charles, A., J. Janeway, P. Travers, M. Walport and M.J. Shlomchik. 2001. Immunobiology: The Immune System in Health and Disease. 5th edition. Garland Science, New York, USA.
Dabbagh, M., E. Moghimipour, A. Ameri and N. Sayfoddin. 2010. Physicochemical characterization and antimicrobial activity of nanosilver containing hydrogels. Iran J. Pharm. Res. 21–28.
Davey, A. and C.S. Ince. 1999. Fundamentals of Operating Department Practice. Cambridge University Press, Cambridge, UK.
Dreifke, M.B., A.A. Jayasuriya and A.C. Jayasuriya. 2015. Current wound healing procedures and potential care. Mater. Sci. Eng. C. 48: 651–662.
Eaglstein, W.H. 2001. Moist wound healing with occlusive dressings: a clinical focus. Dermatologic Surg. 27: 175–182.
Engel, H., J.J. Huang, C.K. Tsao, C.-Y. Lin, P.-Y. Chou, E.M. Brey et al. 2011. Remote real-time monitoring of free flaps via smartphone photography and 3G wireless Internet: a prospective study evidencing diagnostic accuracy. Microsurgery. 31: 589–95.
Erfurt-Berge, C. and R. Renner. 2015. Chronic wounds—Recommendations for diagnostics and therapy. Rev. Vasc. Med. 3: 5–9.
Flanagan, M. 2013. Wound Healing and Skin Integrity: Principles and Practice. John Wiley & Sons, Oxford, UK.
Foster, T. 1996. Staphylococcus. *In*: Baron, S. (ed.). Medical Microbiology. University of Texas Medical Branch at Galveston, Galveston (USA), Chapter 12.
Gong, C., Q. Wu, Y. Wang, D. Zhang, F. Luo, X. Zhao et al. 2013. A biodegradable hydrogel system containing curcumin encapsulated in micelles for cutaneous wound healing. Biomaterials. 34: 6377–87.
Granick, M.S. and L. Teot. 2012. Surgical Wound Healing and Management, 2nd ed. CRC Press, Boca Raton (USA).
Gupta, B., R. Agarwal and M.S. Alam. 2010. Textile-based smart wound dressings. Indian J. Fiber Text. Res. 35: 174–187.
Gurtner, G.C., S. Werner, Y. Barrandon and M.T. Longaker. 2008. Wound repair and regeneration. Nature. 453: 314–21.
Hanna, J.R. and J.A. Giacopelli. 1997. A review of wound healing and wound dressing products. J. Foot Ankle Surg. 36: 2–14.

Harding, K.G., H.L. Morris and G.K. Patel. 2002. Clinical review Healing chronic wounds 160–163.

Harper, D., A. Young and C.-E. McNaught. 2014. The physiology of wound healing. Surg. 32: 445–450.

Hess, C.T. 2008. Skin and Wound Care. Lippincott Williams & Wilkins, Philadelphia (USA).

Hinz, B., S.H. Phan, V.J. Thannickal, A. Galli, M.-L. Bochaton-Piallat and G. Gabbiani. 2007. The myofibroblast: one function, multiple origins. Am. J. Pathol. 170: 1807–16.

Holback, H., Y. Yeo and K. Park. 2011. Hydrogel swelling behavior and its biomedical applications. pp. 3–43. *In*: Rimmer, S. (ed.). Biomedical Hydrogels: Biochemistry, Manufacture and Medical Applications. Woodhead Publishing Materials, Philadelphia, USA.

Huether, S.E. and K.L. McCance. 2013. Understanding Pathophysiology, 5th ed. Elsevier Health Sciences, Saint Louis (USA).

Jones, A. and D. Vaughan. 2005. Hydrogel dressings in the management of a variety of wound types: a review. J. Orthop. Nurs. 9: S1–S11.

Jones, J. 2005. Winter's concept of moist wound healing: a review of the evidence and impact on clinical practice. J. Wound Care. 14: 273–6.

Jones, V., J.E. Grey and K.E. Harding. 2006. Wound dressings. BMJ. 332: 777–80.

Keng Wooi Ng and W.M. Lau. 2015. Skin Deep: The Basics of Human Skin Structure and Drug Penetration, in: Percutaneous Penetration Enhancers 3 Chemical Methods in Penetration Enhancement: Drug Manipulation Strategies and Vehicle Effects. © Springer-Verlag Berlin Heidelberg, pp. 3–11.

Leaper, D.J. 2006. Silver dressings: their role in wound management. Int. Wound J. 3: 282–94.

Loo, Y., Y.-C. Wong, E.Z. Cai, C.-H. Ang, A. Raju, A. Lakshmanan et al. 2014. Ultrashort peptide nanofibrous hydrogels for the acceleration of healing of burn wounds. Biomaterials. 35: 4805–14.

McCulloch, J.M. and L.C. Kloth. 2010. Wound Healing: Evidence-Based Management, 4th ed. F.A. Davis, Philadelphia (USA).

Menon, G.K., G.W. Cleary and M.E. Lane. 2012. The structure and function of the stratum corneum. Int. J. Pharm. 435: 3–9.

Mertz, P.M., D.A. Marshall and M.A. Kuglar. 1986. Povidone-iodine in polyethylene oxide hydrogel dressing. Effect on multiplication of *Staphylococcus aureus* in partial-thickness wounds. Arch. Dermatol. 122: 1133–8.

Michaels, A.S., S.K. Chandrasekaran and J.E. Shaw. 1975. Drug permeation through human skin: Theory and *in vitro* experimental measurement. AIChE J. 21: 985–996.

Miguel, S.P., M.P. Ribeiro, H. Brancal, P. Coutinho and I.J. Correia. 2014. Thermoresponsive chitosan-agarose hydrogel for skin regeneration. Carbohydr. Polym. 111: 366–73.

Mulder, M., N. Small, Y. Botma, L. Ziady and J. MacKenzie. 2002. Basic Principles of Wound Care. Pearson South Africa, Cape Town (South Africa).

Murphy, P.S. and G.R.D. Evans. 2012. Advances in wound healing: a review of current wound healing products. Plast. Surg. Int. 2012: 1–7.

Nicol, N.H. 2005. Anatomy and physiology of the skin. Dermatol. Nurs. 17: 3–11.

Ovington, L.G. 2007. Advances in wound dressings. Clin. Dermatol. 25: 33–8.

Paul, W. and C.P. Sharma. 2004. Chitosan and Alginate Wound Dressings: A Short Review. Trends Biomater. Artif. Organs 18: 18–23.

Peppas, N.A., P. Bures, W. Leobandung and H. Ichikawa. 2000. Hydrogels in pharmaceutical formulations. 50: 27–46.

Ramos, A., J.M. Morillo, N. Gayo, J.E. Tasiguano, E. Munzón and A.S.F. Ribeiro. 2015. Curar o paliar: ¿qué cuesta más? Análisis de costes del tratamiento de una herida crónica en función de su finalidad. Med. Paliativa. 22: 45–51.

Reyes-Ortega, F., A. Cifuentes, G. Rodríguez, M.R. Aguilar, A. González-Gómez, R. Solis et al. 2015. Bioactive bilayered dressing for compromised epidermal tissue regeneration with sequential activity of complementary agents. Acta Biomater.

Rosiak, J.M. 1995. Pergamon radiation formation of hydrogels for biomedical purposeses. Some remarks and comments. Radiat. Phys. Chem. 46: 161–168.

Salcido, R. 1999. Research partnerships: academia, industry, patients, and clinicians. Adv. Wound Care. 12: 231–2.

Schreml, S., R.-M. Szeimies, L. Prantl, M. Landthaler and P. Babilas. 2010. Wound healing in the 21st century. J. Am. Acad. Dermatol. 63: 866–81.

Sen, C.K., G.M. Gordillo, S. Roy, R. Kirsner, L. Lambert, T.K. Hunt et al. 2009. Human skin wounds: a major and snowballing threat to public health and the economy. Wound Repair Regen. 17: 763–71.

Seth, A.K., M.R. Geringer, A.N. Gurjala, S.J. Hong, R.D. Galiano, K.P. Leung et al. 2012. Treatment of *Pseudomonas aeruginosa* biofilm-infected wounds with clinical wound care strategies: a quantitative study using an *in vivo* rabbit ear model. Plast. Reconstr. Surg. 129: 262e–274e.

Shi, L., N. Yang, H. Zhang, L. Chen, L. Tao, Y. Wei et al. 2015. A novel poly(γ-glutamic acid)/silk-sericin hydrogel for wound dressing: Synthesis, characterization and biological evaluation. Mater. Sci. Eng. C. 48: 533–540.

Sood, A., M.S. Granick and N.L. Tomaselli. 2014. Wound dressings and comparative effectiveness data. Adv. Wound Care. 3: 511–529.

Stashak, T.S., E. Farstvedt and A. Othic. 2004. Update on wound dressings: Indications and best use. Clin. Tech. Equine Pract. 3: 148–163.

Thomas, S. 1990. Wound Management and Dressings. Pharmaceutical Press, London (UK).

Timmons, J. 2006. Skin function and wound healing physiology. Wound Essentials. 1: 9–17.

Timmons, J., M. Bertram, G. Pirie and K. Duguid. 2008. Aquaform?? hydrogel—A new formulation for an improved wound care performance. Wounds UK. 4: 69–73.

Tonnesen, M.G., X. Feng and R.A. Clark. 2000. Angiogenesis in wound healing. J. Investig. Dermatol. Symp. Proc. 5: 40–6.

Trudie, Y. 2015. Accurate assessment of different wound tissue types. Wound Essentials. 10: 51–54.

Tsai, C.-Y., L.-C. Woung, J.-C. Yen, P.-C. Tseng, S.-H. Chiou, Y.-J. Sung et al. 2016. Thermosensitive chitosan-based hydrogels for sustained release of ferulic acid on corneal wound healing. Carbohydr. Polym. 135: 308–315.

van Smeden, J., M. Janssens, G.S. Gooris and J.A. Bouwstra. 2014. The important role of stratum corneum lipids for the cutaneous barrier function. Biochim. Biophys. Acta. 1841: 295–313.

Veredas, F.J., R.M. Luque-Baena, F.J. Martín-Santos, J.C. Morilla-Herrera and L. Morente. 2015. Wound image evaluation with machine learning. Neurocomputing. 164: 112–122.

Vernon, T. 2000. Intrasite gel and intrasite conformable: the hydrogel range. Br. J. Nurs. 9: 1083–8.

Vowden, K. and P. Vowden. 2014. Wound dressings: principles and practice. Surg. 32: 462–467.

Williams, A. 2003. Transdermal and Topical Drug Delivery from Theory to Clinical Practice. Pharmaceutical Press, London (UK).

Williams, C. 1994. Intrasite Gel: a hydrogel dressing. Br. J. Nurs. 3: 843–6.

Williams, C. 1996. Granugel: hydrocolloid gel. Br. J. Nurs. 5: 188, 190. doi:10.12968/bjon.1996.5.3.188.

CHAPTER 8

Hydrogels for Imaging, Sensing and Diagnostics

Dietmar Puchberger[1,*] *and Michael J. Vellekoop*[2]

Introduction

By their hydrophilic nature, crosslinked gels are especially suited for applications in moist or liquid environments. The majority of applications can be found within the food industry and medicine. Common medical applications of hydrogels are found in wound dressings, soft contact lenses, drug delivery systems, hygiene products, and tissue engineering (Caló and Khutoryanskiy 2015). Besides these applications, hydrogels have gained considerable attention in sensor development and diagnostics. The three main areas of gel use in sensors are responsive hydrogels, size exclusion membranes, and (bio)chemical reactors. Depending on their application, important features of these gels are their pore size, swelling behavior, mechanical stability, and biocompatibility.

Initiation of the gelation process results in a decreased solubility by linking macromolecular chains. In physically crosslinked gels this process is reversible, while chemical crosslinking yields irreversible covalent bonds. Natural polysaccharides, including agarose are physically crosslinked by cooling of hot solutions. The gel is held together by hydrogen bonds between helical polymer fibers. In contrast, chemical crosslinking commonly is achieved by free radical polymerization. Photochemical gelation is a popular method for hydrogels in drug delivery, tissue engineering, and sensing systems because of the simple temporal and spatial control. Selective curing

[1] Institute of Sensor and Actuator Systems (ISAS), Vienna University of Technology, Gusshausstrasse 27-29/366-ISS, A-1040 Vienna, Austria.
[2] Institute for Microsensors, -actuators and -systems (IMSAS), MCB, University of Bremen, 28359 Bremen, Germany.
   E-mail: mvellekoop@imsas.uni-bremen.de
* Corresponding author: dietmar.puchberger-enengl@tuwien.ac.at

via a mask or focused UV light beam offers great flexibility in the design of sensing hydrogel networks. In tissue engineering and biological sensors, biocompatibility of UV cured gel and its polymerization is an important issue because many monomer and photoinitiator residuals, as well as UV light show cytotoxic effects. Alternative photoinitiators for visible light curing include eosin Y and triethanolamine (Bahney et al. 2011) and, in addition, improved gelation rates by lithium phenyl-2,4,6-trimethylbenzoylphosphinate (LAP) (Fairbanks et al. 2009). Specialized gel systems, including hyaluronic acid vinyl ester (HAVE) (Qin et al. 2014) and gelatin methacrylate (Nichol et al. 2010) were introduced for three-dimensional cellular patterning with improved biocompatibility.

In recent years several excellent reviews on the synthesis and structure of gels (Hoffman 2001), biomedical devices (Deligkaris et al. 2010; Kirschner and Anseth 2013) and sensor applications (Buenger et al. 2012; Yetisen et al. 2015; Le Goff et al. 2015) have been published. In addition to these publications, this chapter provides an overview over the basic principles and especially emphasizes hydrogel applications in diagnostic procedures. The desire for miniaturized diagnostic systems has propelled the research field of lab-on-a-chip and microfluidic devices. Microfluidics is closely related to tissue engineering, in which hydrogels constitute a basic building block. The need to understand the fluidic microenvironment and the application of (soft) lithography techniques in the fabrication of hydrogel scaffolds and vascular networks demonstrates the affinity between these two fields. In addition, microfluidic devices are utilized to fabricate gel fibers and particles (Onoe et al. 2013; Takeuchi 2013) and vice-versa, hydrogels are utilized in lab-on-a-chip devices for sensing and diagnostics. One of the most prominent use for macroscopic gels in biomolecular research is their application in protein and nucleic acid separation by gel electrophoresis with subsequent staining (Magdeldin 2012). Other applications within lab-on-a-chip and diagnostic systems include cell-based biosensors, diffusion membranes, enzyme reactors, and physiochemical gel sensors, which are summarized throughout the following chapter.

Structural Engineering of Gels in Sensing Applications

For the integration of three dimensional hydrogel networks in sensors, several design parameters have to be considered. As the quantity of interest has to interact with the bulk gel, the response time of the sensor is determined by the dimensions of the gel. In addition, the mechanical structure and pore size influence the sensor performance. Important microfabrication and structure tuning techniques for gels in the micrometer range are highlighted in the following.

Microstructuring of gels

In diagnostic devices, the analyte of interest mainly is a chemical species of any kind. The transport of molecules is governed by diffusion, with the diffusion time t:

$$t \approx \frac{l^2}{2D}$$

where *l* is the diffusion length and *D* the diffusion coefficient of the molecule. As an example for the equation above, the diffusion time of glucose ($D = 570$ $\mu m^2/s$) rises from 9 s to 15 min by increasing the length from 100 μm to 1 mm. As a consequence, hydrogels are mainly deposited as thin layers or shaped to particles in the micrometer range to reduce the sensor response time. Fabrication methods for gel microstructuring are summarized in Fig. 1.

The main processes for the fabrication of extended thin layers are spin coating or moulding. Microfabricated structures in silicon or polydimethylsiloxane (PDMS) are used as moulds in soft lithography and embossing processes (Fig. 1b), also offering parallel particle fabrication on a wafer level (Petersen et al. 2015; Guan et al. 2007). Selective exposure of photochemical gels through a photomask or a focused UV beam enables the fabrication of three dimensional structures. Polyethylene glycol diacrylate (PEG-DA) is among the most widely utilized polymers for UV-polymerization. Using this method, shape encoded multi-analyte detection in a sample by simply changing the particle geometry for each enzyme assay, was presented (Jang and Koh 2010a).

Common microfluidic technologies and devices have found applications in engineering of hydrogel particles and fibers. The most important to mention is a droplet generator, in which two immiscible fluids are injected into a micro channel. Depending on the channel dimensions and the ratio of the fluid velocities, the droplet size can be tuned (Weber et al. 2014). By cascading functional fluidic elements, such as micro mixers, multi-laminar stream sections and droplet generators, the fabrication of complex and heterogeneous structures (Janus particles) is feasible (Zhao et al. 2015; Wang et al. 2011; Chung et al. 2012). As an example, Lewis et al. in 2010 fabricated magnetic movable Janus gel particles, containing viruses on one side and magnetic nanoparticles on the other, by using a microfluidic device as shown in Fig. 1d. Although microfluidic fabrication only allows serial particle fabrication, an advantage is that it is not restricted to only photochemical curing.

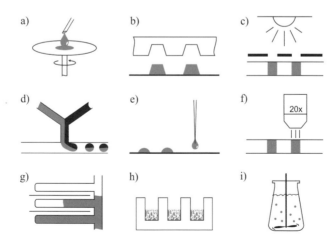

Fig. 1. Hydrogel microstructuring technologies. (a) Spin coating. (b) Casting and soft lithography (c) Mask photolithography. (d) Microfluidic droplet generation in multi-phase flow. (e) Pin dispensing and printing. (f) Focused beam polymerization, stereo lithography, two photon lithography. (g) Hydrophobic patterning by capillary pressure barriers. (h) Introduction of macropores (μm range) for fast diffusion into bulk gel. (f) Emulsion polymerization.

For the simplified structuring of hydrogels in biochemical sensing applications, we developed a microfluidic platform that enables *in situ* polymerization of hydrogel structures in a reaction chamber within a single step (Puchberger-Enengl et al. 2014). The structure dimensions are defined by patterning hydrophobic capillary pressure barriers also referred to as phase guides (Vulto et al. 2011). Parallel arrangement of the gel microstripes with phase guides for interdigitated sample filling allows for macroscopic optical readout while retaining short diffusion lengths (Fig. 1g). Implementing the functional parts in the fabrication process enables rapid assay customization by making surface treatment, curing mask alignment and washing steps obsolete (Puchberger-Enengl et al. 2014). Smaller micro- and nanogel particles are usually fabricated by emulsion and microemulsion polymerization methods, which are discussed elsewhere (Pelton 2000).

Pore size and structure tuning

The degree of interaction between polymer chains determines the mechanical properties of gels. Swelling behavior, pore size and mechanical stability of gels are the main design parameters to consider. A review of experimental molecule diffusivity and mathematical models is given by Amsden (Amsden 1998). Table 1 summarizes literature values of pore size distribution for some common gels, ranging from Å (0.1 nm) to some 100 nm. The pore size, and hence, the solute diffusivity depends on the molecular weight of the gel monomer and its concentration.

The mesh size increases with increasing molecular weight of synthesized PEG-DA chains, allowing for a simple design of diffusion barriers for different proteins (Cruise et al. 1998). A variety of methods and techniques for the customization of the nano and microarchitecture of gels have been developed. Leaching of porogen particles, phase separation, and gas forming are common methods utilized to generate open pores up to the micrometer range (Annabi et al. 2010). Varying the amount and size distribution of leaching salt particles allows adjustment of the macropores (Simms et al. 2005). Polyethylene glycol was successfully used as a simple porogen system for increased hydrogel access in biochemical reactions (Lee et al. 2010). Curing PEG-DA in dichloromethan was presented as a simple method for solvent induced phase separation to fabricate macroporous gels (Bailey et al. 2011). Besides the vast selection of natural and synthetic polymers, the investigation of interpenetrating networks has offered the possibility to tailor mechanical gel properties and their response to external stimuli (Dragan 2014). In order to customize the gel swelling behavior, copolymerization of different polymers has been utilized in the different sensor fabrication routines (Ahn et al. 2008).

Table 1. Literature pore size values for different gels systems.

Gel	Pore size [Å]	Reference
Polyarclyamide (PAM) 4%	100	Park et al. 1990
PEG-DA 20% , 2, 4, 8, 20 kDa	19, 22, 34, 58	Cruise et al. 1998
Calcium alginate 1–5%	250-45	Grassi et al. 2009
Agarose 1–3%	~2000-500	Narayanan et al. 2006
Polyvinyl alcohol 5.2%–11.6%	195-72	Hickey and Peppas 1995

Physically responsive gel sensors

Responsive gels change their physical properties due to an external stimulus that might be a shift in temperature, pH value or chemical concentration (Ahn et al. 2008). By transducing chemical to mechanical energy these gels are attractive for incorporation in sensors. The swelling of gels is converted to an electrical signal by piezoelectric or capacitive readout. Optical transducers include Bragg diffraction in reflection holograms and colloidal photonic crystals, surface plasmon resonance, optical waveguides, and interference measurements (Gawel et al. 2010; Mateescu et al. 2012; Yetisen et al. 2015).

Swelling upon pH change is common in several gels and has been investigated for sensing and drug delivery applications. Swelling occurs due to pH-dependent ionization of network groups, an increased electrostatic repulsion, and a corresponding uptake of water (Ahn et al. 2008). Responsive gels enable the design of pH sensors with high resolution. Chang et al. reported on a gold coated gel diffraction grating with a pH resolution down to 6×10^{-4} units (Chang et al. 2012). Poly(vinyl alcohol) and poly(acrylic acid) (PVA/PAA) copolymer gels were utilized together with a piezoresistive readout in a micro electromechanical system (MEMS) pH sensor. The principle relies on miniaturized pressure sensors, in which swelling of the gel in a chamber results in bending of a micromachined silicon membrane with polysilicon piezoresistive elements for electrical readout as illustrated by Fig. 2a (Gerlach et al. 2005). A similar concept for an implantable glucose sensor uses the swelling of acrylamide and 3-acrylamidophenylboronic acid (PAM/3-AAmPBA) gel by ligation of the sugar at the boronic acid site (Gabai et al. 2001) with the same piezoresistive readout (Guenther et al. 2012). A hybrid integrated system, presented by Kuo et al. 2012 combined capacitive readout (Fig. 2b) of a PDMS membrane, actuated by gel swelling, with a complementary metal oxide semiconductor (CMOS) readout circuit for wireless glucose sensing in a 9 mm² sized package. Integration of ferric particles in gel patterns was utilized for wireless magnetic readout of pH dependent swelling (Fig. 2c). Small gel patches including superparamagnetic iron oxide particles were fabricated on top of a planar coil. By pH induced swelling the magnetic flux to the detector coil was modulated (Song et al. 2014).

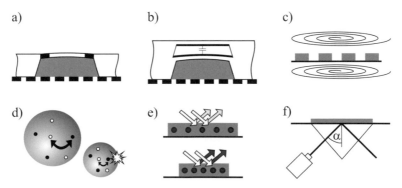

Fig. 2. Transducer principles for responsive gels. (a) MEMS membrane with piezoresistors. (b) Capacitive readout. (c) Magnetic coupling modulation by ferrogel or distance. (d) Fluorescence and FRET. (e) Colloidal photonic crystal hydrogel (CPCH). (f) Surface plasmon resonance (SPR).

Besides pH, thermal swelling in hydrogels has been the most exploited effect for responsive gel sensors. Poly(N-isopropylacrylamide) (PNIPAAm) is among the most studied temperature responsive polymers. Temperature induced swelling is relevant in drug delivery systems and specialized temperature sensing applications at the micro- and nanoscale. Fluorescent readout of stimuli responsive micro- and nanogels is a promising method in a wide range of sensing and imaging applications (Li and Liu 2012). Covalent binding of environment sensitive fluorophores to the polymer fibers results in modulation of the fluorescent signal by changes of the hydrophobic microenvironment upon temperature induce fiber collapse. In addition, the Förster resonance energy transfer (FRET) effect can be employed for sensor readout. Swelling or shrinking of the gel changes the fluorescent donor/acceptor distance, and therefore, the FRET signal (Fig. 2d) (Hu and Liu 2010). With fluorescent nanogel particles intracellular temperature monitoring was presented (Gota et al. 2009).

Ion selective swelling in responsive gels has been achieved by introducing chemical groups to the polymer that selectively bind to an ion. For example, crown ethers bind to metallic ions, increasing the charge in the gel network and swelling occurs due to an increase of osmotic pressure (Holtz and Asher 1997). However, depending on the binding chemistry these systems may lack ion selectivity. A potassium sensor with a potassium selective membrane and a colloidal photonic crystal hydrogel (CPCH) arrangement has been proposed for whole blood potassium measurements (Fenzl et al. 2014). CPCHs include arrays of nanoparticles, which exhibit Bragg diffraction in the visible range. The induced gel shrinking in a CPCH reduces the distance of the nanoparticles and results in a shift of the diffraction peak (Fig. 2e). An ammonia responsive CPCH was suggested for point-of-care diagnostics of blood ammonia levels (Kimble et al. 2006). Similar concepts enable the measurement of toxic heavy metal ions mercury and lead in water samples (Arunbabu et al. 2011; Ye et al. 2012). Alternative methods for the implementation of periodic nanostructures as diffraction gratings in photonic hydrogels include laser interference-based photocuring, and multilayer co-polymerization (Yetisen et al. 2015). Recently, photonic hydrogels have gained interest in the development of diagnostic devices because of their simple colorimetric readout possibilities. A sensitive sensor system, based on a silver nanoparticle Bragg grating in phenylboronic modified acrylamide gel was successfully tested for glucose monitoring in urine samples under fixed pH conditions (Yetisen et al. 2014).

Functionalized (bio)chemical reactors

Despite the slower diffusion dynamics in comparison to free solution, hydrogels have found many applications as reactors in biomedical diagnostics. These gels are functionalized by incorporated biological or chemical probes, including oligonucleotides, enzymes and enzyme substrates, proteins and antibodies, or specific dyes. In contrast to conventional surface-bound assay technologies, the recognition molecules are distributed in three dimensional gel structures. A major advantage of the three dimensional loading is the enhanced signal to noise ratio. Besides reporter molecule, and hence, signal stacking, the low non-specific protein adsorption within the gel matrices increases the signal quality. As an example, Lee et al. 2013 reported on the 1000-fold sensitivity increase of a three dimensional hydrogel assay for Sjögren's syndrome specific marker in comparison to a surface bound version of the same marker. In addition, immobilized proteins exhibit increased stability over time in contrast to surface binding methods (Rubina et al. 2008). An overview of functionalized gel structures in different diagnostic assay formats is given in Table 2. These assays utilize all kinds of gel structuring techniques as previously discussed. Main analytes are nucleic acids from pathogens, protein markers, toxins, enzymes, and glucose. While nucleic acid and protein detection mainly is adopted from classical methods, different enzymes (e.g., secreted by pathogens) can be detected by their digestion of labeled substrates as parts of the gel matrix with a corresponding dye release or FRET signal. These substrates are sometimes also referred to as bioresponsive polymers. A distinct approach for a bioresponsive gel sensor was presented by Wei et al. 2015. Two

Table 2. Biochemical gel sensor overview.

Gel type	Readout	Analyte	Reference
Microfluidic barcoded PEG-DA microparticle sandwich assay	Fluorescent labeling	Interleukin-2 10 pg/ml	Appleyard et al. 2011
Pin dispensed methacrylamide microarrays for hybridization and sandwich assays	Fluorescent labeling	M. tuberculosis, HIV, HBV, HCV virus, protein tumor markers	Gryadunov et al. 2011
Alginate-stained peptidoglycan gel double layer	Dye release upon digestion	Wound infection, lysozyme	Hasmann et al. 2011
Photomask patterned PEG-DA micropatches, immobilized enzyme and quantum dots	QD fluorescence quenching	Phenol 1 μM, glucose 50 μM, alcohol 70 μM	Jang et al. 2010b, 2012
Conjugated enzyme-carboxy seminaphthofluorescein in emulsion polymerized microspheres	Self-referenced dual emission fluorescence	Organophosphate, paraoxon 5 μM	Lee et al. 2009
Macroporous nanofiber-PAM matrix in 96 well plate	Absorbance immunoassay	Sjögren's syndrome, anti-SSB/La antibody 10 pM	Lee et al. 2013
UV beam polymerized PEG-DA enzyme micropatches in microfluidic channels	Colorimetric	Glucose and protein in human urine samples	Lin et al. 2011
Casted PAM micropillars with primers and polymerase	Real-time PCR, fluorescence	Herpes simplex virus from swab samples	Manage et al. 2012
Photopatterned pHEMA enzyme membranes	Electrochemical	Glucose 0.1 mM, lactate 50 μM in whole blood	Moser et al. 2002
In situ polymerized PEG-DA microstructures with labeled substrate/protein specific dye	Fluorescent, colorimetric	Matrix metallo proteinase 470 ng/ml, total protein 20–140 μg/ml, WBC counts	Puchberger-Enengl et al. 2014
Casted PAM gel strips with primers and polymerase	Real-time PCR, fluorescence	Malaria, Plasmodium falciparum from whole blood	Taylor et al. 2014
PNIPAAm waveguide in surface plasmon resonance setup	Label free optical	Imunoglobulin G 10 pM, 17beta-estradiol 50 pg/ml	Zhang et al. 2013

different oligonucleotides are grafted on polyacrylamide fibers. In the presence of a third aptamer, the oligonucleotide-fibers are linked and the formation of the gel stops the sample flow. If a target molecule is present, it forms a complex with the aptamer, subsequently inhibiting gelation. Thus, the sample continues to flow, indicated by food dye which is dragged along. The system was used for the qualitative detection of lead, cocaine, and adenosine.

Whole cell biosensors

In tissue engineering and three dimensional cell studies, different cell types are trapped and cultured in hydrogel scaffolds. Some of these cell cultures have been utilized as biological detectors. Microbial cell-based biosensors have been especially developed for the determination of pollutants in environmental samples and for process monitoring in the food industry (Banerjee et al. 2010). Genetic engineering of microbes for enzyme, and fluorescent protein expression allows the design of versatile biosensors. As an example, green fluorescent protein (GFP) expressing bacteria constitute self-contained sensors in toxicity assays. Engineered yeast cells were immobilized in gelatin for ready-to-use assays of estrogenic activity of environmental samples. The assay was based on estrogen receptor-mediated luminescence of living yeast cells upon exposure to samples without any pre-treatment. Gelatin enabled a superior assay performance over agar gels and showed stable results for 90 days (Bittner et al. 2015). In addition to yeast and bacteria, microalgae have been incorporated in biosensors. Algae are sensitive to environmental changes and can be employed to detect herbicide and heavy metal concentrations. A simple and effective readout is based on the altered chlorophyll fluorescence by these compounds (Ferro et al. 2012).

In addition to microorganisms, mammalian cell lines have been employed in three dimensional gel matrices for the detection of food borne pathogen toxins, viruses, and disease markers by antibody binding (Banerjee et al. 2013). For a simplified readout, the activity of released enzymes from toxin damaged cells can be determined by a color change. This concept was validated with a series of complex food samples and non-toxic background flora (Banerjee et al. 2010). A drawback of mammalian cells in biosensors is the limited shelf life, preventing their extended use in devices for field applications. However, microarrays of gel-encapsulated cells have been proposed for high-throughput multiplexed toxicological assays and drug screening in standard laboratories. These assays mainly use robotic fluid dispensing to spot cellular microhabitats on functionalized surfaces (Berthuy et al. 2016).

Gel membranes for size exclusion and flow control

Flow control and separation of biological species are important sub-tasks in sensing and diagnostic procedures. The degree of freedom in pore size tuning enables hydrogels to be ideal candidates for molecular flow control and size exclusion. As previously mentioned, one of the most important applications of hydrogel membranes is the separation of proteins and nucleic acids in an electric field by size, namely gel electrophoresis. Besides the laboratory-based setups, many miniaturized gel membranes have found their way in sensing applications. A miniaturized electrophoresis system was utilized for protein analysis in a 96-well plate format. Twelve open and free standing gel lanes were photo-polymerized on a substrate with 8 serial 2 x 2 mm wide sample reservoirs at a distance of 9 mm. Proteins were separated within a short timeframe, in the gel between two reservoirs, yielding highly parallel analysis (Duncombe and Herr 2013).

Selective patterning of gel membranes in microchannels for on-chip electrophoresis has been utilized for improved sample handling. Electrophoretic sample and antibody loading against a gel membrane was used in matrix metalloproteinase 8 analysis within saliva samples (Herr et al. 2007). Likewise, we patterned a hydrogel plug in a double-T injector to separate the sample from clean buffer in ion detection of water samples by capacitive contactless conductivity measurement (C4M). Blocking parasitic flows by the gel barrier, allows for a well-defined ion plug in a mobile setup for field applications. The sample and the separation channel were rinsed independently after each experiment, enabling a continuous operation mode (Puchberger-Enengl et al. 2013). Hydrogel barriers were also used in microfluidic chips to capture bacteria and viruses from a continuous flow for sample pre-concentration (Puchberger-Enengl et al. 2011) and subsequent lysis and RNA purification (Hubbe et al. 2013). An electric field perpendicular to the sample flow was applied to direct bacteria and viruses towards a gel membrane. Keeping them away from the electrodes prevents biofouling, lysis and irreversible attachment.

Gel membranes were also implemented in microfluidic chips for diffusion studies without physical contact. In diffusion-based chemical gradient generators the gel is separating cell cultures in a static environment from adjacent continuous flows of a chemical source and sink. Conversely, the gel can be polymerized with a drug concentration gradient and subsequently incubated with a cell culture. Gradient generators are useful tools in chemotaxis studies and high-throughput drug screening (Cheng et al. 2007; Kim et al. 2015; Ostrovidov et al. 2012).

On-chip diffusion membranes have been employed for molecule transport between separated cell cultures to study chemical cell signaling (Bryne et al. 2014). Recently, we developed a device for antibiotic testing of bacteria samples. The design comprises permeable hydrogel culture wells in a glass chip, enabling simple control of culture conditions and analysis. A thin gel barrier, loaded with antibiotics enables oxygen supply and facilitates on-chip analysis by chemical access through the gel while keeping the sample bacteria trapped inside the well. Nutrients and drugs are provided on-chip in the gel for a self-contained and user-friendly handling and rapid antibiotic testing (Puchberger-Enengl et al. 2015).

Gel particles in medical imaging

Responsive and functionalized micro- and nanogel particles have been introduced in medical imaging technologies. Responsive gel coated magnetic nanoparticles possess great potential in combining drug delivery with magnetic resonance imaging (MRI) systems. Magnetic particles add further functionalities to the gel drug delivery systems increasing the possibilities for magnetic targeting, contrast enhancement, and controlled release by heat induction. The gel coating on the other hand reduces particle oxidation, aggregation and increases their blood circulation time (Sundaresan et al. 2014; Sun et al. 2008). Likewise, encapsulation of small molecule contrast agents in gel nanoparticles reduces their toxicity and increases the measurement window and signal in MRI (Soni et al. 2015).

Functionalized and radio labeled acrylamide particles, fabricated by emulsion polymerization were proposed for imaging of lung tissue in PET-CT scans. The particles harbored a cell penetrating peptide and a bovine serum albumin-Alexa fluor dye complex for fluorescence analysis and radiolabeling of tyrosine. Size dependent retention time and inflammatory response were studied for imaging and drug administration in lung diseases (Liu et al. 2009).

Near infrared *in vivo* imaging also benefits from the properties of responsive gel particles. Indocyanin green is a near infrared (NIR) fluorescent probe, approved for clinical imaging but suffers from self-quenching, low circulation time and non-specific protein interaction. In gel nanoparticles the dye is incorporated in the auto-quenched state. If the gel is degraded by an acidic pH or by enzyme digestion, the dye is released and yields a fluorescent signal. These effects can be used in imaging of tumors by the acidic pH of tumor cells and metastasis, which is related to hyaluronidase activity (Soni et al. 2015).

Conclusions

Alongside the advances in regenerative medicine, a multitude of gel-based diagnostic devices and sensors have been proposed in recent years utilizing engineered hydrogel scaffolds. The enormous degree of freedom in designing microgel structures for convenient sample incubation has propelled these developments. Recent efforts in point-of-care diagnostic devices have focused on simple readout strategies to facilitate translation into clinical practice. Cross sensitivities of responsive gels towards pH, ionic strength and other compounds have to be considered and pose obstacles in the development of point-of care diagnostics. Similarly, a low specificity in cell-based toxicological assays has been challenging. Other obstacles to overcome include limited shelf life, and elaborate assay protocol steps. Whilst the first can be tackled by improved immobilization techniques and material science, the latter has led to a number of smart engineered devices for simple operation. For a broader acceptance of these novel sensing technologies the focus of future research has to expand from fundamental principles to validation with complex, clinical specimens.

Acknowledgement

The authors would like to thank Franz Keplinger, Institute of Sensor and Actuator Systems (ISAS), Vienna University of Technology, Austria, and Sander van den Driesche, Institute for Microsensors, -actuators and -systems (IMSAS), MCB, University of Bremen, Germany for proof reading.

References

Ahn, S., R.M. Kasi, S.-C. Kim, N. Sharma and Y. Zhou. 2008. Stimuli-responsive polymer gels. Soft Matter. 4(6): 1151.

Amsden, B. 1998. Solute diffusion within hydrogels. Mechanisms and models. Macromolecules. 31(23): 8382–8395.

Annabi, N., J.W. Nichol, X. Zhong, C. Ji, S. Koshy, A. Khademhosseini et al. 2010. Controlling the porosity and microarchitecture of hydrogels for tissue engineering. Tissue Engineering. Part B, Reviews. 16(4): 371–383.

Appleyard, D.C., S.C. Chapin, R.L. Srinivas and P.S. Doyle. 2011. Bar-coded hydrogel microparticles for protein detection: synthesis, assay and scanning. Nature Protocols. 6(11): 1761–74.

Arunbabu, D., A. Sannigrahi and T. Jana. 2011. Photonic crystal hydrogel material for the sensing of toxic mercury ions (Hg2+) in water. Soft Matter. 7(6): 2592.

Bahney, C.S., T.J. Lujan, C.W. Hsu, M. Bottlang, J.L. West and B. Johnstone. 2011. Visible light photoinitiation of mesenchymal stem cell-laden bioresponsive hydrogels. European Cells and Materials. 22: 43–55.

Bailey, B.M., V. Hui, R. Fei and M.A. Grunlan. 2011. Tuning PEG-DA hydrogel properties via solvent-induced phase separation (SIPS). Journal of Materials Chemistry. 21(46): 18776.

Banerjee, P. and A.K. Bhunia. 2010. Cell-based biosensor for rapid screening of pathogens and toxins. Biosensors and Bioelectronics. 26(1): 99–106.

Banerjee, P., S. Kintzios and B. Prabhakarpandian. 2013. Biotoxin detection using cell-based sensors. Toxins. 5(12): 2366–83.

Berthuy, O.I., L.J. Blum and C.A. Marquette. 2016. Cells on chip for multiplex screening. Biosensors and Bioelectronics. 76: 29–37.

Bittner, M., S. Jarque and K. Hilscherová. 2015. Polymer-immobilized ready-to-use recombinant yeast assays for the detection of endocrine disruptive compounds. Chemosphere. 132: 56–62.

Byrne, M.B., L. Trump, A.V. Desai, L.B. Schook, H.R. Gaskins and P.J.a. Kenis. 2014. Microfluidic platform for the study of intercellular communication via soluble factor-cell and cell-cell paracrine signaling. Biomicrofluidics. 8(4): 044104.

Buenger, D., F. Topuz and J. Groll. 2012. Hydrogels in sensing applications. Progress in Polymer Science. 37(12): 1678–1719.

Caló, E. and V.V. Khutoryanskiy. 2015. Biomedical applications of hydrogels: a review of patents and commercial products. European Polymer Journal. 65: 252–267.

Chang, C., Z. Ding, V.N.L.R. Patchigolla, B. Ziaie and C.A. Savran. 2012. Reflective diffraction gratings From hydrogels as biochemical sensors. IEEE Sensors Journal. 12(7): 2374–2379.

Cheng, S.-Y., S. Heilman, M. Wasserman, S. Archer, M.L. Shuler and M. Wu. 2007. A hydrogel-based microfluidic device for the studies of directed cell migration. Lab on a Chip. 7(6): 763.

Chung, B.G., K.-H. Lee, A. Khademhosseini and S.-H. Lee. 2012. Microfluidic fabrication of microengineered hydrogels and their application in tissue engineering. Lab on a Chip. 12(1): 45–59.

Cruise, G.M., D.S. Scharp and J. Hubbell. 1998. Characterization of permeability and network structure of interfacially photopolymerized poly(ethylene glycol) diacrylate hydrogels. Biomaterials. 19(14): 1287–1294.

Deligkaris, K., T.S. Tadele, W. Olthuis and A. van den Berg. 2010. Hydrogel-based devices for biomedical applications. Sensors and Actuators B: Chemical. 147(2): 765–774.

Dragan, E.S. 2014. Design and applications of interpenetrating polymer network hydrogels. A review. Chemical Engineering Journal. 243(MAY 2014): 572–590.

Duncombe, T.a. and A.E. Herr. 2013. Photopatterned free-standing polyacrylamide gels for microfluidic protein electrophoresis. Lab on a Chip. 13(11): 2115–23.

Fairbanks, B.D., M.P. Schwartz, C.N. Bowman and K.S. Anseth. 2009. Photoinitiated polymerization of PEG-diacrylate with lithium phenyl-2,4,6-trimethylbenzoylphosphinate: polymerization rate and cytocompatibility. Biomaterials. 30(35): 6702–7.

Fenzl, C., M. Kirchinger, T. Hirsch and O. Wolfbeis. 2014. Photonic crystal-based sensing and imaging of potassium ions. Chemosensors. 2(3): 207–218. doi:10.3390/chemosensors2030207.

Ferro, Y., M. Perullini, M. Jobbagy, S. Bilmes and C. Durrieu. 2012. Development of a biosensor for environmental monitoring based on microalgae immobilized *in silica* hydrogels. Sensors. 12(12): 16879–16891.

Gabai, R., N. Sallacan, V. Chegel, T. Bourenko, E. Katz and I. Willner. 2001. Characterization of the swelling of acrylamidophenylboronic acid-acrylamide hydrogels upon interaction with glucose by faradaic impedance spectroscopy, chronopotentiometry, quartz-crystal microbalance (QCM), and surface plasmon resonance (SPR) experiments. Journal of Physical Chemistry B. 105(34): 8196–8202.

Gawel, K., D. Barriet, M. Sletmoen and B.T. Stokke. 2010. Responsive hydrogels for label-free signal transduction within biosensors. Sensors. 10(5): 4381–4409.

Gerlach, G., M. Guenther, J. Sorber, G. Suchaneck, K.-F. Arndt and A. Richter. 2005. Chemical and pH sensors based on the swelling behavior of hydrogels. Sensors and Actuators B: Chemical. 111-112: 555–561.

Gota, C., K. Okabe, T. Funatsu, Y. Harada and S. Uchiyama. 2009. Hydrophilic fluorescent nanogel thermometer for intracellular thermometry. Journal of the American Chemical Society. 131(8): 2766–2767.

Grassi, M., C. Sandolo, D. Perin, T. Coviello, R. Lapasin and G. Grassi. 2009. Structural characterization of calcium alginate matrices by means of mechanical and release tests. Molecules. 14(8): 3003–3017.

Gryadunov, D., E. Dementieva, V. Mikhailovich, T. Nasedkina, A. Rubina, E. Savvateeva et al. 2011. Gel-based microarrays in clinical diagnostics in Russia. Expert Review of Molecular Diagnostics. 11(8): 839–853.

Guan, J., H. He, L.J. Lee and D.J. Hansford. 2007. Fabrication of particulate reservoir-containing, capsule like, and self-folding polymer microstructures for drug delivery. Small. 3(3): 412–8.

Guenther, M., G. Gerlach, T. Wallmersperger, M.N. Avula, S.H. Cho, X. Xie et al. 2012. Smart hydrogel-based biochemical microsensor array for medical diagnostics. Advances in Science and Technology. 85: 47–52.

Hasmann, A., E. Wehrschuetz-Sigl, G. Kanzler, U. Gewessler, E. Hulla, K.P. Schneider et al. 2011. Novel peptidoglycan-based diagnostic devices for detection of wound infection. Diagnostic Microbiology and Infectious Disease. 71(1): 12–23.

Herr, A.E., A.V. Hatch, D.J. Throckmorton, H.M. Tran, J.S. Brennan, W.V. Giannobile et al. 2007. Microfluidic immunoassays as rapid saliva-based clinical diagnostics. Proceedings of the National Academy of Sciences of the United States of America. 104(13): 5268–73.

Hickey, A.S. and N.A. Peppas. 1995. Mesh size and diffusive characteristics of semicrystalline poly(vinyl alcohol) membranes prepared by freezing/thawing techniques. Journal of Membrane Science. 107(3): 229–237.

Hoffman, A.S. 2001. Hydrogels for biomedical applications. Advanced Drug Delivery Reviews. 64: 18–23.

Holtz, J.H. and S.A. Asher. 1997. Polymerized colloidal crystal hydrogel films as intelligent chemical sensing materials. Nature. 389: 829–832. doi:10.1016/S0956-5663(97)84356-4.

Hu, J. and S. Liu. 2010. Responsive polymers for detection and sensing applications: Current status and future developments. Macromolecules. 43: 8315–8330.

Hubbe, H., S. Hakenberg, G. Dame and G.A. Urban. 2013. Phaseguide-chip for point-of-care diagnostic of bacteria with integrated enrichment, lysis, and nucleic acid purification. In 2013 Transducers & Eurosensors XXVII: The 17th International Conference on Solid-State Sensors, Actuators and Microsystems (TRANSDUCERS & EUROSENSORS XXVII) (pp. 2134–2136). IEEE.

Jang, E. and W.-G. Koh. 2010a. Multiplexed enzyme-based bioassay within microfluidic devices using shape-coded hydrogel microparticles. Sensors and Actuators B: Chemical. 143(2): 681–688.

Jang, E., K.J. Son, B. Kim and W.-G. Koh. 2010b. Phenol biosensor based on hydrogel microarrays entrapping tyrosinase and quantum dots. The Analyst. 135(11): 2871–8.

Jang, E., S. Kim and W.-G. Koh. 2012. Microfluidic bioassay system based on microarrays of hydrogel sensing elements entrapping quantum dot-enzyme conjugates. Biosensors & Bioelectronics. 31(1): 529–36.

Kim, B.J., L.V. Richter, N. Hatter, C. Tung, B.A. Ahner and M. Wu. 2015. An array microhabitat system for high throughput studies of microalgal growth under controlled nutrient gradients. Lab Chip. 15(18): 3687–3694.

Kimble, K.W., J.P. Walker, D.N. Finegold and S.a. Asher. 2006. Progress toward the development of a point-of-care photonic crystal ammonia sensor. Analytical and Bioanalytical Chemistry. 385(4): 678–85.

Kirschner, C.M. and K.S. Anseth. 2013. Hydrogels in healthcare: from static to dynamic material microenvironments. Acta Materialia. 61(3): 931–944.

Kuo, P., S. Lu, J.-C. Kuo, Y.-J. Yang, T. Wang, Y.-L. Ho et al. 2012. A hydrogel-based implantable wireless CMOS glucose sensor SoC. In 2012 IEEE International Symposium on Circuits and Systems (pp. 994–997). IEEE.

Lee, A.G., C.P. Arena, D.J. Beebe and S.P. Palecek. 2010. Development of macroporous poly(ethylene glycol) hydrogel arrays within microfluidic channels. Biomacromolecules. 11(12): 3316–24.

Lee, Y., D. Choi, W.-G. Koh and B. Kim. 2009. Poly(ethylene glycol) hydrogel microparticles containing enzyme-fluorophore conjugates for the detection of organophosphorus compounds. Sensors and Actuators B: Chemical. 137(1): 209–214.

Lee, D.-S., J.-S. Park, E.J. Lee, H.J. Kim and J. Lee. 2013. A protein nanofiber hydrogel for sensitive immunoassays. The Analyst. 138(17): 4786–94.

Le Goff, G.C., R.L. Srinivas, W. Adam Hill and P.S. Doyle. 2015. Hydrogel microparticles for biosensing. European Polymer Journal. 72: 386–412.

Lewis, C.L., Y. Lin, C. Yang, A.K. Manocchi, K.P. Yuet, P.S. Doyle et al. 2010. Microfluidic fabrication of hydrogel microparticles containing functionalized viral nanotemplates. Langmuir: The ACS Journal of Surfaces and Colloids. 26(16): 13436–41.

Li, C. and S. Liu. 2012. Polymeric assemblies and nanoparticles with stimuli-responsive fluorescence emission characteristics. Chemical Communications. 48(27): 3262.

Lin, L., Z. Gao, H. Wei, H. Li, F. Wang and J.-M. Lin. 2011. Fabrication of a gel particle array in a microfluidic device for bioassays of protein and glucose in human urine samples. Biomicrofluidics. 5(3): 34112–3411210.

Liu, Y., A. Ibricevic, J.A. Cohen, J.L. Cohen, S.P. Gunsten, J.M.J. Fréchet et al. 2009. Impact of hydrogel nanoparticle size and functionalization on *in vivo* behavior for lung imaging and therapeutics. Molecular Pharmaceutics. 6(6): 1891–902.

Magdeldin, S. (ed.). 2012. Gel Electrophoresis— Principles and Basics. InTech, Rijeka.

Manage, D.P., J. Lauzon, A. Atrazhev, Y.C. Morrissey, A.L. Edwards, A.J. Stickel et al. 2012. A miniaturized and integrated gel post platform for multiparameter PCR detection of herpes simplex viruses from raw genital swabs. Lab on a Chip. 12(9): 1664–71.

Mateescu, A., Y. Wang, J. Dostalek and U. Jonas. 2012. Thin hydrogel films for optical biosensor applications. Membranes. 2(4): 40–69.

Moser, I., G. Jobst and G.A. Urban. 2002. Biosensor arrays for simultaneous measurement of glucose, lactate, glutamate, and glutamine. Biosensors and Bioelectronics 17(4): 297–302.

Narayanan, J., J.-Y. Xiong and X.-Y. Liu. 2006. Determination of agarose gel pore size: absorbance measurements vis a vis other techniques. Journal of Physics: Conference Series. 28: 83–86.

Nichol, J.W., S.T. Koshy, H. Bae, C.M. Hwang, S. Yamanlar and A. Khademhosseini. 2010. Cell-laden microengineered gelatin methacrylate hydrogels. Biomaterials. 31(21): 5536–5544.

Onoe, H., T. Okitsu, A. Itou, M. Kato-Negishi, R. Gojo, D. Kiriya et al. 2013. Metre-long cell-laden microfibres exhibit tissue morphologies and functions. Nature Materials. 12(6): 584–90.

Ostrovidov, S., N. Annabi, A. Seidi, M. Ramalingam, F. Dehghani, H. Kaji et al. 2012. Controlled release of drugs from gradient hydrogels for high-throughput analysis of cell–drug interactions. Analytical Chemistry. 84(3): 1302–1309.

Park, I.H., C.S. Johnson and D.A. Gabriel. 1990. Probe diffusion in polyacrylamide gels as observed by means of holographic relaxation methods: search for a universal equation. Macromolecules. 23(5): 1548–1553.

Pelton, R. 2000. Temperature-sensitive aqueous microgels. Advances in Colloid and Interface Science. 85(1): 1–33.

Petersen, R.S., S.S. Keller and A. Boisen. 2015. Lab on a Chip microstructures for drug delivery. Lab on a Chip. 15: 2576–2579.

Puchberger-Enengl, D., S. Podszun, H. Heinz, C. Hermann, P. Vulto and G.A. Urban. 2011. Microfluidic concentration of bacteria by on-chip electrophoresis. Biomicrofluidics. 5(4): 44111–4411110.

Puchberger-Enengl, D., M. Bipoun, M. Smolka, C. Krutzler, F. Keplinger and M.J. Vellekoop. 2013. Hydrogel plug for independent sample and buffer handling in continuous microchip capillary electrophoresis. *In*: Schmid, U., J.L. Sánchez de Rojas Aldavero and M. Leester-Schaedel (eds.). Proc. SPIE 8763, Smart Sensors, Actuators, and MEMS VI (Vol. 8763, p. 87631B).

Puchberger-Enengl, D., C. Krutzler, F. Keplinger and M.J. Vellekoop. 2014. Single-step design of hydrogel-based microfluidic assays for rapid diagnostics. Lab on a Chip. 14(2): 378–83.

Puchberger-Enengl, D., S. van den Driesche, C. Krutzler, F. Keplinger and M.J. Vellekoop. 2015. Hydrogel-based microfluidic incubator for microorganism cultivation and analyses. Biomicrofluidics. 9(1): 014127.

Qin, X.-H., P. Gruber, M. Markovic, B. Plochberger, E. Klotzsch, J. Stampfl et al. 2014. Enzymatic synthesis of hyaluronic acid vinyl esters for two-photon microfabrication of biocompatible and biodegradable hydrogel constructs. Polym. Chem. 5(22): 6523–6533.

Rubina, A.Y., A. Kolchinsky, A.a. Makarov and A.S. Zasedatelev. 2008. Why 3-D? Gel-based microarrays in proteomics. Proteomics. 8(4): 817–831.

Simms, H.M., C.M. Brotherton, B.T. Good, R.H. Davis, K.S. Anseth and C.N. Bowman. 2005. *In situ* fabrication of macroporous polymer networks within microfluidic devices by living radical photopolymerization and leaching. Lab on a Chip. 5(2): 151–7.

Song, S.H., J.H. Park, G. Chitnis, R.a. Siegel and B. Ziaie. 2014. A wireless chemical sensor featuring iron oxide nanoparticle-embedded hydrogels. Sensors and Actuators B: Chemical. 193: 925–930.

Soni, K.S., S.S. Desale and T.K. Bronich. 2015. Nanogels: An overview of properties, biomedical applications and obstacles to clinical translation. Journal of Controlled Release. doi:10.1016/j.jconrel.2015.11.009.

Sun, C., J. Lee and M. Zhang. 2008. Magnetic nanoparticles in MR imaging and drug delivery. Advanced Drug Delivery Reviews. 60(11): 1252–1265.

Sundaresan, V., J.U. Menon, M. Rahimi, K.T. Nguyen and A.S. Wadajkar. 2014. Dual-responsive polymer-coated iron oxide nanoparticles for drug delivery and imaging applications. International Journal of Pharmaceutics. 466(1-2): 1–7.

Takeuchi, S. 2013. Cell-laden hydrogel beads, fibers and plates for 3D tissue construction. 2013 Transducers & Eurosensors XXVII: The 17th International Conference on Solid-State Sensors, Actuators and Microsystems (TRANSDUCERS & EUROSENSORS XXVII) (pp. 1515–1518). IEEE.

Taylor, B.J., A. Howell, K.A. Martin, D.P. Manage, W. Gordy, S.D. Campbell et al. 2014. A lab-on-chip for malaria diagnosis and surveillance. Malaria Journal. 13(1): 179.

Vulto, P., S. Podszun, P. Meyer, C. Hermann, A. Manz and G.a. Urban. 2011. Phaseguides: a paradigm shift in microfluidic priming and emptying. Lab on a Chip. 11(9): 1596–602.

Wang, J.-T., J. Wang and J.-J. Han. 2011. Fabrication of advanced particles and particle-based materials assisted by droplet-based microfluidics. Small. 7(13): 1728–54.

Weber, E., D. Puchberger-Enengl, F. Keplinger and M.J. Vellekoop. 2014. In-line characterization and identification of micro-droplets on-chip. Optofluidics, Microfluidics and Nanofluidics. 1(1): 11–18.

Wei, X., T. Tian, S. Jia, Z. Zhu, Y. Ma, J. Sun et al. 2015. Target-responsive DNA hydrogel mediated "stop-flow" microfluidic paper-based analytic device for rapid, portable and visual detection of multiple targets. Analytical Chemistry. 87(8): 4275–4282.

Ye, B.-F., Y.-J. Zhao, Y. Cheng, T.-T. Li, Z.-Y. Xie, X.-W. Zhao et al. 2012. Colorimetric photonic hydrogel aptasensor for the screening of heavy metal ions. Nanoscale. 4(19): 5998–6003.

Yetisen, A.K., Y. Montelongo, F. da Cruz Vasconcellos, J.L. Martinez-Hurtado, S. Neupane, H. Butt et al. 2014. Reusable, robust, and accurate laser-generated photonic nanosensor. Nano Letters. 14(6): 3587–3593.

Yetisen, A.K., H. Butt, L.R. Volpatti, I. Pavlichenko, M. Humar, S.J.J. Kwok et al. 2015. Photonic hydrogel sensors. Biotechnology Advances.

Zhao, Y., Y. Cheng, L. Shang, J. Wang, Z. Xie and Z. Gu. 2015. Microfluidic synthesis of barcode particles for multiplex assays. Small. 11(2): 151–74.

Zhang, Q., Y. Wang, A. Mateescu, K. Sergelen, A. Kibrom, U. Jonas et al. 2013. Biosensor based on hydrogel optical waveguide spectroscopy for the detection of 17β-estradiol. Talanta. 104(7): 149–154.

CHAPTER 9

Engineering Hyaluronan (HA) Hydrogels with Bioactive and Mechanical Signals

Helena S. Azevedo

Introduction

Interest in hyaluronic acid (HA), also known as hyaluronan, as a biomaterial has increased dramatically since the early 1980s with major clinical applications in ophthalmology (ocular surgery), in the treatment of degenerative joint disease (viscosupplementation for arthritis), and in adhesion prevention (anti-adhesive component in plastic surgery), combined with production of the polymer on an industrial scale. HA offers many unique advantages as a starting material to obtain hydrogels for regenerative medicine. First and foremost, is the ubiquitous distribution of HA in nature. It is found in virtually every species in the animal kingdom, as well as in the capsule of certain microorganisms, and in every tissue in the human body (Viola et al. 2015). Moreover, the HA repeating unit disaccharide (Fig. 1A) is identical in all species and all tissues and is therefore never itself recognized as immunologically foreign within its respective host. HA preparations with varying properties (molecular weight) and quality (ultrapure, non-pyrogenic, sterile) are now widely available from many manufacturers.

The second attribute of HA that is advantageous for preparing hydrogels is its unique physicochemical properties. HA solutions can be extremely elastoviscous, yet pseudoplastic enough to be extruded through narrow gauge needles. The third important factor underlying the biomedical utility of HA derives from the magnitude and pathways available for systemic HA metabolism. In the human body, the disposal of HA is almost

School of Engineering & Materials Science and Institute of Bioengineering, Queen Mary University of London, Mile End Road, London E1 4NS, UK.
E-mail: h.azevedo@qmul.ac.uk

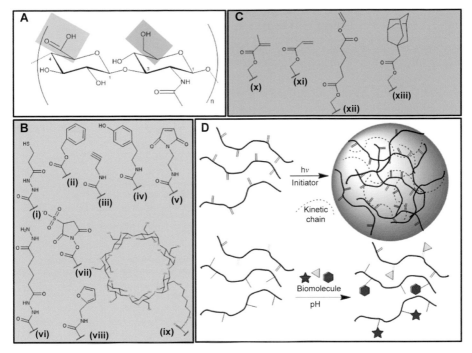

Fig. 1. Strategies for the chemical derivatization of HA for crosslinking and functionalization with biomolecules. (A) Chemical structure of HA (native) disaccharide repeating unit highlighting the chemical groups targeted for chemical derivatization: carboxylic groups (light grey) and primary hydroxyl groups (brown). (B) (i) Thiopropionyl hydrazide (DTPH), (ii) Benzyl esther, (iii) Alkyne (AL), (iv) Tyramide, (Tyr), (v) Maleimide (MA), (vi) Adipic dihydrazide (ADH), (vii) 3,3'-*N*-(ε-maleimidocaproic acid) hydrazide (EMCH), (viii) Furan, (ix) β-cyclodextrin (CD). (C) (x) Methacrylate (ME), (xi) Acrylate (AC), (xii) Divinyl adipate (DVA), (xiii) Adamantane (Ad). (D) Hydrogel formation by photopolymerization and biomolecule conjugation using HA derivatives.

entirely effected by the complete catabolism rather than excretion. Its degradation to monosaccharides is carried out by hyaluronidase to large oligosaccharides, which are then hydrolyzed to single sugars by N-acetyl-D-hexosaminidase. Due to its water solubility, unmodified HA is eliminated too rapidly from the human body. Therefore, many methods have been developed for HA derivatization to improve rheological properties or to create new physical forms (hydrogels with decreased water solubility), while maintaining its natural biocompatibility and thereby expanding its therapeutic applications. HA derivatization has been achieved by chemical modification methods (mainly crosslinking and attachment of pendant groups). Chemical modification of HA has been obtained exploiting the reactivity of its carboxylic groups (Fig. 1B) and primary hydroxyl groups (Fig. 1C). Subsequently, different crosslinking methods (Table 1) have been investigated to obtain hydrogels with different crosslinking kinetics and densities, thus providing hydrogels with tailorable properties. The review by Oh and colleagues (Oh et al. 2010) describes several chemically-modified HA derivatives that can be used to form covalently crosslinked hydrogels.

Table 1. Functionalized HA for hydrogel formation via different crosslinking mechanisms.

HA-derivative(s)	Crosslinker(s)	Crosslinking mechanism/Gel formation	References
Native HA (Fig. 1A)	Diepoxybutane (DEB) Divinyl sulfone (DVS)	Reaction of HA hydroxyl groups with diepoxides under basic conditions. Hydroxyl groups of HA.	(Neffe et al. 2011) (Borzacchiello et al. 2015)
Aldehyde- or oxidized-HA (Oxi-HA, obtained by periodate oxidation)	Adipic acid dihydrazide (ADH)	Schiff-base addition reaction (reaction between aldehydes in oxi-HA with amines of ADH to form imine bond).	(Shoham et al. 2013; Su et al. 2010)
Hydrazide-modified HA (ADH-HA, Fig. 1B-vi) conjugated with *N*-acryloxysuccinimide (AC-NHS) (AC-ADH-HA) AC-HA (Fig. 1C-xi) MA-HA (Fig. 1B-v)	PEG tetra-thiols (PEG-SH$_4$) MMP-degradable peptide crosslinker GCRE*GPQGIWGQ*ERCG GCRDVPMSQMRGGDRCG Dithiothreitol (DTT)	Michael-type addition (reaction of acrylates with thiols of PEG-SH$_4$ or cysteine (C) from the peptide linkers. Maleimide groups react with thiols (6.5 < pH < 7.5) forming a stable thioether linkage that is not reversible (i.e., the bond cannot be cleaved with reducing agents).	(Kim et al. 2007; Hong et al. 2013) (Lam and Segura 2013; Lei et al. 2011) (Feng et al. 2014)
(Methacrylated HA (ME-HA, AC-HA, Fig. 1C-x) Vinyl esters HA (VE-HA, Fig. 1C-xii)	DTT	Reaction of acrylate groups with thiols at the ends of DTT (Michael-type addition polymerisation). UV/Vis-photopolymerization with single (Irgacure 2959, TEOA/eosin Y/NVP) or two-photon initiator (P2CK).	(Qin et al. 2014; Lei et al. 2011) (Park et al. 2003) (Guvendiren and Burdick 2012)
Thiolated HA (SH-HA, Fig. 1B-i)	Poly(ethylene glycol) divinyl sulfone (PEGDVS), PEG diacrylate (PEGDA)	Michael-type addition (reaction of vinyl groups with free thiols).	(Addington et al. 2015; Pike et al. 2006)
Tyramine-HA (Tyr-HA, Fig. 1B-iv)	Horseradish peroxidase (HRP)/H$_2$O$_2$	Enzyme-mediated oxidative coupling of Tyr with formation of di-Tyr.	(Loebel et al. 2015; Xu et al. 2015)

Furan-modified HA (Fig. 1B-viii) Azido-modified HA (N$_3$-HA) Alkyne-modified HA (AL-HA, Fig. 1B-iii)	Dimaleimidepoly(ethylene glycol) (MI)$_2$ PEG Propiolic acid-modified gelatin 4,4'-diazidostilbene, 2,2'-disulfonic acid, 1,8-diazidooctane, PEGdiazide (MW = 1108 g·mol^{-1})	Diels-Alder click reaction. Azido groups in HA react with alkynyl groups of modified gelatin catalyzed by CuCl. Reaction of terminal acetylene groups in AL-HA and azides from the crosslinker.	(Hu et al. 2011; Nimmo et al. 2011; Owen et al. 2013; Piluso et al. 2011)
β-clycodextrin-modified HA (CD-HA, Fig. 1B-ix) Adamantane-modified HA (Ad-HA, Fig. 1C-xiii) CB[6]-HA DAH-HA or SPM-HA	-	Supramolecular (guest–host) interactions.	(Rodell 2013; Rodell et al. 2015a; Rodell et al. 2015b) (Jung et al. 2014; Park et al. 2012)

Covalently Crosslinked HA Hydrogels

Covalent crosslinking is necessary to impart stability and improve functions of HA hydrogels. HA can be directly crosslinked without any chemical modifications via hydroxyl groups using bisepoxide or divinyl sulfone (DVS) (Table 1). However, carboxyl groups have been selected as the preferred site for derivatization due to their superior reactivity and hydrogels have been obtained via 1-ethyl-3-(3-dimethylaminopropyl) carbodiimide hydrochloride (EDC) and N-hydroxysuccinimide (NHS) chemistry, biscarbodiimide and multifunctional hydrazides under acidic conditions (Xu et al. 2012). Some of these methods require toxic reagents and harsh conditions that are not suitable for cell and protein encapsulation.

Schiff base reaction

Schiff base reaction can be formed between an amine group and aldehyde group without additional chemical crosslinking reagents. HA can be oxidized with sodium periodate ($NaIO_4$) to produce aldehyde functionalities (Burdick and Prestwich 2011). Combinations of oxidized HA with adipic acid dihydrazide (ADH) hydrogels can be readily obtained by Schiff base reaction forming a hydrazine linkage (Su et al. 2010). Cell viability and cytotoxicity assays using nucleus pulposus (NP) cells showed good biocompatibility of these hydrogels, as well as an ability to promote gene expression of aggrecan and type II collagen, which are the major ECM components of NP cells. Computational finite element studies of the mechanical behaviour of ADH-HA hydrogels showed that the stiffness of the hydrogels were not affected by the presence of encapsulated adipocytes, indicating the application of these hydrogels for the delivery of preadipocytes in tissue reconstruction (Shoham et al. 2013).

Despite being a simple method to form hydrogels, the use of periodate oxidation to obtain aldehyde-modified HA causes degradation of the polymer chain. Thus, more chemo-selective chemistries for the synthesis of HA hydrogels that occur under physiological conditions without generating any toxic by-products have been explored.

Michael-type addition

The Michael addition reaction results in the nucleophilic addition of a nucleophile or a carbonation (e.g., amines and thiols) to an α,β-unsaturated carbonyl compound (Yang et al. 2014). This reaction has high selectivity, enabling efficient coupling under physiological conditions, without producing side products or toxic compounds. For example, the Michael addition reaction can occur between thiol and vinyl sulfone (VS) or aminoethyl methacrylate (Table 1). Cells and growth factors can be encapsulated by simply mixing them with the polymer precursor solutions.

Thiolated HA (DTPH-HA, Fig. 1B-i) can be readily crosslinked in contact with air via the formation of disulphide bond. To better control crosslinking kinetics and density, several crosslinkers have also been used, such as polyethylene glycol diacrylate (PEGDA), PEG divinyl sulfone (PEGDVS), PEG tetra-thiols (PEG-SH_4) (Table 1). SH-HA has been used to form covalently crosslinked hydrogels which have been utilized to control the release of growth factors (Pike et al. 2006; Burdick and Prestwich 2011), for culturing different cell types, including neural stem cells (Addington et al. 2015), adult human dermal fibroblasts (Ghosh et al. 2006) and epidermal keratinocytes. When implanted *in vivo* (on forelimbs of dogs and horses), they enhanced the rate of wound healing (Yang et al. 2011). HyStem® Hydrogels is a commercial product that uses Michael addition reaction between SH-HA and PEGDA (Table 3). Gelation properties, including gelation time and hydrogel stiffness, can be controlled by varying the concentration and pH of the polymer precursor solutions.

Conversely, HA has been modified with acrylate groups (AC-HA, Fig. 1C-xi) and then crosslinked with PEG-SH$_4$ (Kim et al. 2007) or through bis-cysteine (C) containing peptide crosslinker (Lam and Segura 2013; Lei et al. 2011) via Michael addition chemistry. AC-HA can be obtained by coupling acrylic acid to tetrabutylammonium salt of HA in the presence of dimethylamino pyridine and di-tert-butyl-dicarbonate in dimethyl sulfoxide (DMSO) (Khetan and Burdick 2010) or via two-step reactions: introduction of an amine group using ADH (Fig. 1B-vi) followed by acrylation with *N*-acryloxysuccinimide (AC-NHS). These HA hydrogels were used to culture mesenchymal stem cells (MSCs) in 3D (Kim et al. 2007; Lam et al. 2014; Lei et al. 2011; Khetan and Burdick 2010) and study their behaviour to different biochemical signals, such as cell adhesive peptides (Lam et al. 2014; Lei et al. 2011) and bone morphogenetic protein-2 (Kim et al. 2007).

Dual functionalized HA derivative, possessing orthogonal thiol and hydrazide groups were obtained to form a doubly crosslinked network (Ossipov et al. 2010) and used for bio-conjugation of a fibronectin (FN) fragment to SH-HA (Table 2) and the subsequent hydrazone network formation, respectively (Ossipov et al. 2010).

The results from these studies suggest the potential of these *in situ* crosslinked hydrogels to deliver stem cells, as well as growth factors, to promote tissue regeneration.

Photopolymerizable HA Hydrogels

(Meth)acrylated polymers have been used for *in situ* hydrogel formation by photocrosslinking with a photoinitiator (Fig. 1D). Photopolymerization reactions are driven by chemicals that produce free radicals when exposed to specific wavelengths of light. The most extensively used photoinitiator for hydrogel formation has been Irgacure 2959 (2-methyl-1[4-(hydroxyethoxy)phenyl]-2-methyl-1-propanone), which is water-soluble and uses ultraviolet (UV) light, whereas the eosin Y/triethanolamine (TEOA)/1-vinyl-2-pyrrolidinone (NVP) photoinitiator system uses visible light. When light excites the photoinitiator, radicals are produced which then initiate the formation of kinetic chains through the double bonds in the macromer (i.e., propagation, Fig. 1D) (Kim et al. 2011). Thus, the hydrogel precursor solution can be injected into the body and then exposed to visible or UV light. Photopolymerization can be used to rapidly convert macromer solutions to a crosslinked network under physiological conditions. Important advantages of photopolymerizable systems include powerful spatial and temporal control of reaction kinetics, minimal heat production, ability to uniformly encapsulate biomolecules, and significant adaptability for *in situ* polymerization by adapting light sources.

The primary hydroxyl groups on the HA backbone (Fig. 1A) can easily be modified to include methacrylate (ME-HA, Fig. 1C-x) or acrylate (AC-HA,

Table 2. Bioengineering HA hydrogels with bioactive and mechanical signals.

HA-derivative	Biomolecule	Functionalization method	Application	References
ME-HA	-	Different crosslinking strategies to control hydrogel stiffness.	Photocrosslinkable ME-HA hydrogels promoted the retention of the chondrocytic phenotype and cartilage matrix synthesis for encapsulated chondrocytes *in vitro* and accelerated healing in an *in vivo* osteochondral defect model. Study chondrogenesis of MSCs under dynamic compressive loading. Spatially control hydrogel mechanics to direct stem cells differentiation into specific phenotype.	(Bian et al. 2012; Nettles et al. 2004, Guvendiren and Burdick 2012)
AC-HA ME-HA MA-HA	GCY*GRGDSPG* CGGNGEP*RGDTYRAY* C*RGDSP* (peptides containing the *cell adhesive sequence*) GCRD*VPMS↓MRGGDRCG* (*MMP-2 degradable peptide,* ↓indicates the site of proteolytic cleavage) GCRDG*PQG↓IWGQDRCG* GCRE*PQG↓IWGQERCG* (*MMP-1 degradable peptide*) C*QPQGLAKC* (*MMP-13-cleavable peptide sequence*)	Michael addition via thiol of cysteine (C) in the oligopeptides (Michael donor) with acrylate groups on ME-HA or PEG acrylates, or maleimides on MA-HA (Michael acceptors).	Study the effect of RGD clustering on mouse MSCs encapsulated in 3D ME-HA hydrogels. Modulation of ME-HA hydrogel properties from cell (human dermal fibroblasts) non-adhesive to adhesive via the incorporation of RGD peptide. Direct stem differentiation by the generation of degradation-mediated cellular traction. Investigate the effect of MMP-mediated hydrogel degradation on the chondrogenesis of encapsulated hMSCs. Generate functional human microvasculature by culturing endothelial colony-forming cells (ECFCs) within 3D HA hydrogels. Sequester growth factors to improve survival of transplanted cardiac progenitor cells.	(Lam and Segura 2013; Lei et al. 2011) (Park et al. 2003) (Khetan et al. 2013; Khetan and Burdick 2010; Feng et al. 2014) (Hanjaya-Putra et al. 2011; Hanjeya-Putra et al. 2012) (Jha et al. 2015)
AC-HA	NH_2-L_{15} (polypeptide)	Michael addition via primary amine of polypeptide N-terminal to AC-HA.	Gel formation driven by β-sheet formation rendered by the polypeptide chain.	(Wang et al. 2010)

EMCH-HA (Fig. 1B-vii)	Ephrin-B2 protein (ectodomain)	Activation of HA with EDC/Sulfo-NHS followed by EMCH functionalization. Maleimide groups react with thiols from the protein C-terminal cysteine to form stable thioether linkages.	Promote neuronal differentiation of neural stem cells both *in vitro* (in culture) and *in vivo* (within the brain).	(Conway et al. 2013)
SH-HA	FNfds (Fibronectin (FN) functional domains) FN III9*-10 (FN fragment)	Cysteine-tagged FNfds were first coupled to a homobifunctional PEGs (PEGDA, PEGDVS) by Michael-type addition and then coupled to SH-HA. Michael-type addition between SH-HA and VS-terminated FN fragment.	To promote migration of human dermal fibroblasts (HDF) and stimulate wound healing of porcine cutaneous wounds. Improve the osteogenic potential of BMP-2 by supporting MSCs attachment and spreading.	(Ghosh et al. 2006) (Kisiel et al. 2013)
SH-HA	Laminin (cell adhesive protein)	Laminin was conjugated to PEGDVS via Michael addition of thiol groups and then reacted with SH-HA.	Culture of neural progenitor/stem cells and probe the chemotactic effect of stromal cell-derived factor-1α.	(Addington et al. 2015)
MA-HA	CGG*AGTFALRGDNPQG* CGG*RKRLQVQLSIRT* (*laminin-derived cell-adhesive peptides*)	Maleimide groups on MA-HA react with thiol of cysteine (C) in the oligopeptides to form stable thioether linkages.	Mimic basement membrane (BME). The 3D peptide-HA matrices promoted HDF spreading and PC12 cell neurite outgrowth similar to that observed on 3D BME matrices.	(Yamada et al. 2013)
ME-HA	CD34 antibody (recognizes the CD34 antigen present on the cell surface of EPCs)	Activation of free carboxylate groups on ME-HA by EDC/NHS followed by coupling with amine groups of the antibody.	To promote the endothelialisation by selective capturing of endothelial progenitor cells (EPCs).	(Camci-Unal et al. 2010)
Tyr-HA	Phenol2–PEG–*RGD* (cell adhesive peptide)	The phenol2–PEG–*RGD* was conjugated to Tyr-HA hydrogels during gel formation process by the HRP-mediated crosslinking reaction.	Encapsulation of HUVECs and HFF1 fibroblasts within Tyr-HA hydrogels. Subcutaneous implantation showed the formation of functional vasculature inside the cell-laden gel after 2 weeks.	(Wang et al. 2014a)

A: Alanine; C: Cysteine; D: Aspartic acid; E: Glutamic acid; F: Phenylalanine; G: Glycine; I: Isoleucine; K: Lysine; L: Leucine; M: Methionine; N: Asparagine; P: Proline; Q: Glutamine; R: Arginine; S: Serine; T: Threonine; V: Valine; W: Tryptophan.

Fig. 1C-xi) functional groups that allow for photoinitiated crosslinking, but different methods have been used to introduce meth(acrylate) groups on HA. For example, ME-HA was obtained via free carboxylic groups using N-(3-aminopropyl) methacrylamide as an acrylating agent and the water soluble EDC as a coupling agent (Park et al. 2003) whereas methacrylate groups were introduced via primary hydroxyl groups using methacrylic anhydride (Nettles et al. 2004; Burdick et al. 2005) or glycidyl methacrylate (GMA) in the presence of excess triethylamine and tetra-butyl ammonium bromide (Baier Leach et al. 2003). Molecular weight, ME-HA concentration, and crosslink density can be varied to optimize mechanical, and degradation properties of ME-HA hydrogels. More recently, the synthesis of HA vinyl esters (VE-HA, Fig. 1C-xii) was reported using lipase-catalysed transesterification reaction between hydroxyl groups in HA and divinyl adipate (DVA) (Qin et al. 2014). The VE-HA macromers were explored for fabricating 3D hydrogels by two-photon lithography and compared with ME- and AC-HA, in terms of cytotoxicity and photoreactivity. VE-HA showed low cytotoxicity on L929 fibroblasts, high reactivity and degradability, either by enzyme or by hydrolysis. Crosslinking efficiency of VE-HA was comparable to AC-HA and much higher than ME-HA.

Photocrosslinked hydrogels can present some limitations for biomedical applications including: toxicity associated with some photoinitiators, long exposure to UV light and short penetration depth of light sources (Yang et al. 2014). Nevertheless, ME- and AC-HA have been widely exploited to engineer hydrogels with ECM signals (Table 2) and these photocrosslinked hydrogels have been applied in numerous studies, including controlled expansion and differentiation of human embryonic stem cells (hESCs) (Gerecht et al. 2007), promoting chondrogenesis of MSCs (Bian et al. 2011), localization and sustained delivery of stromal cell-derived factor-1 alpha (SDF-1α) and HA homing cues to the remodelling heart for enhanced engraftment of circulating bone marrow derived cells (BMCs) in the myocardium (Purcell et al. 2012).

"Click" HA Hydrogels

Most of the crosslinking chemistries described above require a coupling agent, catalyst, or photoinitiator, which may be cytotoxic, or involve a multistep synthesis of functionalized-HA, increasing the complexity of the system. Click chemistry is a Cu(I)-catalysed reaction between azide ($-N_3$) and terminal acetylene groups, forming 1,2,3-triazoles. This reaction has been applied to the formation of hydrogels due to: rapid reactivity under physiological conditions; absence of toxic by-products; high yield and regiospecificity (Yang et al. 2014).

To design simpler one-step, aqueous-based crosslinking system, the Shoichet group developed HA hydrogels via Diels-Alder "click" chemistry (Nimmo et al. 2011; Owen et al. 2013). Using 4-(4,6-dimethoxy-1,3,5-triazin-2-yl)-4-methylmorpholinium chloride (DMTMM), they synthesized furan-modified HA (Fig. 1B-viii) and used dimaleimide poly(ethyleneglycol) as a crosslinker. By controlling the furan to maleimide molar ratio, both the mechanical and degradation properties of the resulting Diels-Alder crosslinked hydrogels could be tuned. These HA crosslinked hydrogels were shown to be cytocompatible.

To obtain azide-modified HA (N$_3$-HA), azido-3,6,9-trioxaundecan-1-amine was grafted onto HA by EDC/NHS chemistry (Hu et al. 2011). To form a hydrogel, the –N$_3$ groups of N$_3$-HA were reacted with the acetylene groups of gelatin modified with propiolic acid, catalyzed by Cu(I), to form triazole rings. Chondrocytes seeded on the surface of the hydrogels were shown to remain viable and proliferate.

Alkyne-functionalized HA (obtained via EDC/NHS-mediated coupling of propargylamine to the HA carboxylic groups, Fig. 1B-iii) was crosslinked with linkers possessing two terminal azide functionalities (Piluso et al. 2011). Variation of the crosslinker density and crosslinker type (length and rigidity) created hydrogels with elastic moduli in the range of 0.5–4 kPa. Cytotoxicity assays did not show toxic effects on L929 cells.

Thermoreversible poly(N-isopropylacrylamide)-hyaluronan (PNIPAM-HA) hydrogels were synthesized through "click" chemistry and RAFT polymerization (Mortisen et al. 2010) using copper-catalyzed azide-alkyne cycloaddition of AL-HA with azido-terminated PNIPAM (N$_3$-PNIPAM). PNIPAM-HA hydrogels were shown to be cytocompatible to hTERT-BJ1 fibroblasts.

Enzyme-Mediated HA-Tyramine Hydrogels

As described previously, covalent crosslinking has been widely used to obtain HA hydrogels with precise control over crosslinking density. However, many of the crosslinking reagents used are toxic, precluding their use for cell encapsulation applications. Enzyme-mediated crosslinking reactions are finding increasing applications for developing hydrogels due to their mild conditions and enzyme specificity. Tyramine-modified HA (Fig. 1B-iv) has been used to induce covalent crosslinking (Loebel et al. 2015; Wang et al. 2014a; Lee et al. 2009) by horseradish peroxidase (HRP) and hydrogen peroxide (H$_2$O$_2$). HA derivatization with tyramine has been obtained through EDC/NHS chemistry (Lee et al. 2009; Lee et al. 2008), but the use of DMTMM was also recently reported (Loebel et al. 2015). The later method was shown to provide several advantages, compared with conventional method, such as accurate control of the degree of substituted (DS) tyramine (Tyr) on HA and consequently better control over the viscoelastic properties, *in vitro* swelling and enzymatic degradation of the crosslinked hydrogels. The mechanical strength of the HA-Tyr hydrogel was shown to be tuned solely by the H$_2$O$_2$ amount without affecting the gelation rate. Subcutaneous injections of HA-Tyr with H$_2$O$_2$ and HRP demonstrated that rapid gelation could prevent diffusion of the injected polymer solution and ensure localized gelation at the injection site (Lee et al. 2008). HA-tyramine hydrogels conjugated with the bioactive peptide epitope arginine-glycine-aspartic acid (RGD) promoted the adhesion, proliferation and migration of human umbilical vein endothelial cells (HUVECs), as well as capillary-like network formation and extension, in combination with co-culture of HUVECs and human fibroblasts (HFF1) *in vitro*, compared to an unmodified hydrogel. *In vivo* formation of vasculature in the cell-laden hydrogel constructs confirmed the anastomosis with the host vasculature (Wang et al. 2014a). By changing the polymer and H$_2$O$_2$ concentrations, Tyr-HA hydrogels with different mechanical properties (soft, medium and stiff) were obtained and tested for their ability to support the expansion of hESCs in 3D (Xu et al. 2015). Tyr-HA hydrogels with compressive modulus of ~350 Pa best supported the proliferation of hESCs and maintained their pluripotency.

The Corgel® BioHydrogel from Lifecore Biomedical (Table 3) is a typical hydrogel obtained by enzymatic crosslinking reaction with HRP and H_2O_2. Corgel® offers a range of physical properties depending on the tyramine substitution (TS) percentage and the tyramine substituted hyaluronan (TS-NaHy) concentration.

Supramolecular HA Hydrogels

Self-assembling hydrogels are formed through specific supramolecular (noncovalent) interactions between pendant or end group functionalities and do not require the use of triggers such as chemical initiators or heat. Furthermore, because many of these supramolecular interactions are reversible, supramolecular self-assembly allows ease of injection without potential premature gel formation and near-instantaneous reassembly for hydrogel retention at the target site. The use of supramolecular interactions to form HA hydrogels by self-assembly has been explored through guest-host interactions, such as the interaction between or adamantane (Ad, guest) and cyclodextrin (CD, host). Ad associates strongly with CD (association constant on the order of 1×10^5 M^{-1}) by hydrophobic interactions. The Burdick group has separately conjugated HA with Ad (Fig. 1C-xiii) and CD (Fig. 1B-ix) to form injectable HA hydrogels (Rodell et al. 2013). Mixing both components resulted in rapid formation of a supramolecular hydrogel displaying shear-thinning and near-instantaneous self-healing (shear recovering) properties. The hydrogel's physical properties, including mechanics ($G' \approx 300$ Pa at 1 Hz) and flow characteristics, were dependent on crosslink density and network structure, controlled through: macromer concentration; the extent of guest macromer modification and the molar ratio of guest and host functional groups. They have further upgraded these supramolecular hydrogels via the introduction of secondary covalent crosslinking (addition of thiols and Michael-acceptors on HA: e.g., methacrylates, acrylates, vinyl sulfones) to increase hydrogel moduli (E = 25.0+/−4.5 kPa) and *in vivo* stability (>3.5 fold at 28 days) (Rodell et al. 2015a). Inclusion of proteolytically degradable peptides make these hydrogels responsive to enzymatic degradation *in vitro* and *in vivo* (Rodell et al. 2015b). The rational and selective modification of amino acid residues near the proteolytic site enabled selective protease susceptibility and control over hydrogel degradation kinetics.

The macrocyclic host molecule cucurbituril (CB) was also conjugated to HA to obtain supramolecular hydrogels upon interaction with HA monofunctionalized with polyamines (PAs) of diaminohexane (DAH) or spermine (SPM) (Jung et al. 2014; Park et al. 2012). CB[n] has exceptionally high binding affinity and selectivity toward alkylammonium ions in aqueous solution. In particular, it tightly binds PAs, like DAH or SPM in their protonated forms, to make stable 1:1 host–guest complexes with a binding constant up to 10^{10} or 10^{12} M^{-1}. MonoCB[6]-HA was obtained by thiolene "click" photoreaction between monoallyloxy CB[6] and SH-HA (Fig. 1B-i), while DAH-HA or SMP-HA were obtained by activation of HA carboxyl groups with EDC followed by reaction with amines of DAH and SMP (Oh et al. 2010). MonoCB[6]/DAH-HA or MonoCB[6]/SPM-HA hydrogels were obtained by simply mixing DAH-HA or SPM-HA and monoCB[6]-HA solutions driven by the host–guest interaction between CB[6] and DAH or SPM molecules in the precursor solutions. Hydrogel formation occurs at mild conditions, allowing the direct encapsulation of cells and sensitive molecules, like growth factors. These gels showed *in vivo* stability up to 11 days after subcutaneous injection in nude mice (Park et al. 2012) and encapsulation of human MSCs (hMSCs) and differentiation agents (transforming growth factor-β3 and/or dexamethasone) within these gels showed effective chondrogenic differentiation of hMSCs (Jung et al. 2014).

These supramolecular hydrogels show potential as a minimally invasive injectable hydrogels for therapeutic delivery of cells or growth factors and may have great utility in many regenerative medicine applications, such as artificial environments for the controlled differentiation of stem cells, soft tissue reconstruction, nucleus pulpous replacement or mechanical stabilization of myocardial infarct.

(Bio)Engineering HA Hydrogels to Control Cell Behaviour

HA hydrogels can be engineered in several ways to control the behaviour of encapsulated cells. Tuning their mechanical properties, through controlled degradation and/or degree of crosslinking, can regulate cell mechanosensing and topographical patterns can be used to direct cell migration. However, regardless of the crosslinking mechanism, bioactive molecules must be incorporated into the hydrogel matrix to help direct cell behaviour. These biomolecules can be full-length extracellular matrix proteins, like collagen, fibronectin (FN) and laminin, or small peptide sequences derived from these proteins (Table 2). In addition, a variety of bioconjugation techniques (Ahadian et al. 2015) can be used to couple one or more biomolecules to obtain controllable bioconjugates (Fig. 1D) for specific interactions with cells (gel formation for cell encapsulation, binding sites for cell adhesion, matrix degradation for cell migration). Bioconjugated HA hydrogels with multiple chemical, biological and physical functionalities have been developed (Table 2) to mimic different aspects of the ECM (Lam et al. 2014; Guvendiren and Burdick 2013).

Applications of HA Hydrogels in Regenerative Medicine

HA hydrogels have broad utility within regenerative medicine. They have been integrated with 3D bioprinting (Skardal and Atala 2015; Hong et al. 2013) and used for: engineering the stem cell niche; delivery of growth factors and cells; wound healing and cartilage tissue engineering (Burdick and Prestwich 2011; Cai et al. 2005; Kim et al. 2011; Prestwich 2008; 2011).

Previously described HA-based hydrogels have been optimized to address clinical needs and provide reliable 3D matrices with controlled viscoelasticity for cell culture. Some of these hydrogel technologies have been translated into commercial products (Table 3). These commercially available hydrogels have permitted the development of numerous studies where they were used as 3D scaffolds for capillary-like structure formation from endothelial colony-forming cells to generate vascularized tissue constructs (Yee et al. 2011), co-culture of MSCs and macrophages in 3D (Hanson et al. 2011), 3D culture and maintenance of hepatocyte function *in vitro* (Skardal et al. 2012), culture of human astrocytes in defined 3D microenvironment to recapitulate

Table 3. Commercially available HA-based hydrogels.

HA-based hydrogel	Crosslinking mechanism	Commercial name	Supplier
Tyramine-substituted sodium hyaluronate (TS-NaHy)	TS-NaHy hydrogels are formed by using the oxidative coupling of tyramine moieties catalyzed by hydrogen peroxide (H_2O_2) and horseradish peroxidase (HRP).	Corgel® BioHydrogel	Lifecore Biomedical, LCC has licensed this technology from the Cleveland Clinic.
Thiol-modified hyaluronan (Gycosil®), thiol-reactive PEGDA crosslinker (Extralink®)	The hydrogel is formed when the crosslinking agent, Extralink®-Lite (PEGDA) is added to a mixture of Glycosil® (thiol-modified hyaluronan).	HyStem® Hydrogels	Developed by Gycosan BioSystems, Inc which was acquired by BioTime in 2011. HyStem® Hydrogels are commercialized by ESI BIO—A Division of BioTime, Inc. The product is licensed for selling by other suppliers (Sigma-Aldrich, Advanced Biomatrix, Thermo Scientific).
Thiol-modified hyaluronic acid, thiol-modified gelatin (Gelin-S®), PEG-norbornene (UVlink™), Irgacure 2959 for photoinitiation	Photopolymerization by UV light.	HyStem® Hydrogel UV	ESI BIO—A Division of BioTime, Inc.

the brain ECM (Placone et al. 2015), 3D culture of human skin-derived precursors for dermal stem cell expansion *in vitro* (Wang et al. 2014b), 2-D plating of human dermal fibroblasts on top of hydrogel (Ferreira et al. 2013). The availability of HA hydrogels able to provide consistent and physiologically relevant environments for cell culture will facilitate their preclinical and clinical application.

Acknowledgment

H.S. Azevedo acknowledges the financial support of the European Union under the Marie Curie Career Integration Grant SuprHApolymers (PCIG14-GA-2013-631871).

References

Addington, C.P., J.M. Heffernan, C.S. Millar-Haskell, E.W. Tucker, R.W. Sirianni and S.E. Stabenfeldt. 2015. Enhancing neural stem cell response to SDF-1 alpha gradients through hyaluronic acid-laminin hydrogels. Biomaterials. 72: 11–9.

Ahadian, S., R.B. Sadeghian, S. Salehi, S. Ostrovidov, H. Bae, M. Ramalingam et al. 2015. Bioconjugated hydrogels for tissue engineering and regenerative medicine. Bioconjug. Chem. 26(10): 1984–2001.

Baier Leach, J., K.A. Bivens, C.W. Patrick Jr and C.E. Schmidt. 2003. Photocrosslinked hyaluronic acid hydrogels: Natural, biodegradable tissue engineering scaffolds. Biotechnol. Bioeng. 82(5): 578–589.

Bian, L., D.Y. Zhai, E. Tous, R. Rai, R.L. Mauck and J.A. Burdick. 2011. Enhanced MSC chondrogenesis following delivery of TGF-beta3 from alginate microspheres within hyaluronic acid hydrogels *in vitro* and *in vivo*. Biomaterials. 32(27): 6425–34.

Bian, L., D.Y. Zhai, E.C. Zhang, R.L. Mauck and J.A. Burdick. 2012. Dynamic compressive loading enhances cartilage matrix synthesis and distribution and suppresses hypertrophy in hMSC-laden hyaluronic acid hydrogels. Tissue Eng. Part A. 18(7-8): 715–24.

Borzacchiello, A., L. Russo, B.M. Malle, K. Schwach-Abdellaoui and L. Ambrosio. 2015. Hyaluronic acid based hydrogels for regenerative medicine applications. Biomed. Res. Int. 2015: 871218.

Burdick, J.A., C. Chung, X. Jia, M.A. Randolph and R. Langer. 2005. Controlled degradation and mechanical behavior of photopolymerized hyaluronic acid networks. Biomacromolecules. 6(1): 386–91.

Burdick, J.A. and G.D. Prestwich. 2011. Hyaluronic acid hydrogels for biomedical applications. Adv. Mater. 23(12): H41–56.

Cai, S., Y. Liu, X. Zheng Shu and G.D. Prestwich. 2005. Injectable glycosaminoglycan hydrogels for controlled release of human basic fibroblast growth factor. Biomaterials. 26(30): 6054–67.

Camci-Unal, G., H. Aubin, A.F. Ahari, H. Bae, J.W. Nichol and A. Khademhosseini. 2010. Surface-modified hyaluronic acid hydrogels to capture endothelial progenitor cells. Soft Matter. 6(20): 5120–5126.

Conway, A., T. Vazin, D.P. Spelke, N.A. Rode, K.E. Healy, R.S. Kane et al. 2013. Multivalent ligands control stem cell behaviour *in vitro* and *in vivo*. Nat. Nanotechnol. 8(11): 831–8.

Feng, Q., M. Zhu, K. Wei and L. Bian. 2014. Cell-mediated degradation regulates human mesenchymal stem cell chondrogenesis and hypertrophy in mmp-sensitive hyaluronic acid hydrogels. PLoS ONE. 9(6): e99587.

Ferreira, D.S., A.P. Marques, R.L. Reis and H.S. Azevedo. 2013. Hyaluronan and self-assembling peptides as building blocks to reconstruct the extracellular environment in skin tissue. Biomater. Sci. 1(9): 952–964.

Gerecht, S., J.A. Burdick, L.S. Ferreira, S.A. Townsend, R. Langer and G. Vunjak-Novakovic. 2007. Hyaluronic acid hydrogel for controlled self-renewal and differentiation of human embryonic stem cells. Proc. Natl. Acad. Sci. USA. 104(27): 11298–303.

Ghosh, K., X.D. Ren, X.Z. Shu, G.D. Prestwich and R.A. Clark. 2006. Fibronectin functional domains coupled to hyaluronan stimulate adult human dermal fibroblast responses critical for wound healing. Tissue Eng. 12(3): 601–13.

Guvendiren, M. and J.A. Burdick. 2012. Stiffening hydrogels to probe short- and long-term cellular responses to dynamic mechanics. Nat. Commun. 3: 792.

Guvendiren, M. and J.A. Burdick. 2013. Engineering synthetic hydrogel microenvironments to instruct stem cells. Curr. Opin. Biotechnol. 24(5): 841–6.

Hanjaya-Putra, D., V. Bose, Y.I. Shen, J. Yee, S. Khetan, K. Fox-Talbot et al. 2011. Controlled activation of morphogenesis to generate a functional human microvasculature in a synthetic matrix. Blood. 118(3): 804–15.

Hanjaya-Putra, D., K.T. Wong, K. Hirotsu, S. Khetan, J.A. Burdick and S. Gerecht. 2012. Spatial control of cell-mediated degradation to regulate vasculogenesis and angiogenesis in hyaluronan hydrogels. Biomaterials. 33(26): 6123–31.

Hanson, S.E., S.N. King, J. Kim, X. Chen, S.L. Thibeault and P. Hematti. 2011. The effect of mesenchymal stromal cell-hyaluronic acid hydrogel constructs on immunophenotype of macrophages. Tissue Eng. Part A. 17(19-20): 2463–71.

Hong, S., S.J. Song, J.Y. Lee, H. Jang, J. Choi, K. Sun et al. 2013. Cellular behavior in micropatterned hydrogels by bioprinting system depended on the cell types and cellular interaction. J. Biosci. Bioeng. 116(2): 224–30.

Hu, X., D. Li, F. Zhou and C. Gao. 2011. Biological hydrogel synthesized from hyaluronic acid, gelatin and chondroitin sulfate by click chemistry. Acta Biomater. 7(4): 1618–26.

Jha, A.K., K.M. Tharp, J. Ye, J.L. Santiago-Ortiz, W.M. Jackson, A. Stahl et al. 2015. Enhanced survival and engraftment of transplanted stem cells using growth factor sequestering hydrogels. Biomaterials. 47: 1–12.

Jung, H., J.S. Park, J. Yeom, N. Selvapalam, K.M. Park, K. Oh et al. 2014. 3D tissue engineered supramolecular hydrogels for controlled chondrogenesis of human mesenchymal stem cells. Biomacromolecules. 15(3): 707–14.

Khetan, S., M. Guvendiren, W.R. Legant, D.M. Cohen, C.S. Chen and J.A. Burdick. 2013. Degradation-mediated cellular traction directs stem cell fate in covalently crosslinked three-dimensional hydrogels. Nat. Mater. 12(5): 458–65.

Khetan, Sudhir and J.A. Burdick. 2010. Patterning network structure to spatially control cellular remodeling and stem cell fate within 3-dimensional hydrogels. Biomaterials. 31(32): 8228–8234.

Kim, I.L., R.L. Mauck and J.A. Burdick. 2011. Hydrogel design for cartilage tissue engineering: a case study with hyaluronic acid. Biomaterials. 32(34): 8771–82.

Kim, J., I.S. Kim, T.H. Cho, K.B. Lee, S.J. Hwang, G. Tae et al. 2007. Bone regeneration using hyaluronic acid-based hydrogel with bone morphogenic protein-2 and human mesenchymal stem cells. Biomaterials. 28(10): 1830–7.

Kisiel, M., M.M. Martino, M. Ventura, J.A. Hubbell, J. Hilborn and D.A. Ossipov. 2013. Improving the osteogenic potential of BMP-2 with hyaluronic acid hydrogel modified with integrin-specific fibronectin fragment. Biomaterials. 34(3): 704–12.

Lam, J. and T. Segura. 2013. The modulation of MSC integrin expression by RGD presentation. Biomaterials. 34(16): 3938–47.

Lam, J., N.F. Truong and T. Segura. 2014. Design of cell-matrix interactions in hyaluronic acid hydrogel scaffolds. Acta Biomater. 10(4): 1571–80.

Lee, F., J.E. Chung and M. Kurisawa. 2009. An injectable hyaluronic acid-tyramine hydrogel system for protein delivery. J. Control. Release. 134(3): 186–93.

Lee, F., J.E. Chung and M. Kurisawa. 2008. An injectable enzymatically crosslinked hyaluronic acid-tyramine hydrogel system with independent tuning of mechanical strength and gelation rate. Soft Matter. 4(4): 880–887.

Lei, Y., S. Gojgini, J. Lam and T. Segura. 2011. The spreading, migration and proliferation of mouse mesenchymal stem cells cultured inside hyaluronic acid hydrogels. Biomaterials. 32(1): 39–47.

Loebel, C., M. D'Este, M. Alini, M. Zenobi-Wong and D. Eglin. 2015. Precise tailoring of tyramine-based hyaluronan hydrogel properties using DMTMM conjugation. Carbohydr. Polym. 115: 325–33.

Mortisen, D., M. Peroglio, M. Alini and D. Eglin. 2010. Tailoring thermoreversible hyaluronan hydrogels by "click" chemistry and RAFT polymerization for cell and drug therapy. Biomacromolecules. 11(5): 1261–72.

Neffe, A.T., K.A. Kobuch, M. Maier, N. Feucht, C.P. Lohmann, A. Wolfstein et al. 2011. *In vitro* and *in vivo* evaluation of a multifunctional hyaluronic acid based hydrogel system for local application on the retina. Macromol. Symp. 309-310(1): 229–235.

Nettles, D.L., T.P. Vail, M.T. Morgan, M.W. Grinstaff and L.A. Setton. 2004. Photocrosslinkable hyaluronan as a scaffold for articular cartilage repair. Ann. Biomed. Eng. 32(3): 391–397.

Nimmo, C.M., S.C. Owen and M.S. Shoichet. 2011. Diels-alder click crosslinked hyaluronic acid hydrogels for tissue engineering. Biomacromolecules. 12(3): 824–30.

Oh, E.J., K. Park, K.S. Kim, J. Kim, J-A. Yang, J-. Kong et al. 2010. Target specific and long-acting delivery of protein, peptide, and nucleotide therapeutics using hyaluronic acid derivatives. J. Control. Release. 141(1): 2–12.

Ossipov, D.A., X. Yang, O. Varghese, S. Kootala and J. Hilborn. 2010. Modular approach to functional hyaluronic acid hydrogels using orthogonal chemical reactions. Chem. Comm. 46(44): 8368–8370.

Owen, S.C., S.A. Fisher, R.Y. Tam, C.M. Nimmo and M.S. Shoichet. 2013. Hyaluronic acid click hydrogels emulate the extracellular matrix. Langmuir. 29(24): 7393–400.

Park, K.M., J.A. Yang, H. Jung, J. Yeom, J.S. Park, K.-H. Park et al. 2012. *In situ* supramolecular assembly and modular modification of hyaluronic acid hydrogels for 3d cellular engineering. ACS Nano. 6(4): 2960–2968.

Park, Y.D., N. Tirelli and J.A. Hubbell. 2003. Photopolymerized hyaluronic acid-based hydrogels and interpenetrating networks. Biomaterials. 24(6): 893–900.

Pike, D.B., S. Cai, K.R. Pomraning, M.A. Firpo, R.J. Fisher, X.Z. Shu et al. 2006. Heparin-regulated release of growth factors *in vitro* and angiogenic response *in vivo* to implanted hyaluronan hydrogels containing VEGF and bFGF. Biomaterials. 27(30): 5242–51.

Piluso, S., B. Hiebl, S.N. Gorb, A. Kovalev, A. Lendlein and A.T. Neffe. 2011. Hyaluronic acid-based hydrogels crosslinked by copper-catalyzed azide-alkyne cycloaddition with tailorable mechanical properties. Int. J. Artif. Organs. 34(2): 192–7.

Placone, A.L., P.M. McGuiggan, D.E. Bergles, H. Guerrero-Cazares, A. Quinones-Hinojosa and P.C. Searson. 2015. Human astrocytes develop physiological morphology and remain quiescent in a novel 3D matrix. Biomaterials. 42: 134–43.

Prestwich, G.D. 2008. Engineering a clinically-useful matrix for cell therapy. Organogenesis. 4(1): 42–7.

Prestwich, G.D. 2011. Hyaluronic acid-based clinical biomaterials derived for cell and molecule delivery in regenerative medicine. J. Control. Release. 155(2): 193–9.

Purcell, B.P., J.A. Elser, A. Mu, K.B. Margulies and J.A. Burdick. 2012. Synergistic effects of SDF-1alpha chemokine and hyaluronic acid release from degradable hydrogels on directing bone marrow derived cell homing to the myocardium. Biomaterials. 33(31): 7849–57.

Qin, X.-H., P. Gruber, M. Markovic, B. Plochberger, E. Klotzsch, J. Stampfl et al. 2014. Enzymatic synthesis of hyaluronic acid vinyl esters for two-photon microfabrication of biocompatible and biodegradable hydrogel constructs. Polym. Chem. 5(22): 6523–6533.

Rodell, C.B., A.L. Kaminski and J.A. Burdick. 2013. Rational design of network properties in guest-host assembled and shear-thinning hyaluronic acid hydrogels. Biomacromolecules. 14(11): 4125–34.

Rodell, C.B., J.W. MacArthur, S.M. Dorsey, R.J. Wade, Y.J. Woo and J.A. Burdick. 2015a. Shear-thinning supramolecular hydrogels with secondary autonomous covalent crosslinking to modulate viscoelastic properties. Adv. Funct. Mater. 25(4): 636–644.

Rodell, C.B., R.J. Wade, B.P. Purcell, N.N. Dusaj and J.A. Burdick. 2015b. Selective proteolytic degradation of guest–host assembled, injectable hyaluronic acid hydrogels. ACS Biomater. Sci. Eng. 1(4): 277–286.

Shoham, N., A.L. Sasson, F.-H. Lin, D. Benayahu, R. Haj-Ali and A. Gefen. 2013. The mechanics of hyaluronic acid/adipic acid dihydrazide hydrogel: towards developing a vessel for delivery of preadipocytes to native tissues. J. Mech. Behav. Biomed. Mater. 28: 320–331.

Skardal, A., L. Smith, S. Bharadwaj, A. Atala, S. Soker and Y. Zhang. 2012. Tissue specific synthetic ECM hydrogels for 3-D *in vitro* maintenance of hepatocyte function. Biomaterials. 33(18): 4565–75.

Skardal, A. and A. Atala. 2015. Biomaterials for integration with 3-D bioprinting. Ann. Biomed. Eng. 43(3): 730–46.

Su, W.Y., Y.C. Chen and F.H. Lin. 2010. Injectable oxidized hyaluronic acid/adipic acid dihydrazide hydrogel for nucleus pulposus regeneration. Acta Biomater. 6(8): 3044–55.

Viola, M., D. Vigetti, E. Karousou, M.L. D'Angelo, I. Caon, P. Moretto et al. 2015. Biology and biotechnology of hyaluronan. Glycoconj. J. 32(3-4): 93–103.

Wang, L.S., F. Lee, J. Lim, C. Du, A.C. Wan, S.S. Lee et al. 2014a. Enzymatic conjugation of a bioactive peptide into an injectable hyaluronic acid-tyramine hydrogel system to promote the formation of functional vasculature. Acta Biomater. 10(6): 2539–50.

Wang, X., S. Liu, Q. Zhao, N. Li, H. Zhanga, X. Zhang et al. 2014b. Three-dimensional hydrogel scaffolds facilitate *in vitro* self-renewal of human skin-derived precursors. Acta Biomater. 10(7): 3177–87.

Wang, X., J. Messman, J.W. Mays and D. Baskaran. 2010. Polypeptide grafted hyaluronan: synthesis and characterization. Biomacromolecules. 11(9): 2313–20.

Xu, K., K. Narayanan, F. Lee, K.H. Bae, S. Gao and M. Kurisawa. 2015. Enzyme-mediated hyaluronic acid-tyramine hydrogels for the propagation of human embryonic stem cells in 3D. Acta Biomater. 24: 159–71.

Xu, X., A.K. Jha, D.A. Harrington, M.C. Farach-Carson and X. Jia. 2012. Hyaluronic acid-based hydrogels: from a natural polysaccharide to complex networks. Soft Matter. 8(12): 3280–3294.

Yamada, Y., K. Hozumi, F. Katagiri, Y. Kikkawa and M. Nomizu. 2013. Laminin-111-derived peptide-hyaluronate hydrogels as a synthetic basement membrane. Biomaterials. 34(28): 6539–47.

Yang, G., G.D. Prestwich and B.K. Mann. 2011. Thiolated carboxymethyl-hyaluronic-acid-based biomaterials enhance wound healing in rats, dogs, and horses. ISRN Vet. Sci. 2011: 851593.

Yang, J.A., J. Yeom, B.W. Hwang, A.S. Hoffman and S.K. Hahn. 2014. *In situ*-forming injectable hydrogels for regenerative medicine. Prog. Polym. Sci. 39(12): 1973–1986.

Yee, D., D. Hanjaya-Putra, V. Bose, E. Luong and S. Gerecht. 2011. Hyaluronic acid hydrogels support cord-like structures from endothelial colony-forming cells. Tissue Eng. Part A. 17(9-10): 1351–61.

CHAPTER 10

Hydrogel Nanomaterials for Cancer Diagnosis and Therapy

Ricardo A. Pires,[1,2,]* *Yousef M. Abul-Haija,*[3]
Rui L. Reis,[1,2] *Rein V. Ulijn*[3,4] *and Iva Pashkuleva*[1,2]

Introduction

Cancer remains a major burden for our modern society. Despite the tremendous advances made in the understanding and fighting against different cancers, the deaths caused by them continue to grow significantly each year: it is estimated that, worldwide, this number will reach 13 million per year within the next two decades (WHO 2014). Conventional therapies based on specific ligand-receptor interactions are compromised by the great complexity of cancer cells and their resistance to current therapeutic drug regimens (Zhou and Xu 2015). Thus, new paradigms are urgently needed to change this devastating pattern. In the last few years, self-assembly of small molecules has emerged as a powerful tool to develop novel selective and functional nanomaterials that enhance our understanding about disease specific pathways and, thus, aid both cancer treatment and diagnosis. The main rationales for using such systems is their ability to operate in the cellular environment; the unique properties that these systems have upon organization in ordered nanostructures; and their intrinsic dynamic nature related to their rapid responsiveness to physiological signals (e.g., pH, enzymatic activity, etc.)

[1] 3B's Research Group - Biomaterials, Biodegradables and Biomimetics, University of Minho, Headquarters of the European Institute of Excellence on Tissue Engineering and Regenerative Medicine, AvePark, 4806-909 Taipas, Guimarães, Portugal.
[2] ICVS/3B's - PT Government Associate Laboratory, Braga/Guimarães, Portugal.
[3] Pure and Applied Chemistry Department/WestCHEM and Technology and Innovation Centre, University of Strathclyde, 99 George Street, Glasgow, G1 1RD, UK.
[4] Advanced Science Research Center (ASRC) and Hunter College, 85 St Nicholas Terrace, City University of New York, NY10027, USA.
* Corresponding author

associated with the malignant transformation. Among different approaches that make use of the self-assembly, the biocatalytic self-assembly (BSA) concept has emerged as a new approach in cancer research and is the focus of this chapter. BSA makes use of an enzyme sensitive moiety (group or bond) that is incorporated in a peptide amphiphile (PA) to prevent the PA self-assembly. This moiety is transformed (e.g., cleaved) under the action of the respective enzyme typically resulting in a rebalancing of the amphiphilicity of the PA. As a result, the obtained molecules are able to self-assemble into nanofibers that can further generate two-dimensional networks or localized supramolecular gels under physiological conditions (Yang et al. 2004; Ulijn 2006; Gao et al. 2009; Hirst et al. 2010). This concept, and the fact that cancers present an overexpression of different enzymes, led to the development of BSA approach as: a cancer diagnostic and imaging methodology; a direct anti-cancer strategy (due to the cytotoxicity of the nanofibers themselves or their network); and to induce the controlled release of drugs or pro-drugs. All these strategies will be discussed in the following sections.

Self-Assembling Hydrogels for the Diagnosis of Cancer

Malignant transformation and tumour metastasis are associated with altered expression of a number of biomolecules, such as proteins and glycans. Some of these biomolecules have been identified and nowadays are used as hallmarks for certain cancers, aiding the staging, monitoring and prognosis (invasion and metastasis) of these diseases. Many others remain to be discovered. Thus, the development of molecular tools for selective detection of these biomarkers is of fundamental importance for both basic cancer research and cancer diagnosis. Approaches, involving different fluorescent probes together with non-invasive methods for their detection (e.g., endoscopic molecular imaging), are quite attractive as they can avoid unnecessary biopsies. Moreover, they are cost effective and allow real time observation. The main challenge in these approaches is the design of a probe that is sufficiently selective (cancer cells share many common features with the normal host cells from which they derive) and sensitive (easily distinguished from the background signal). During the last five years, supramolecular self-assembly of small molecules has been applied in several strategies for design of fluorescent probes that meet such criteria. These probes are typically composed of a core self-assembling unit—such as a short PA derivative of diphenylalanine (Fig. 1, blue), and a biologically sensitive unit (functional group or bond, Fig. 1, green). The amphiphile capping groups are polycyclic aromatic hydrocarbons (R in Fig. 1), which not only provide driving force for the self-assembly via aromatic interactions (π-π interactions) but also endows the obtained supramolecular structure with intrinsic fluorescent signal. Depending on the chosen approach, the design of the probe can include additional fluorescent units (e.g., 4 in Fig. 1).

The principle that drives the self-assembly dependent imaging is that the properties of a fluorophore incorporated into the probe-gelator are quite different if the molecules bearing them are assembled or not. Characteristic shifts are observed for different molecular organisations: hypsochromic shift (blue shift) is typical for the H-assemblies, in which the transition moments of the monomers are organized in a "face-to-face" manner, i.e., aligned parallel but perpendicular to the line joining their centres. In

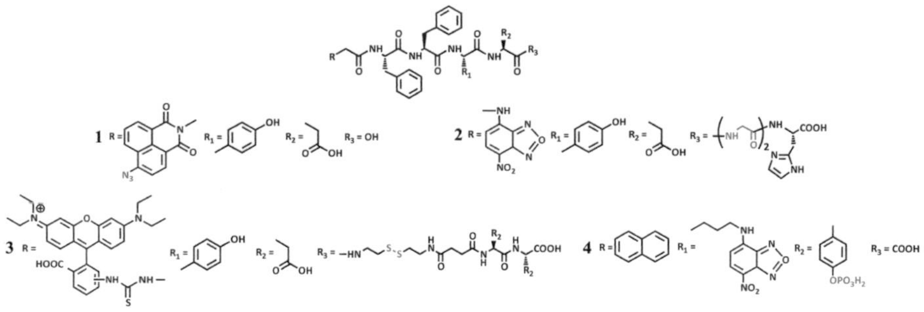

Fig. 1. Chemical structure of probes used in self-assembly dependent imaging. The unit that drives the self-assembly is presented in blue, the fluorophore in red and the biologically sensitive groups are marked in green: they can be incorporated in the fluorescent group (Cai et al. 2016), in the peptide portion of the amphiphile (Cai et al. 2014; Wang et al. 2015) or attached as a separate unit (Gao et al. 2012; Gao et al. 2013a; Gao et al. 2013b).

J-aggregate assemblies an end-to-end arrangement is observed, i.e., the transition moments of the monomers are aligned parallel to the line joining their centres, and this organisation results in a narrow bathochromic shift (red shift), known as J-band (Zhai et al. 2014). Besides these shifts, the self-assembly is generally associated with the quenching of the fluorescence signal (weakens the read out signal). Although this may seem to be a drawback, the aggregation induced quenching is often used in the development of probes (Kiyonaka et al. 2004; Zhai et al. 2014). The opposite process—disassembly—has received much less attention as a sensing mechanism (Mizusawa et al. 2010; Zhai et al. 2014). This process, however, is quite relevant in the case of approaches using supramolecular structures, for which the disassembly results in enhancing the read-out signal and can be used for the design of turn-on probes (Mizusawa et al. 2010). In addition to these changes in the fluorescent properties, the self-assembly process influences dramatically the contrast in fluorescent imaging (Gao et al. 2012). Upon excitation, the dissolved unassembled probe emits identically in each direction within the optical thickness of the focal plan resulting in little contrast for imaging. The directional self-assembly of the probes leads to localization of the fluorophores within the assembled nanofibers and thus, provide excellent contrast for imaging of these assemblies. These changes in the fluorescence read-out signal upon self-assembly have inspired the development of several approaches for cancer diagnosis and imaging *in vitro* and *in vivo*.

Biocatalytic self-assembly (BSA) for diagnosis and imaging

BSA merges the efficiency and selectivity of an enzymatic transformation with the sensitivity of the self-assembly process. The concept was first introduced in 2004 by Xu's group (Yang et al. 2004; Yang and Xu 2004). In these first studies, the sol-gel transition state that is easily visible by naked eye was applied as a simple detection method for the presence of an enzyme—phosphatase and its inhibitors. This pioneering work was vastly explored in the following years (Thornton et al. 2009; Thornton et al. 2013) and used in different analytical methodologies involving phosphatases (Gao et al. 2013a; Du et al. 2015a; Gao et al. 2013b; Gao et al. 2012; Zhou and Xu 2015; Yang and Xu 2004; Yang et al. 2004; Yang et al. 2007a) (e.g., alkaline phosphatase, ALP that is overexpressed in several cancers, such as, prostatic and bone cancers) but also extended to other enzymes such as proteases, specifically matrix metalloproteinases (MMPs) (Cai et al. 2014; Bremmer et al. 2012; Zhou and Xu 2015; Yang et al. 2009; Kalafatovic et al. 2015), caspases (Shi et al. 2012; Cai et al. 2014) and several proteases, including thermolysin (Toledano et al. 2006; Williams et al. 2009) and subtilisin (Hirst et al. 2010). The BSA-based detection and imaging uses a precursor molecule (e.g., Fig. 1) that can diffuse freely inside the cell (Fig. 2A) where it is converged by the targeted enzyme into a gelator (by acting on the group/bond marked in green, Fig. 1.

Once transformed, the gelator molecules self-assemble into fibers that have reduced diffusion—they are entrapped into the cell compartment in which the enzyme is overexpressed; and can be visualized because of the enhanced fluorescence contrast discussed above (Gao et al. 2012; Gao et al. 2013a). This approach can be also used to detect the enzyme inhibitors (Fig. 2B). Those will bind competitively to the active side of the enzyme and thus, the conversion of the precursor will be blocked and no self-assembly will occur (Yang and Xu 2004). Currently, different precursors are emerging, including the ones that are sensitive to cell-surface markers (e.g., ectoenzymes (Du et al. 2015a)), and self-assemble on the cell surface; or result in gelators that bind specifically to cellular receptors (Shi et al. 2015) (Fig. 2D).

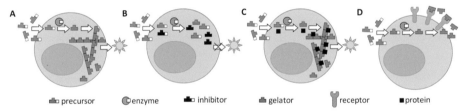

Fig. 2. Different methodologies that use BSA for the detection of cancer markers such as: enzymes (A), enzyme inhibitors (B), proteins (C) or cell surface receptors (D).

Enhancement of fluorescence probes

The peculiar properties of self-assembling materials can be also applied to optimize already existing probes by enhancing their properties. Stability in aqueous solution, enhanced cellular uptake, low background, high spatiotemporal resolution and higher specificity are some of the properties that have been targeted (Shi et al. 2012; Cai et al. 2016; Dong et al. 2015; Kiyonaka et al. 2004; Cai et al. 2014; Huang et al. 2015; Wang et al. 2015; Yoshimura et al. 2004). As an example, ratiometric probes (these emit at several wavelengths upon excitation) can be enhanced by incorporating a self-assembling motif (e.g., diphenylalanine) in the same molecule. This subtle change of their structure results in enhanced values of the fluorescence ratio by lowering the short-wavelength and/or enhancing the long-wavelength fluorescence (Cai et al. 2016). Moreover, the incorporated peptide also enhances the cellular uptake by endocytosis and, as a result, the probe has much better performance *in vitro*. Ordered nanostructures of short peptides can also enhance the quenching effect (Kiyonaka et al. 2004) or enhance the brightness of an environmentally sensitive fluorophore by hosting it in the hydrophobic pockets formed as a result of the self-assembly (Cai et al. 2014; Gao et al. 2012).

High-throughput screening

Hydrogels offer unique wet environment that retains protein activity. Thus, molecular probes that have prolonged preserved recognition properties can be developed based on supramolecular gels. Arrays that allow high-throughput screening are one example of such application (Yamaguchi et al. 2005; Kiyonaka et al. 2004; Yoshimura et al. 2004). The semi-wet arrays overcome the main drawback of classical screening platforms in which the bioactivity of the protein is compromized as a result of its immobilisation to the solid support. Indeed, enzymes (Kiyonaka et al. 2004) and artificial receptors (Yoshimura et al. 2004) can be entrapped in supramolecular hydrogel matrices where many nanofibers are entangled to form aqueous microcavities, which can host the biomolecules and, the hydrophobic domains of the fibers are used as a site for monitoring the reaction (by enhancing the fluorescence as previously described). Besides the advantages mentioned above, the signal/noise ratio in such systems is improved because the microcavities are accumulated in a 3D manner and changes can be observed both by naked eye or simple digital camera (Yoshimura et al. 2004).

Biocatalytic Self-Assembling Systems as Cancer Therapeutic Tools

In 2007, Xu and co-workers demonstrated that the PA naphthalene-diphenylalanine-$NHCH_2CH_2OH$, modified to include a butyric diacid motif (cleavable by esterase), self-assemble upon biocatalytic conversion and regulate the death of HeLa cells (Yang et al. 2007b) without affecting NIH3T3 fibroblasts that presented a lower esterase activity. These results demonstrated the very promising impact of BSA for selective cancer treatment. Indeed, the concept was expanded to include other enzymes that are overexpressed in cancers and also initiate the downstream apoptosis pathway using PAs specifically designed to be sensitive to those enzymes (Zorn et al. 2011; Tanaka et al. 2015). While the trigger of apoptosis by PAs may be different for different cancer types, the mechanism of action was found to be the same in each case and related to the intracellular presence of nanofibers but not with the un-assembled PA itself (Julien et al. 2014). Indeed, internalization of self-assembled nanofibers was shown to disrupt the self-assembly of crucial cell components, e.g., microtubules, leading to cellular death (Kuang and Xu 2013) (Fig. 3).

The pericellular space is also rich in bio-entities and there are different ecto-enzymes that have been identified as cancer markers. Indeed, these can be also used under BSA (Kuang et al. 2014; Pires et al. 2015). The mechanism in this case is different as the sol-gel transformation takes place in the pericellular space. The formed self-assembled nanofibers generate a network of fibers that block cell-matrix interactions (including metabolite exchange), leading to apoptosis and cell death (Fig. 4).

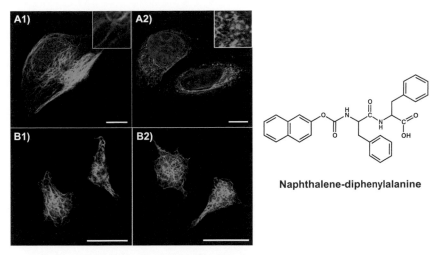

Naphthalene-diphenylalanine

Fig. 3. Confocal images of the (A) T89G and (B) PC12 cells in the (A1, B1) absence and (A2, B2) presence of 400 μM of naphthalene-diphenylalanine, showing the disruption of the microtubules in the case of T89G cells. The insets are expansions (three times) of the cell surfaces and scale bars correspond to 10 μm. Adapted with permission from (Kuang and Xu 2013).

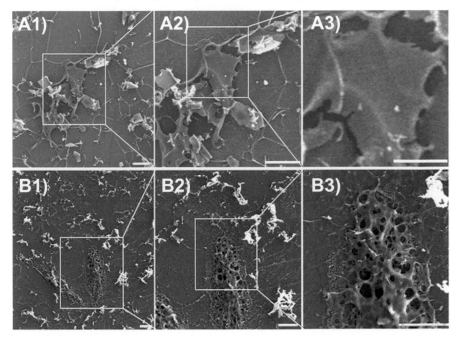

Fig. 4. SEM micrographs of HeLa cells cultured in the (A) absence and (B) presence of naphthalene-diphenylalanine-tyrosine phosphate. Adapted with permission from (Kuang et al. 2014).

So far, most of the BSA based anti-cancer systems are composed of a peptide motif that assure the bioactivity of the PA and its self-assembly via H-bonding and van der Waals interactions, and an aromatic moiety, which strengthens the assembly via aromatic interactions. However, carbohydrates are the second most widespread biomolecules in living systems and are relatively unexplored as a platform for the design of bioactive amphiphiles. Moreover, carbohydrates in the form of glycosaminoglycans are able to interact directly with cellular machinery or indirectly through the activation of proteins as a part of their bioactive cascade. When compared with the PA, the carbohydrate amphiphiles (CA) present a much larger structural diversity (regio- and stereoisomers) and capacity for encoding bioinformation (Pashkuleva and Reis 2010). We, therefore, proposed a phosphorylated CA Fluorenylmethoxycarbonyl-(Fmoc)-glucosamine-6-phosphate, chemical structure depicted in Fig. 5, as a biocatalytic system able to selectively target osteosarcoma cells (SaOs2) triggering apoptotic pathways that lead to their death (Pires et al. 2015). We selected SaOs2 due to the known overexpression of alkaline phosphatase (ALP), which we hypothesized would lead to the localized biocatalytic transformation of the phosphorylated precursor into Fmoc-glucosamine. The accumulation of the latter in the pericellular space of SaOs2 caused cell death (Fig. 5). However, when ATDC5 cells (that present an ALP activity ~15–20 times lower than SaOs2) were tested under the same conditions, their metabolic activity was not affected. Moreover, the addition of a phosphatase inhibitor in the SaOs2 culture medium increased drastically the cell survival. These results demonstrated that SaOs2 cells can be targeted through their ALP overexpression.

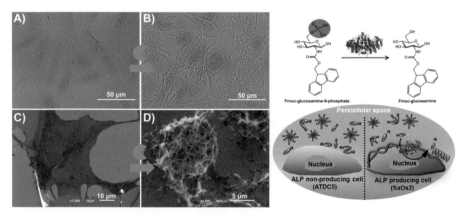

Fig. 5. (A, B) Brightfield and (C, D) SEM images of the SaOs2 cells cultured in the presence of the CA Fmoc-glucosamine-6-phosphate (0.5 mM and 7 hr of cell culture) (adapted with permission from Pires et al. 2015. Copyright 2015. American Chemical Society).

Stimuli-Responsive Systems for the Delivery of Cancer Therapeutics

Supramolecular self-assembly is considered as an important approach to design and fabricate controlled drug release materials. Drug delivery systems are typically used to enhance the efficiency of the desirable drug and overcome the toxic effects at non-target sites. Researchers have designed variant responsive materials to develop such systems including materials, which are responsive to changes in their environment (pH, temperature) and/or host-guest complexations (Mura et al. 2013; Webber et al. 2016; Du et al. 2015b). Another approach takes advantage of locally over-expressed enzymes to help dissociation (following hydrolysis) of the supramolecular nanostructures and subsequently release the drug in the desired location. This approach is of particular importance for anti-cancer therapeutics where enzymes are considered as cancer biomarkers, which is the focus of this section. In this context, there are mainly two routes to deliver a drug from gel matrices; the first is based on drugs, which are covalently conjugated with therapeutics (i.e., pro-drug based materials); the second is based on drugs' encapsulation within the gel matrix.

Pro-drug based hydrogels

There has been a great interest to deliver therapeutics using this route; drugs (or model drugs) are modified in such a way that they have the correct hydrophobic and hydrophilic balance to allow them to self-assemble and form supramolecular structures. The formed structures (i.e., pro-drugs) might then entangle to form a gel. Ideally, this chemical modification should include a covalent conjugation of an enzyme cleavable linker. This allows for specific bond cleavage upon enzymatic exposure, leading to the release of the therapeutic molecule.

Up to this end, Cisplatin (cis-diamminedichloroplatinum II) (a chemotherapeutic agent used in treating different cancers such as testicular, ovarian and bladder cancers, as well as, lymphoma and glioma) was conjugated with a PA (comprising an MMP-2 sensitive derivative GTAGLIGQRGDS) (Kim et al. 2009). The new compound (i.e., pro-drug) was developed so it can self-assemble to form nanofibers that eventually gel (Fig. 6A). Cisplatin derivative release from the pro-drug gel was a consequence of MMP-2 cleavage of the PA (between glycine (G) and leucine (L)). TEM analysis was used (before and after enzymatic treatment) to confirm the hydrolysis process (Fig. 6A). The drug release was found to be dependent on the enzyme concentration. It was also found that the higher the MMP-2 concentration the more drug can be released from the gel matrix (Fig. 6B).

Using a similar approach, Escuder and Miravet have prepared a pro-drug through the conjugation of a low-molecular weight gelator (containing lysine) to model anti-cancer drugs (benzylamine or phenethylamine). The drug and self-assembling units were connected through a self-immolative linker (p-aminobenzoylcarbonyl) which is stable under physiological conditions (Fig. 7A) (Sáez et al. 2010). This pro-drug molecule forms a stable hydrogel with a minimum gelator concentration of 0.1% w/v. Cryo-SEM image showed that the gels have a sponge-like morphology with micrometre sized cavities filled with the solvent (Fig. 7B). Upon trypsin treatment, the amide bond of the molecule is hydrolysed, the amino group of p-aminobenzoylcarbonyl becomes free and undergoes a rapid 1,6-elimination to carbamic acids that are unstable and decompose to release the model drug (Fig. 7C).

Another interesting supramolecular design of a pro-drug conjugate was reported by Gao et al. (Gao et al. 2009). In this work, an anti-cancer drug (taxol) was modified so it can form nanofibers and finally entangled to form a supramolecular hydrogel. Taxol

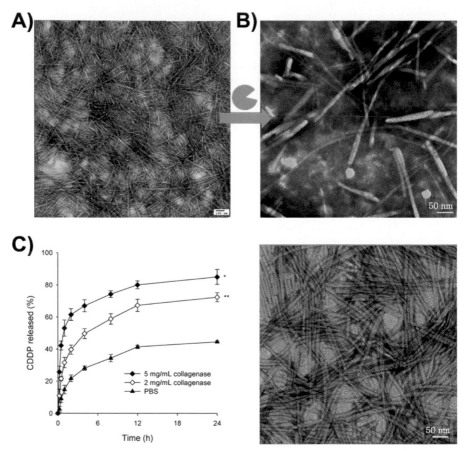

Fig. 6. (A) TEM images of pro-drug nanofiber networks before and after hydrolysis with 2 mg/mL MMP-2 enzyme. (B) Release profiles of the drug at different concentrations MMP-2. (C) TEM image of a control sample (in PBS). Adapted with permission from (Kim et al. 2009).

was covalently conjugated to a precursor, which has a part cleavable by phosphatase. Hydrolysis of the phosphate group occurs upon exposure to ALP leading to hydrogel formation with a subsequent release of the taxol derivative. Importantly, both taxol and its derivative (developed in this study) were found to present similar toxicity.

Drug encapsulation within a hydrogel matrix

More recently, Kalafatovic et al. designed an MMP-9 responsive PA to control the release of doxorubicin (an anti-cancer drug) (Kalafatovic et al. 2015). When MMP-9 cleaves the peptide, micelle to fibre structural transformation occurs. Localized fibre formation allows for encapsulating the drug within these fibers and consequently slows its release (Fig. 8).

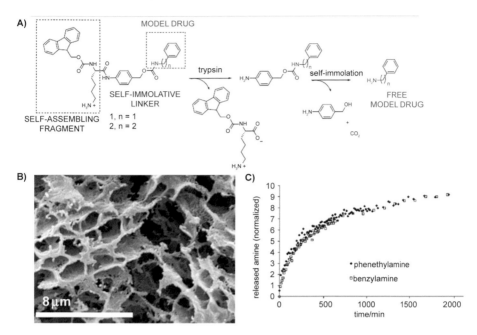

Fig. 7. (A) Schematic representation of possible mechanism of enzymatic cleavage and self-immolative hydrolysis of the pro-drugs. (B) Cryo-SEM image of sponge-like hydrogel (n = 1) and (C) Kinetic profile of the release of model drug amines. Adapted with permission from (Sáez et al. 2010).

In another study, Gao et al. exploited a tyrosinase enzyme to control a supramolecular disassembly process, which was considered to be potentially useful for controlled drug release in the case of elevated tyrosinase activity in malignant melanoma. Congo red (as a model drug) was incorporated within the hydrogel matrix assembled from aromatic tetrapeptide methyl esters, Ac-YYYY-OMe and Ac-FYYY-OMe (Gao et al. 2011). Upon treatment with tyrosinase, tyrosine residues were converted to quinone. This oxidation process resulted in the loss of π-π interactions between phenol rings and ultimately a gel-to-sol transition, which in turn resulted in release of model drug molecules. The incorporated model drug could be released in a controllable manner by using different enzyme concentrations.

In an interesting study, Vemula and co-workers combined both routes (pro-drug and drug encapsulation) to design a (dual) drug delivery system. Initially, they conjugated acetaminophen drug to fatty acids to form a hydrogelator, which is able to form a hydrogel. Upon enzymatic treatment (with lipolase), the hydrogel disassembled leading to single drug release. They also encapsulated curcumin (a hydrophobic anti-cancer drug) in the hydrogel matrix described above (Vemula et al. 2009). The formed hydrogel was degraded completely to form two non self-assembling components by the enzyme, lipolase, while releasing the encapsulated chemopreventive hydrophobic drug curcumin which is monitored by time depended UV-Vis spectroscopy. It was possible to control the drug release by manipulation of both the enzyme concentration the temperature.

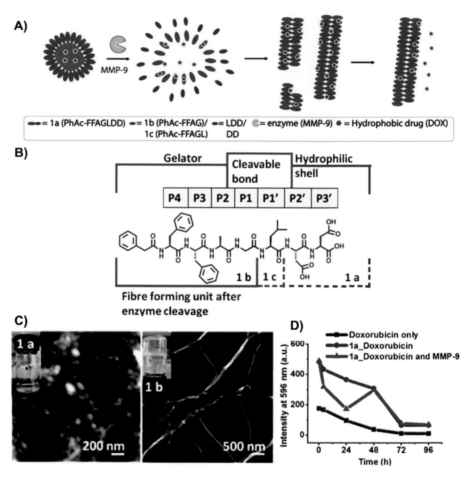

Fig. 8. (A) Schematic representation of micelle-to-fibre transition induced by MMP-9 cleavage showing disassembly of micelles and the re-assembly into fibers after the removal of the hydrophilic group enabling prolonged drug release. (B) Chemical structure of the biocatalytic gelation system and its components. (C) AFM showing the micellar aggregates (solution) for 1a and fibers (hydrogels at 20 mM) for 1b. (D) Fluorescence intensities of doxorubicin monitored over time for doxorubicin only, doxorubicin loaded into precursor peptide (1a) micelles and MMP-9 treated precursor peptide (1a) micelles loaded with doxorubicin. Adapted with permission from Kalafatovic et al. 2015.

Conclusions

BSA and their ensuing 2D nanoscale networks or hydrogels have been exploited in recent years to develop different strategies for advanced diagnosis, enhanced imaging and selective therapies for cancer treatment. Undoubtedly, we are witnessing a critical period in this field that brought already tremendous advances in understanding and controlling the BSA process as demonstrated by the numerous *in vitro* studies. Now, the field is shifting to an applied perspective as demonstrated by the most recent *in vivo* studies. These most recent examples demonstrate the feasibility of BSA as a localized anti-cancer therapy that can be used alone or in combination with other methodologies to improve the prognosis of the patients by enhancing the efficacy of the treatment, while minimizing the typical side effects of anti-cancer drugs. We believe that the next few years will transform the generated knowledge in efficient diagnostic tools and therapies and thus, will generate the expected social impact.

Acknowledgement

This work was supported by the European Research Council grant agreement ERC-2012-ADG 20120216-321266—project ComplexiTE. IP acknowledges the Portuguese Foundation for Science and Technology (IF/00032/2013). YMA and RVU would like to thank the BBSRC (BB/K007513/1) for funding.

References

Bremmer, S.C., J. Chen, A.J. McNeil and M.B. Soellner. 2012. A general method for detecting protease activity via gelation and its application to artificial clotting. Chem. Commun. 48(44): 5482–5484.

Cai, Y., J. Zhan, H. Shen, D. Mao, S. Ji, R. Liu et al. 2016. Optimized ratiometric fluorescent probes by peptide self-assembly. Anal. Chem. 88(1): 740–745.

Cai, Y.B., Y. Shi, H.M. Wang, J.Y. Wang, D. Ding, L. Wang et al. 2014. Environment-sensitive fluorescent supramolecular nanofibers for imaging applications. Anal. Chem. 86(4): 2193–2199.

Dong, L., Q.Q. Miao, Z.J. Hai, Y. Yuan and G.L. Liang. 2015. Enzymatic hydrogelation-induced fluorescence turn-off for sensing alkaline phosphatase *in vitro* and in living cells. Anal. Chem. 87(13): 6475–6478.

Du, X.W., J. Zhou and B. Xu. 2015a. Ectoenzyme switches the surface of magnetic nanoparticles for selective binding of cancer cells. J. Colloid. Interf. Sci. 447: 273–277.

Du, X.W., J. Zhou, J. Shi and B. Xu. 2015b. Supramolecular hydrogelators and hydrogels: from soft matter to molecular biomaterials. Chem. Rev. 115(24): 13165–13307.

Gao, J., W. Zheng, D. Kong and Z. Yang. 2011. Dual enzymes regulate the molecular self-assembly of tetra-peptide derivatives. Soft Matter. 7(21): 10443–10448.

Gao, Y., Y. Kuang, Z.F. Guo, Z.H. Guo, I.J. Krauss and B. Xu. 2009. Enzyme-instructed molecular self-assembly confers nanofibers and a supramolecular hydrogel of taxol derivative. J. Am. Chem. Soc. 131(38): 13576–13577.

Gao, Y., J.F. Shi, D. Yuan and B. Xu. 2012. Imaging enzyme-triggered self-assembly of small molecules inside live cells. Nat. Commun. 3: 1033.

Gao, Y., C. Berciu, Y. Kuang, J.F. Shi, D. Nicastro and B. Xu. 2013a. Probing nanoscale self-assembly of nonfluorescent small molecules inside live mammalian cells. Acs Nano. 7(10): 9055–9063.

Gao, Y., Y. Kuang, X.W. Du, J. Zhou, P. Chandran, F. Horkay et al. 2013b. Imaging self-assembly dependent spatial distribution of small molecules in a cellular environment. Langmuir. 29(49): 15191–15200.

Hirst, A.R., S. Roy, M. Arora, A.K. Das, N. Hodson, P. Murray et al. 2010. Biocatalytic induction of supramolecular order. Nat. Chem. 2(12): 1089–1094.

Huang, P., Y. Gao, J. Lin, H. Hu, H.S. Liao, X.F. Yan et al. 2015. Tumor-specific formation of enzyme-instructed supramolecular self-assemblies as cancer theranostics. Acs Nano. 9(10): 9517–9527.

Julien, O., M. Kampmann, M.C. Bassik, J.A. Zorn, V.J. Venditto, K. Shimbo et al. 2014. Unraveling the mechanism of cell death induced by chemical fibrils. Nat. Chem. Biol. 10(11): 969–976.

Kalafatovic, D., M. Nobis, N. Javid, P.W.J.M. Frederix, K.I. Anderson, B.R. Saunders et al. 2015. MMP-9 triggered micelle-to-fibre transitions for slow release of doxorubicin. Biomater. Sci. 3(2): 246–249.

Kim, J.-K., J. Anderson, H.-W. Jun, M.A. Repka and S. Jo. 2009. Self-Assembling peptide amphiphile-based nanofiber gel for bioresponsive cisplatin delivery. Mol. Pharm. 6(3): 978–985.

Kiyonaka, S., K. Sada, I. Yoshimura, S. Shinkai, N. Kato and I. Hamachi. 2004. Semi-wet peptide/protein array using supramolecular hydrogel. Nat. Mater. 3(1): 58–64.

Kuang, Y. and B. Xu. 2013. Disruption of the dynamics of microtubules and selective inhibition of glioblastoma cells by nanofibers of small hydrophobic molecules. Angew. Chem. Int. Edit. 52(27): 6944–6948.

Kuang, Y., J. Shi, J. Li, D. Yuan, K.A. Alberti, Q. Xu et al. 2014. Pericellular hydrogel/nanonets inhibit cancer cells. Angew. Chem. Int. Edit. 53(31): 8104–8107.

Mizusawa, K., Y. Ishida, Y. Takaoka, M. Miyagawa, S. Tsukiji and I. Hamachi. 2010. Disassembly-driven turn-on fluorescent nanoprobes for selective protein detection. J. Am. Chem. Soc. 132(21): 7291–7293.

Mura, S., J. Nicolas and P. Couvreur. 2013. Stimuli-responsive nanocarriers for drug delivery. Nat. Mater. 12(11): 991–1003.

Pashkuleva, I. and R.L. Reis. 2010. Sugars: burden or biomaterials of the future? J. Mater. Chem. 20(40): 8803–8818.

Pires, R.A., Y.M. Abul-Haija, D.S. Costa, R. Novoa-Carballal, R.L. Reis, R.V. Ulijn et al. 2015. Controlling cancer cell fate using localized biocatalytic self-assembly of an aromatic carbohydrate amphiphile. J. Am. Chem. Soc. 137(2): 576–579.

Sáez, J.A., B. Escuder and J.F. Miravet. 2010. Supramolecular hydrogels for enzymatically triggered self-immolative drug delivery. Tetrahedron. 66(14): 2614–2618.

Shi, H.B., R.T.K. Kwok, J.Z. Liu, B.G. Xing, B.Z. Tang and B. Liu. 2012. Real-time monitoring of cell apoptosis and drug screening using fluorescent light-up probe with aggregation-induced emission characteristics. J. Am. Chem. Soc. 134(43): 17972–17981.

Shi, J., X. Du, D. Yuan, R. Haburcak, D. Wu, N. Zhou et al. 2015. Enzyme transformation to modulate the ligand-receptor interactions between small molecules. Chem. Commun. 51(23): 4899–4901.

Tanaka, A., Y. Fukuoka, Y. Morimoto, T. Honjo, D. Koda, M. Goto et al. 2015. Cancer cell death induced by the intracellular self-assembly of an enzyme-responsive supramolecular gelator. J. Am. Chem. Soc. 137(2): 770–775.

Thornton, K., A.M. Smith, C.L.R. Merry and R.V. Ulijn. 2009. Controlling stiffness in nanostructured hydrogels produced by enzymatic dephosphorylation. Biochem. Soc. Trans. 37(4): 660–664.

Thornton, K., Y.M. Abul-Haija, N. Hodson and R.V. Ulijn. 2013. Mechanistic insights into phosphatase triggered self-assembly including enhancement of biocatalytic conversion rate. Soft Matter. 9(39): 9430–9439.

Toledano, S., R.J. Williams, V. Jayawarna and R.V. Ulijn. 2006. Enzyme-triggered self-assembly of peptide hydrogels via reversed hydrolysis. J. Am. Chem. Soc. 128(4): 1070–1071.

Ulijn, R.V. 2006. Enzyme-responsive materials: a new class of smart biomaterials. J. Mater. Chem. 16(23): 2217–2225.

Vemula, P.K., G.A. Cruikshank, J.M. Karp and G. John. 2009. Self-assembled prodrugs: an enzymatically triggered drug-delivery platform. Biomaterials. 30(3): 383–393.

Wang, H.M., D. Mao, Y.Z. Wang, K. Wang, X.Y. Yi, D.L. Kong et al. 2015. Biocompatible fluorescent supramolecular nanofibrous hydrogel for long-term cell tracking and tumor imaging applications. Sci. Rep. 5: 16680.

Webber, M.J., E.A. Appel, E.W. Meijer and R. Langer. 2016. Supramolecular biomaterials. Nat. Mater. 15(1): 13–26.

WHO. 2014. World Cancer Report 2014: IARC Nonserial Publication.

Williams, R.J., A.M. Smith, R. Collins, N. Hodson, A.K. Das and R.V. Ulijn. 2009. Enzyme-assisted self-assembly under thermodynamic control. Nat. Nanotechnol. 4(1): 19–24.

Yamaguchi, S., L. Yoshimura, T. Kohira, S. Tamaru and I. Hamachi. 2005. Cooperation between artificial receptors and supramolecular hydrogels for sensing and discriminating phosphate derivatives. J. Am. Chem. Soc. 127(33): 11835–11841.

Yang, Z.M. and B. Xu. 2004. A simple visual assay based on small molecule hydrogels for detecting inhibitors of enzymes. Chem. Commun. (21): 2424–2425.

Yang, Z.M., H.W. Gu, D.G. Fu, P. Gao, J.K. Lam and B. Xu. 2004. Enzymatic formation of supramolecular hydrogels. Adv. Mater. 16(16): 1440–1444.

Yang, Z.M., G.L. Liang, M.L. Ma, Y. Gao and B. Xu. 2007a. *In vitro* and *in vivo* enzymatic formation of supramolecular hydrogels based on self-assembled nanofibers of a beta-amino acid derivative. Small. 3(4): 558–562.

Yang, Z.M., K.M. Xu, Z.F. Guo, Z.H. Guo and B. Xu. 2007b. Intracellular enzymatic formation of nanofibers results in hydrogelation and regulated cell death. Adv. Mater. 19(20): 3152–3156.

Yang, Z.M., M.L. Ma and B. Xu. 2009. Using matrix metalloprotease-9 (MMP-9) to trigger supramolecular hydrogelation. Soft Matter. 5(13): 2546–2548.

Yoshimura, I., Y. Miyahara, N. Kasagi, H. Yamane, A. Ojida and I. Hamachi. 2004. Molecular recognition in a supramolecular hydrogel to afford a semi-wet sensor chip. J. Am. Chem. Soc. 126(39): 12204–12205.

Zhai, D.T., W. Xu, L.Y. Zhang and Y.T. Chang. 2014. The role of "disaggregation" in optical probe development. Chem. Soc. Rev. 43(8): 2402–2411.

Zhou, J. and B. Xu. 2015. Enzyme-instructed self-assembly: a multistep process for potential cancer therapy. Bioconjugate. Chem. 26(6): 987–999.

Zorn, J.A., H. Wille, D.W. Wolan and J.A. Wells. 2011. Self-assembling small molecules form nanofibrils that bind procaspase-3 to promote activation. J. Am. Chem. Soc. 133(49): 19630–19633.

CHAPTER 11

Thermosensitive Hydrogels for Drug Delivery and Tissue Engineering

Manisha Sharma,[1,*] *Long Jingjunjiao*[2] *and*
Ali Seyfoddin[2]

Introduction

Thermosensitive hydrogels are categorized as second generation hydrogels as they have the ability to respond to a change in environmental condition, the temperature. They show a significant change in properties upon a small or modest change in temperature. Because of this unique characteristic they are also called "smart" hydrogels and have attracted increasing interest in wide range of pharmaceutical and biomedical applications such as drug delivery, protein and gene delivery, tissue engineering and tissue regeneration (Gandhi et al. 2015; Hrubý et al. 2015). Thermosensitive hydrogels maintain a solution status at or below room temperature, which allows easy handling, allowing easy administration through syringe and needle and transform into gel state at body temperature forming a high viscosity and sustained release depot (Ruel-Gariépy and Leroux 2004; Lai et al. 2014). The sol-to-gel transition of these polymers is described typically by phase diagram as a function of concentration and temperature (Fig. 1).

Phase diagram on the left (Fig. 1) is characterized by the lower critical solution temperature (LCST) suggesting that the transition from sol-to-gel occurs with increasing temperature. Whereas, the phase diagram on right (Fig. 1) represents phase transition occurring upon cooling and therefore are characterized by upper critical

[1] School of Pharmacy, Faculty of Medical and Health Sciences, University of Auckland, New Zealand.
[2] School of Applied Sciences, Auckland University of Technology Auckland, New Zealand.
* Corresponding author: manisha.sharma@auckland.ac.nz

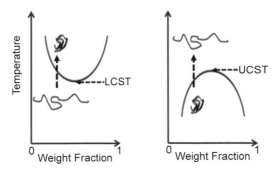

Fig. 1. Schematic representation of phase diagram showing lower critical solution temperature (LCST) and upper critical solution temperature (UCST) behaviour of thermosensitive polymers. (Adopted from (Gibson and O'Reilly 2013)).

solution temperature (UCST). LCST and UCST are the two critical temperature points, below and above which the polymer and solvent are in one phase. Polymers dissolved in organic solvent commonly show UCST, whereas those dissolved in aqueous solvents show LCST (Peppas et al. 2000; Hrubý et al. 2015). This phase transition is typically energy driven phenomena and can be explained by Gibbs equation: $\Delta G = \Delta H - T\Delta S$ (G: Gibbs free energy, H: Enthalpy and S: Entropy) (Ward and Georgiou 2011). Hydrogel systems showing LCST, the driving force is entropy of water, at higher temperature the water is less ordered and has higher entropy producing a "hydrophobic effect" and resulting in a formation of gel (Southall et al. 2002; Klouda and Mikos 2008).

Most polymers discussed in this chapter represent LCST. The LCST of such polymeric systems is close to the body temperature (37°C) and therefore is of much interest to pharmaceutical and biomedical scientists due to numerous potential applications in the respective fields.

Mechanism of thermogelation

There are different mechanisms reported in the literature responsible for thermogelation of aqueous polymer solutions. These include coil-to-helix transition, hydrophobic interaction, micelle packing and micelles entanglements. These transitions are mainly associated with the hydrophobicity and hydrophilicity of the polymer chains. Polymers exhibiting LCST commonly consists of hydrophobic functional groups such as methyl, ethyl and propyl groups. Because of the presence of these groups, three basic interactions within the aqueous polymer solution are possible: polymer-water, polymer-polymer and water-water (Klouda and Mikos 2008; Matanović et al. 2014). As mentioned above the change in the solubility of the polymer with respect to changes in temperature is governed by the Gibbs free energy rule. The increase in environment temperature results in formation of free negative energy in the system, which in turn makes polymer-water interactions unfavourable and promotes polymer-polymer interaction, thereby converting the solution to a more hydrophobic gel form (Ruel-Gariépy and Leroux 2004; Klouda and Mikos 2008). However, it is important to note that all the mechanisms mentioned are reversible and the sol form is retained on removing the gelling stimulus. Thermogelation mechanism will be discussed further in this chapter alongside the different polymer types.

Classification of Thermosensitive Hydrogels

Thermosensitive hydrogels based on natural polymers

Natural polymers such as polysaccharides (cellulose, chitosan, xyloglucan, agarose, alginates), cellulose derivatives, carrageenans and polypeptides (gelatin) (Fig. 2) exhibit phase transition in response to changes in environmental temperatures (Arnott et al. 1974; Rees and Jane 1977; Franz 1986; Rozier et al. 1989; Meeting et al. 1990; Li and Guan 2011). These naturally occurring materials have excellent biocompatible and biodegradable properties and therefore are widely explored.

Cellulose and its derivatives are widely explored for its thermosensitive properties. Methylcellulose (MC) (Fig. 2a) shows thermogelation in the temperature range of 40 to 50°C. The thermogelation mechanism is mainly due to the hydrophobic interactions among methoxy groups present in the polymer chains.

However, the phase transition temperature of MC is far above the body temperature limiting its biomedical application. The gelation temperature of MC can be modified by physical and chemical alterations. The thermosensitivity of cellulose-based

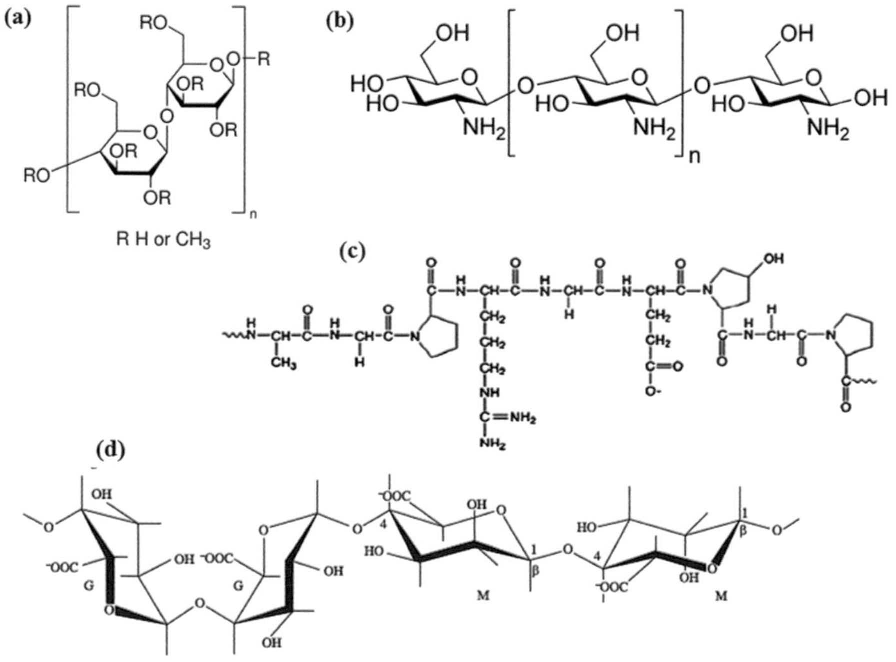

Fig. 2. Chemical structure of selected naturally occurring thermosensitive polymers, (a) methyl cellulose, (b) chitosan, (c) gelatin, (d) alginates.

hydrogels could also be modified by the addition of other thermosensitive components. For instance, cellulose hydrogels could become thermosensitive by chemically introducing alkyl groups to cellulose and blending cellulose hydrogels with some other thermosensitive polymers (Chen and Fan 2008; Zhang et al. 2014). Liu et al. grafted MC with synthetic polymer PNIPAAm and was able to produce a fast gelling system by varying the percentage compositions of the two polymers (Liu et al. 2004).

Chitosan (Fig. 2b) is a natural polysaccharide sourced from the exoskeleton of crustaceans. Chitosan is formed from the alkaline deacetylation of chitin and is composed of glucosamine and acetyl glucosamine units making it a cationic polymer. Chitosan is approved by US Food and Drug Administration (FDA) as pharmaceutical excipient due to its non-toxic, biodegradable, biocompatible and bio adhesive properties (Ruel-Gariépy and Leroux 2004; Bhattarai et al. 2010). Chitosan has low solubility in water and is maintained in solution state up to a pH of 6.2. Gelation occurs at body temperature when the pH of the solution is further increased to 7.2. Basically, chitosan is pH sensitive and can be transformed into thermogelling solutions by the incorporation of polyol- or sugar-phosphate salts such as glycerol, sorbitol or glycerophosphate (Tahrir et al. 2015). Chenite et al. reported a thermogelling chitosan system by incorporation of β-glycerophosphate (β-GP) (Chenite et al. 2000). The developed system was stable at neutral pH, remained liquid at or below room temperature, and formed gels at body temperature. The gelation processes is mainly attributed to the presence of hydrophobic interactions between chitosan chains, neutralisation of the cationic charge by β-GP and hydrogen bonding as a consequence of reduced electrostatic repulsion (Ruel-Gariépy and Leroux 2004).

Gelatin (Fig. 2c) is another natural polymer which shows temperature dependent phase transition. The gelation is mainly achieved through coil-to-helix transition (Fig. 3).

At temperatures below 25°C, an aqueous solution of gelatin transforms into a highly viscous gel structure due to the aggregation of triple helix structure. As the solution is heated above 30°C, the conformation changes from helix to flexible coil, converting back, gel to a solution form (Matanović et al. 2014). However, this transition of the gelatin solution is opposite to what is desired for biomedical application and therefore scientists have developed various combinations of gelatin with other

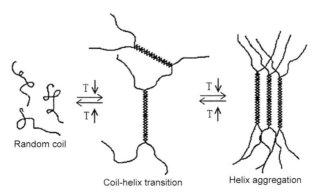

Random coil

Coil-helix transition   Helix aggregation

Fig. 3. Thermoreversible gelation of gelatin by coil-to triple helix transition (Adopted from (Matanović et al. 2014)).

polymers to obtain thermogelation close to body temperature. Modification of gelatin is easily achieved at amino acid end points. Yang and Kao conjugated poly(ethylene glycol)-poly(D, L-lactide) with gelatin and developed a rapidly forming gel at 37°C (Yang and Kao 2006).

Alginate is a naturally occurring anionic polysaccharide composed of 1,4-linked β-D-mannuronte (M) and 1,4-linked α-L-guluronate (G) (Fig. 2d) in various compositions. Generally, in the presence of divalent cations such as ca^{2+}, alginate forms hydrogels. Thermosensitive alginates were prepared by conjugating alginate with other thermosensitive polymers such as poly(N-isopropylacrylamide) (PNIPAAm) and were explored for drug delivery and tissue engineering applications. Tan et al. developed thermosensitive aminated alginate-g-PNIPAAm by coupling carboxylic end capped PNIPAAm through amide bond linkages. The copolymer developed exhibited sol-to-gel transition with LCST around 35°C (Tan et al. 2012). Figure 4 represents the gelation mechanism of the hydrogel at physiological temperature which mainly involves dehydration of the PNIPAAm block. As a result of increased temperature, water molecules bound to the isopropyl side of PNIPAAm is released, which enhances inter- and intra-molecular hydrophobic interactions between isopropyl groups forming a gel structure.

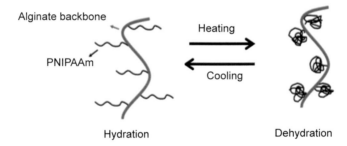

Fig. 4. Schematic representation of the gelation mechanism of alginate-g-PNIPAAm thermosensitive hydrogels (Adopted from (Sun and Tan 2013)).

Thermosensitive hydrogels based on synthetic polymers

Even though naturally derived thermosensitive hydrogels have excellent biocompatibility and biodegradability, the polypeptides or sugar rings have limited space for further modifications to fit various requirements for biomedical applications. To overcome this limitation, synthetic polymers have been used, as they offer capability of chemical modification.

N-isopropylacrylamide based systems

Thermosensitive hydrogels based on poly(N-isopropylacrylamide) (PNIPAAm) (Fig. 5a) are the most extensively investigated systems. PNIPPAm exhibits LCST, which is around 32°C in aqueous solutions. At temperatures above LCST the solution becomes cloudy and transforms into a gel due to hydrophobic interactions and coil-

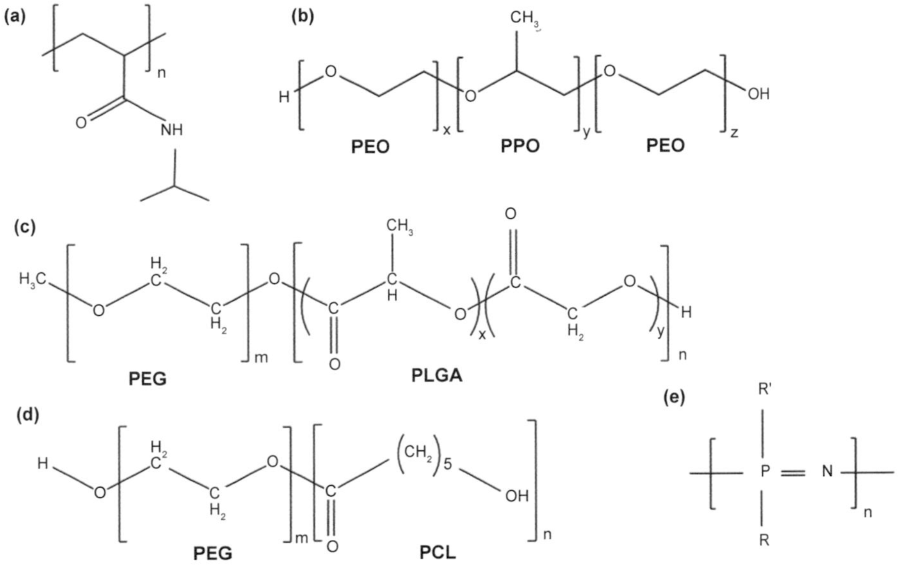

Fig. 5. Chemical structure of selected synthetic thermosensitive polymers.

to-globule transformation. Temperature below LCST results in the dissolution of the polymer due to hydrogen bonding between polar amide groups in PNIPAAm and water molecules.

Below 32°C, the enthalpy from hydrogen bonding between polar groups of the copolymers and water molecules contributes to the dissolution of the PNIPAAm. At or above LCST, the entropy from hydrophobic interactions leads to gelation in water (Jeong et al. 2012). Phase transition in PNIPAAm can be controlled by altering the hydrophilic/hydrophobic balance. Grafting additional hydrophobic monomer (such as butyl methacrylate) on PNIPAAm results in a reduced LCST whereas, LCST can be elevated by attaching more hydrophilic monomer (such as acrylic acid or hydroxyethyl methacrylate) (Yoshida et al. 1994; Kim et al. 2009).

For the synthesis of PNIPAAm-based thermosensitive hydrogels, several methods have been explored such as free radical polymerization (Zhang et al. 2004a; Zhang et al. 2004b; Ankareddi and Brazel 2007), UV photocrosslinking and UV irradiation (Zhang et al. 2004b; Wei et al. 2005). PNIPAAm has been conjugated with many natural polymers such as chitosan (Chen and Cheng 2006; Mu and Fang 2008), collagen (Chen and Lee 2008) and hyaluronic acid (Tan et al. 2009) to adjust its gelation temperature and mechanical properties for various biomedical applications.

PEO/PPO/PEO based systems

Poloxamers, also known as Pluronics® or Lutrol® are commercially available thermosensitive triblock copolymer based on poly(ethylene oxide)-poly(propylene oxide)-poly(ethylene oxide) (PEO–PPO–PEO) backbone (Fig. 5b). As numbers of each PEO/PPO block is adjustable, a wide range of Pluronics can be achieved. They are available as liquids, pastes or solids and include polymers with various molecular weights and PEO/PPO ratios (Bromberg and Ron 1998). Pluronics show reversible phase transitions when the polymer concentration is above a critical value (Jeong et al. 2012). The gelation mechanism in poloxamers is highly investigated but the actual mechanism is still a point of debate. Most studies support dehydration of the PPO block as the main driving force behind the gelation process (Cabana et al. 1997; Jia et al. 2010; Matanović et al. 2014). Poloxamers are amphiphilic in nature and at low temperatures are soluble in water. They contain hydrophilic, EO block which favour solubilization in cold water. Hydrogen bonding between the EO and PO blocks with water molecules at colder temperatures keeps the poloxamer blocks separate and so it remains in solution. A previous study demonstrated that the micellization process of the triblock co-polymers in water is endothermic (Alexandridis and Hatton 1995). The polarity of EO and PO segments decrease with the increase in temperature. Thus, the poloxamers become less soluble in water causing the hydrogen bonds to destabilize and the hydrophobic PO blocks to assemble together and form a gel. The gelation process occurs through micellization and dehydration of the hydrophobic PO core. As the temperature increases and reaches the critical micelle temperature (CMT), the solubility of the PO block reduces, causing the poloxamer structures to aggregate and self-assemble into a spherical micelle. The size of the micelles grow until the PO

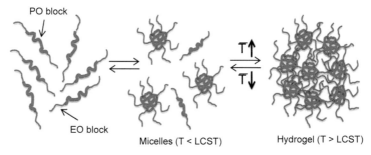

Fig. 6. Schematic representation of the micellization and gel formation of aqueous poloxamers solution (Adopted from (Matanović et al. 2014)).

core becomes dehydrated, then the outer EO chains swell and interacts with other EO chains to form a cubic 3D structure (the gel) (Fig. 6).

PEG/PLGA copolymers based systems

Thermosensitive hydrogels discussed in above sections are not all completely biodegradable and therefore can have toxicity concerns when used *in vivo*. Therefore, attempts were made to enhance the biodegradability of these thermoresponsive systems. Novel composite hydrogels were prepared by conjugating biodegradable polyesters, such as poly(L-lactic acid) (PLA) (Suk et al. 2004; Loh and Li 2007), poly(D,L-lactic acid-co-glycolic acid) (PLGA) (Alexander et al. 2013) to biocompatible poly(ethylene glycol) (PEG).

PEG/PLA di/tri-block copolymers exhibits sol-to-gel phase transition with increasing temperature (Danafar et al. 2014). The phase transition temperature could be adjusted by changing the concentration of PEG-PLA copolymers in solution or the composition of the di/tri-block copolymers (Loh and Li 2007).

The sol-gel transition of PEG/PLGA triblock copolymers also occurs with increase in temperature. For PEG-PLGA-PEG copolymers, the increased size of micelles results in their gelation transition. The attractions between polymers get stronger with increasing temperature that makes the total volume fraction of micelles larger than the maximum packing fraction (Fig. 7A) (Velthoen 2008). For PLGA-PEG-PLGA copolymers, the hydrogel is formed in a PLGA core and a PEG shell. The polymers form bridges between the micelles and the number of bridges increases consequently resulting into the formation of compact gel (Fig. 7B) (Velthoen 2008).

Polycaprolactone (PCL) is a hydrophobic and crystalline copolymer, which when conjugated to PEG exhibits excellent thermosensitivity and the transition temperature can be adjusted by changing the ratio of PEG/PCL components (Kim et al. 2004; Suk et al. 2004). For the synthesis of PEG-based thermosensitive hydrogels, ring-opening copolymerisation method has been widely used (Piao et al. 2003; Liu et al. 2007; Fu et al. 2009; Gong et al. 2009a). Copolymerization occurs in the presence of catalysts such as stannous octoate (Fu et al. 2009; Gong et al. 2009a) and calcium ammoniate (Piao et al. 2003) followed by crosslinking with hexamethylene diisocyanate (HMDI) to prepare PEG-PCL-PEG (PECE) or PCl-PEG-PCL (PCEC) or other PEG-based thermosensitive hydrogels.

PEG-based hydrogels are generally biodegradable, however, the main limitation of these composite hydrogels is that the degradation products of PLA, PLGA, PCL and

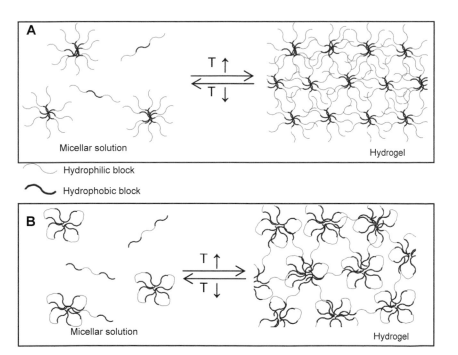

Fig. 7. Gelation of (A) PEG-PLGA-PEG, and (B) PLGA-PEG-PLGA triblock copolymers in water upon a temperature increase (Adopted from (Velthoen 2008)).

the copolymers themselves are acids, which often trigger inflammatory and fibrotic reactions *in vivo* (Jiang et al. 2007).

Other synthetic hydrogels

Poly(oligo (ethylene glycol) methacrylate) (POEGMA), and poly(organo) phosphazene, based hydrogels are emerging thermosensitive hydrogels and exhibits excellent biocompatibility (Li and Guan 2011). For POEGMA polymers, the LCST could be adjusted by controlling the ethylene oxide chain length of the oligo (ethylene glycol) methacrylate (OEGMA) monomer (Lutz and Hoth 2006; Sun and Wu 2012). The transition temperature of POEGMA hydrogel ranges from 23°C to 90°C (Lutz 2008; Sun and Wu 2012). The gelation of poly(organo) phosphazene-based gel also depends on the balance between the hydrophobic and hydrophilic substituents in the polymer chains (Cho et al. 2012) and therefore can be modified as per the desired application.

Thermosensitive Hydrogels Characterization Parameters

Sol-gel transition temperature

Phase transition is the most attractive feature of thermosensitive hydrogels. Different methods have been proposed in the literature to determine the gelation temperature. Ideal hydrogel for biomedical application should be liquid at ambient or room temperature and transform into a gel structure at body temperature. Tube inversion test is the most widely used method to determine the sol-gel transition temperature particularly of LCST systems (Boffito et al. 2015). In this method the copolymer aqueous solution is prepared in various compositions. A known part of the prepared solution is then taken in a tube/vial and is subjected to a controlled heating system in which the temperature can be increased in small increments. Formulations are maintained at a set temperature for specified amount of time, after which the tube is inverted to observe the phase change. The gel state is assessed, when formulations stopped flowing upon inversion of the tube (Fig. 8). Various factors such as sample

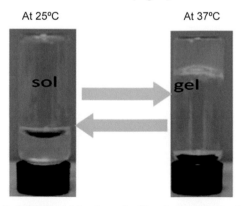

Fig. 8. Sol-gel transition determined by tube inversion method.

weight/volume, tube dimensions (ChangYang et al. 2007; Jeong et al. 2012) and heating method could influence the accurate measurement of the sol-gel transition temperature and therefore it is important to keep these parameters constant to obtain comparable results.

Other factors such as copolymer concentration, copolymer chemical composition, presence of salts and other additives affects the phase transition temperature and therefore the performance of the hydrogel system. The effects of these factors are covered by Boffito et al. in their review (Boffito et al. 2015). Other method described in the literature is the stirrer bar method. A formulation containing a magnetic stirrer bar is heated up slowly and the gelation temperature is defined as the temperature at which the stirrer bar stops rotating (Yong et al. 2001; Dumortier et al. 2006; Yuan et al. 2012). However the mechanical force offered by the rotating stirrer bar might interfere with the accurate measurement of the gelation temperature. The gelation temperature of thermosensitive hydrogels could be modulated by chemical modification: adjusting the ratio of the hydrophobic/hydrophilic components results in the change in their gelation temperature (Sang et al. 2005; Jiang et al. 2007).

Thermal properties

Thermal properties of thermosensitive hydrogels can be studied by differential scanning calorimetry (DSC) (Ankareddi and Brazel 2007; Fu et al. 2009; Gai et al. 2015; Gong et al. 2009a; Liu et al. 2007; Piao et al. 2003; Wei et al. 2005; Zhang et al. 2004a). DSC is a thermoanalytical technique that is widely used for testing polymer thermodynamic properties by detecting the heat transition. Glass transition temperature (T_g) and melting temperature (T_m) of thermosensitive hydrogels can be determined by the heat changes of endothermic or exothermic reactions when the phase transition (sol-to-gel) occurs. T_g of the hydrogels is determined by subjecting the polymer sample to heat/cool/heat cycle. The inflection point of the endothermic drift in the second heating curve of thermograms gives the T_g of the sample (Gai et al. 2015). It is important to know the thermal characteristics of copolymers as it helps in understanding and adopting the correct method for their solubilization, particularly in case of semicrystalline polymers. It also provides information about the presence of interactions and interference from copolymer crystallization with gelation temperature (Lee et al. 2001). LCST of the polymer can also be determined by DSC analysis. A temperature ramp is performed at a defined heating rate under a flow of nitrogen; the temperature of the endothermic maximum obtained is referred as the LCST of the polymer. The effect of the crosslinking agents and other additives can also be investigated by this technique (Petrusic et al. 2012).

Rheological characterization

Rheological characterization of thermogelling systems is important as it will be helpful in determining their performance *in vivo*. The two main prerequisites of an *in situ* thermoresponsive system are viscosity and gelling capacity. The formulation should have optimum viscosity, which will allow easy administration as a solution and should show rapid change in viscosity at body temperature to transform into gel form. The flow characteristics of these systems will affect the injectability, syringibility, residence time and maintenance of the gel form at the administration site (Baloglu et al. 2011). Most of the rheological studies done in the past used the viscosity as a parameter to study these properties. However, conventional methods employed for viscosity measurements, destroy the gel structure resulting into false interpretation (Deasy and Quigley 1991). Hence to keep the gel structure intact, oscillatory measurements at low oscillatory angle were proposed to study the viscoelastic properties of the hydrogel (Chang et al. 2002; Baloglu et al. 2011). Advanced stress and strain controlled rheometers are now available which allow the measurements in oscillatory mode without destroying the microstructure of the gel. Oscillatory measurements are conducted in the linear viscoelastic range from which storage/elastic modulus (G') and viscous/loss modulus (G'') can be calculated, the two moduli are characteristic of the stored elastic energy and the viscous dissipated energy, respectively (Dumortier et al. 2006).

Sol-gel phase transition of LCST systems can also be determined by rheological studies (Gong et al. 2009a; Boffito et al. 2015). Phase transition is determined by performing temperature sweep test at defined rates and analyzing the behavior of the G' and G'' as a function of temperature. In sol state, at low temperatures, the value of G' is relatively low than G'' ($G' < G''$). With increase in temperature, the value of G' increases and at the temperature when G' exceeds the value of G'' ($G' < G''$) phase transition is said to occur. The temperature at which G' is higher than G'' is referred as sol-gel transition temperature (Lin et al. 2013). G' reflects the solid like behavior of the elastic component of the formulation and is the measure of the energy stored and regained at each deformation.

Gelation time could also be determined through rheological studies. Gelation time describes time-dependent gelation mechanism. It is defined as the time after which the G' becomes higher than the G'' at a constant temperature. Gelation time is important to understand the effect of dilution with biological fluids after *in vivo* administration. Rapidly gelled formulation exhibiting short gelation time have less risk of dilution with physiological fluids and the possibility of drainage from the administration site (Chang et al. 2002; Dumortier et al. 2006).

Mechanical properties

The mechanical properties of thermosensitive hydrogels play a significant role in predicting the behavior and performance of these systems. It gives valuable information to formulate a preparation with adequate gel strength, consistency, acceptable viscosity and ease of administration. The mechanical strength of the hydrogels is important both in drug delivery and tissue engineering application. The mechanical properties of the thermosensitive hydrogels is usually studied with the help of a texture analyser (Sinem Yaprak et al. 2012; Singh et al. 2014). Texture profile analysis (TPA) permits to evaluate the textural properties of these hydrogels under different environmental and physiological conditions. Mechanical properties such as hardness, compressibility, adhesiveness, cohesiveness and elasticity are derived from the resultant force-time curve obtained from the TPA. These characteristics are used to quantify sample deformation under compression (Jones et al. 1996; Jones et al. 1997). The mechanical properties of hydrogels are known to be dependent upon the chemical composition and concentration of the polymers (Baloglu et al. 2011). Chen et al. reported the mechanical properties enhancing effect of natural borneol/(2-hydroxypropyl)-β-cyclodextrin (NB/HP-β-CD) on the thermosensitive composite hydrogel which might be due to the changes in the micelle packing and poloxamer entanglements of the composite hydrogel (Chen et al. 2013). TPA can also be utilized to determine the syringeability (ease of withdrawal of a product from a container) and injectability (injection into the intended administration site) of the *in situ* gelling systems (Madan et al. 2009; Cilurzo et al. 2011).

Most thermosensitive hydrogels are also used for the development of mucoadhesive systems to deliver to specific mucosal surface such as nasal (Balakrishnan et al. 2015), rectal (Yuan et al. 2012), vaginal (Sinem Yaprak et al. 2012), periodontal (Jones et al. 1997; Singh et al. 2014) and ocular (Edsman et al. 1998). Mucoadhesion is defined as the force, with which the formulation binds to the mucous membrane at body temperature. To achieve mucoadhesive characteristics the formulation should show a prolonged residence time and minimum drainage from the application site. The mucoadhesive strength of the hydrogel can also be determined by TPA by operating in a tension mode. Mucoadhesion is then measured by determining the area under the curve (AUC) from force-distance plot (Baloglu et al. 2011; Hurler et al. 2012).

Applications of Thermosensitive Hydrogels

Drug delivery

Along with the growing understanding of disease principle and development of new therapies, more and more attentions have been given to the efficient delivery of drugs so that therapeutic concentration could be attained at the desired location for specific duration. Thermosensitive hydrogels exhibit excellent properties for drug delivery as their ability of sol-to-gel transition at body temperature can be used as the trigger for efficient drug encapsulation within the hydrogel matrix. Initially hydrogels were used to deliver hydrophilic, small-molecule drugs due to their high affinity to water molecules. However, various approaches to modify the chemical/physical properties of hydrogels have been investigated to expand the range of drugs that could be loaded within hydrogels matrix. The hydrophobic and macromolecule drugs can be loaded by adopting one of the following three approaches. Firstly, hydrophobic domains can be created within the hydrogel networks by co-polymerizing with hydrophobic monomers (Yin et al. 2002). Secondly, hydrogels grafted with hydrophobic side chains could self-assemble to form hydrophobic domains during gelation that could incorporate hydrophobic drugs (Legros et al. 2008). Thirdly, cyclodextrin can be used to maintain the hydrophilic surface and hydrophobic core of hydrogels, which enables both water affinity of hydrogels and the payload and controlled release of hydrophobic drugs (Siemoneit et al. 2006).

The drug release from thermosensitive hydrogels can be affected by several parameters, including pore size, degradability of hydrogel, drug hydrophobicity, drug concentration and the presence of specific interactions between hydrogels and drugs (Jeong et al. 2000). Typically, the drug release mechanism from hydrogel is diffusion-controlled at an initial stage followed by a combination of diffusion and gel degradation at later stages. As reported by Jeong et al. hydrophilic drug has greater tendency to be partitioned into the hydrophilic domain of thermosensitive hydrogels, while the hydrophobic drug tends to be partitioned into the hydrophobic core of the hydrogel. This property results in faster release rate of hydrophilic drugs compared with that of hydrophobic drugs. To reduce the release rate of drugs from hydrogels, there are several approaches to be applied, such as enhancing the physical and chemical interactions between loaded drug and the hydrogel matrix, modifying the microstructure of the hydrogel (including interpenetrating polymer networks (IPNs)), surface diffusion control and composite hydrogels (Hoare and Kohane 2008). The drug release kinetics can also be tailored by adjusting gelation temperature, altering mechanical properties and incorporating additives (Li and Guan 2011).

Several advantages of thermosensitive hydrogels such as biocompatibility, biodegradability and non-toxic nature contribute to their wide application in drug delivery. Multiple routes of administration have been investigated for drugs loaded within thermosensitive hydrogels: ocular delivery (Gao et al. 2010), periodontal delivery (Ji et al. 2010), nasal delivery (Wu et al. 2007) and transdermal delivery (Muzzarelli and Muzzarelli 2005). For ocular administration, Hao et al. (2014) fabricated a poloxamers based composite thermosensitive hydrogel containing drug loaded solid lipid nanoparticles to achieve a sustained release of Resina Draconis. Also, Gao et al. (2010) investigated that the ocular delivery of dexamethasone acetate (DXA) via PLGA-PEG-PLGA thermosensitive hydrogel matrix has promising potential for the treatment of eye diseases. β-GP chitosan-based thermosensitive hydrogel loaded with 0.1% chlorhexidine (Chx) was applied for periodontal therapy where over 18 h release of Chx was observed which efficaciously inhibited primary periodontal pathogens (Ji et al. 2010). Thermosensitive hydrogels could also offer sustained release of the anti-cancer drugs at specific targets (Li and Guan 2011). PEG-based thermosensitive hydrogels (PLGA-PEG-PLGA triblock copolymers) have been reported as carriers for anticancer drug, such as ricin and paclitaxel, and was able to provide sustained release for 18 and 50 days respectively (Zentner et al. 2001; Chang et al. 2011; Alexander et al. 2013). In addition, thermosensitive hydrogels are also applied for insulin therapy (Kwon and Kim 2003), growth factor delivery (Mattioli-Belmonte et al. 1999) and enzyme immobilisation (Shiroya et al. 1995). Chitosan-based thermosensitive hydrogels have also sparked great interest in local tumor therapy (Bhattarai et al. 2010). The drug delivery manners are particularly important for cancer treatment as most of anticancer drugs are nonspecific and have shown toxicity to normal cells thereby causing serious side effects. Chitosan-based thermosensitive hydrogel is one of the most important natural hydrogels in drug delivery application. An injectable thermosensitive chitosan-β-GP based hydrogel was prepared to deliver the antineoplastic drug paclitaxel and exhibited excellent efficacy in a site-directed, controlled-release of paclitaxel (Ruel-Gariépy et al. 2004).

The chitosan-β-GP system has been reported to deliver bone morphogenetic protein (BMP) *in vivo* and normal cartilage formation was observed for over 3 weeks (Chenite et al. 2000). However, some limitations of chitosan-β-GP system have restrained their applications. One of the limitations is its fast release rate of proteins and low molecular weight drugs (Gordon et al. 2010), whereas, this problem could be solved by encapsulating the drug with liposome and then incorporating it in chitosan-β-GP hydrogel (Ruel-Gariépy et al. 2002). Another disadvantage of chitosan-β-GP thermosensitive hydrogels is their potential toxicity as they were found to cause inflammatory response *in vivo* (Molinaro et al. 2002).

Pluronics thermosensitive hydrogels have been applied for drug delivery over the past decades. Pluronic F127 is one of the most widely used copolymer, which has lower critical gelation concentration (CGC) and least toxicity among pluronic series (Gong et al. 2013). Pluronics have been used to deliver anticancer drugs *in situ* (Li and Guan 2011) and several protein/peptide drugs, such as insulin, protein (BMP), fibroblastic growth factor (FGF), and endothelial cell growth factor (ECGF) (Jeong et al. 2012a). However, several drawbacks of pluronic F127 have limited its application in drug delivery, such as short duration in subcutaneous layer, fast dissolution rate and non-biodegradability. To overcome these limitations, Yang et al. (2009) have investigated a novel mixed micelle system composed of both pluronic F127 and Tween 80 to deliver chemotherapeutic agent docetaxel for gynecological tumors. Docetaxel loaded in the mixed hydrogel exhibited a sustained release for more than 156 h. Pluronic F127 also has the ability to promote the cytotoxicity of chemotherapeutic agents by enhancing the sensitisation of malignant cells to anti-tumor drugs (Batrakova et al. 1999). Li et al. (2015) has reported that pluronic F127 mediated with aptamer AS1411 was used for targeted delivery of anticancer drug doxorubicin (DOX) to human breast tumor. *In vivo* study has illustrated that the formulation was able to achieve enhance drug accumulation in tumor, improved antitumor activity, and decreased cardiotoxicity.

The synthetic thermosensitive hydrogel PNIPAAm has gained great interest for its LCST around 32°C while its poor biodegradability has greatly limited its applications as drug delivery system, as it cannot be easily removed from the body once transform into gel at physiological conditions (Li and Guan 2011). One of the approaches to address this drawback is to conjugate the PNIPAAm polymers with the natural hydrogel chitosan. A thermosensitive hydrogel chitosan-g-PNIPAAm with better biocompatibility and biodegradability to delivery an anti-tumor drug curcumin was prepared. The study demonstrated that the chitosan-g-PNIPAAm containing curcumin could induce apoptosis to tumor cells with lower cytotoxicity to normal cells (Sanoj et al. 2011).

Poly (organo) phosphazene-based hydrogels have also attracted great interests in drug delivery for cancer therapy due to their fast gelation rate, nontoxic degradation products (Teasdale and Brüggemann 2014) and low protein adsorption (Zhou et al. 2010).

Tissue engineering and tissue regeneration

Tissue engineering involves the application of the engineering and biomedical principles towards the development of biological surrogates to improve and restore tissue function (Langer and Vacanti 1993). The unique 3D network structure of hydrogels and its hydrophilic properties resembles the biological tissue's actual environments, making them highly biocompatible. Thermosensitive hydrogels in tissue engineering are commonly used either as substrates to enable cell growth and proliferation or as *in situ* injectable gels. When used as substrates the thermoresponsive ability of the hydrogel is used to regulate the cell attachment and detachment from the surface (Kumashiro et al. 2010; Reed et al. 2010; Varghese et al. 2010). The cells are mixed with the thermosensitive polymer at room temperature and then injected into the body. Upon injection the LCST of the polymer is exceeded at body temperature and the polymer solution transforms into a gel, encapsulating the cells within the 3D network scaffold (Ward and Georgiou 2010). The encapsulated cells grow within the hydrogel scaffold, proliferate and differentiate to restore the damaged tissue. A variety of naturally or synthetically derived thermosensitive hydrogels have been utilised for tissue engineering applications. Natural polymers such as collagen, chitosan, gelatin, alginates and agarose show excellent biocompatibility but often undergo rapid degradation upon contact with body fluids (Tan and Marra 2010).

Chitosan and its derivatives have been extensively investigated for tissue engineering due to their biocompatibility, biodegradability, low immunogenicity and cationic nature (Berger et al. 2004; Ganji et al. 2007). To develop an *in situ* injectable hydrogel, chitosan is usually combined with β-GP that enhances its solubility at physiological neutral pH and changes its gelation temperature to 37°C. This chitosan-β-GP composite has shown application in cartilage tissue engineering (Jin et al. 2009), due to chitosan structural resemblance with the glycosaminoglycans present in cartilage providing good cytocompatibility with cartilage tissues, the chondrocytes. Additionally β-GP also acts as an osteogenic supplement, promoting cartilage growth (Moreira et al. 2016). Chitosan-β-GP scaffolds have also been explored for nerve and bone tissue engineering (Tahrir et al. 2015). Chitosan have shown good nerve affinity and enhanced neurite growth with up-regulation of neurofilament-H mRNA (Yang et al. 2009). Neural stem cells differentiate either into astrocytes or as oligo-dencrocytes. Hence to achieve differentiation of neural cells into particular desired phenotypes, hydrogel chitosan-β-GP scaffolds have been surface modified with extracellular matrix (ECM) derived peptides to target specific nerve tissue regeneration and to enhance the efficiency of stem cell differentiation (Kuraitis et al. 2012; Hsu et al. 2013). This approach was utilized to target specific neurological disorders.

Another potential application of thermosensitive hydrogels is in bone tissue engineering. Bone tissues have very limited self-healing ability and therefore bone tissue repair remains a challenge. Moreover the most important requisite for bone tissue engineering application is that the scaffold should provide appropriate mechanical properties along with ECM properties to serve as temporary skeletal framework. To improve the mechanical properties of hydrogel a composite hydrogel of chitosan has been developed by incorporating collagen (Wang and Stegemann 2010). The incorporation of collagen provided the desired mechanical strength and the composite exhibited approximately three times higher stiffness compared to hydrogel without collagen. The composite was also able to retain 90% of cell viability. Dessi et al. reported development of novel composite hydrogels based on chitosan reinforced by β-tricalcium phosphate for bone tissue engineering application (Dessì et al. 2013). This hydrogel exhibited gel phase transition at body temperature and the presence of inorganic component provided a strong gel structure that mimicked natural bone tissue favouring enhanced cellular activity. PEG/PCL hydrogels, due to their extensively porous structure and biocompatibility have also been extensively investigated for bone tissue engineering (Fu et al. 2012; Ni et al. 2012; Ni et al. 2014).

However, compared to natural polymers, synthetic polymers are more attractive, because of the efficient control over their physical and chemical properties. Synthetic polymers offer improved control over the architecture of the hydrogel structure, by utilising specific block copolymers with defined molecular weight and compositions. Synthetic polymer PNIPAAm has been widely used as cell culture substrates. Physiological cells preferentially adhere to hydrophobic surfaces due to their high affinity. PNIPAAm being a thermosensitive polymer, its hydrophobicity can be switched with change in temperature. PNIPAAm exhibits its hydrophobic behaviour above its LCST and therefore is an ideal substrate for cell/tissue culture. PNIPAAm is used to coat tissue culture plates and when exposed to physiological temperature it promotes cell attachment and proliferation. Cultured cells can then be easily detached from the substrate by lowing the temperature below LCST making the substrate more hydrophilic (Klouda and Mikos 2008). Surface modification of PNIPAAm with cell adhesive peptides resulted in increased cell adhesion and proliferation thereby reducing the culture time (Hatakeyama et al. 2006). It also enhanced the interaction of the hydrogels with the cells at molecular level (Stile and Healy 2001).

Injectable PEG/PCL hydrogels have been used as antiadhesive materials, specifically to prevent post-surgical abdominal adhesion (Yang et al. 2010; Gao et al. 2013). Postsurgical tissue adhesion is common problem after abdominal surgeries and is associated with pain, functional obstruction and difficulties in re-operative procedures. A novel thermosensitive PEG/PCL/PEG hydrogel composite was developed which combined dual properties, anti-adhesion barrier with controlled release of anti-adhesion drug dexamethasone (Wu et al. 2015). As mentioned earlier, synthetic hydrogels provide the flexibility for chemical and structural modifications to enhance the overall performance of the hydrogel network. Imran et al. (2014) reported the development of extremely stretchable PNIPAAm hydrogels composite with enhanced toughness by using polyrotaxane derivatives composed of α cyclodextrin and PEG as crosslinkers. The excellent mechanical properties of this novel composite hydrogel showed promising applications in tissue engineering and as artificial muscles (Bin Imran et al. 2014).

Commercial Formulations at a Glance

ReGel™

ReGel is based on a triblock copolymer, composed of PLGA-PEG-PLGA (Ramesh and Kirk 2008). The polymer composite is specifically designed to achieve an adequate hydrophilic/hydrophobic balance, making it free flowing at or below room temperature for easy handling and transform into a stable gel at body temperature (Zentner et al. 2001). It is available in various grades that offer a range of gelation temperatures, degradation rates and release profiles as a function of molecular weight, degree of hydrophobicity and polymer concentration. The availability of various grades provides broad formulation capability. ReGel formulations have been developed to deliver various small molecules, hydrophobic drugs, proteins and peptides (Choi and Kim 2003; Vukelja et al. 2007). The drug release mechanism through this formulation is primarily by diffusion followed by diffusion and erosion of the gel. The gel erosion/ degradation can be tailored over a duration of 1–6 weeks (Ramesh and Kirk 2008).

OncoGel™ is the formulation of drug paclitaxel in ReGel for local delivery to solid tumours to achieve therapeutic cytotoxic concentration at tumour site without causing systemic toxicities (Elstad and Fowers 2009). OncoGel™ provides constant release of paclitaxel for a period of 4 to 6 weeks.

Cytoryn™ is a peri-tumoral, injectable depot formulation based on ReGel technology to deliver interleukin-2 (IL-2) for cancer immunotherapy. With Cytoryn™ the effect of IL-2 on tumour regression was enhanced four fold as compared to conventional therapy. The stability and bioactivity of IL-2 was also enhanced by the ReGel system (Madan et al. 2009).

InGell gamma™

InGell Gamma is an aliphatically modified triblock copolymer composed of PCL-PEG-PCL (Jo et al. 2006). Both hydrophilic and hydrophobic drugs can be delivered using this copolymer. The sol-to-gel transition is through micelles formation. At lower temperatures, the micelles are dispersed in an aqueous solution and therefore easily administered. At body temperature the hydrophobic character of the amphiphilic tri-block copolymers dominates and consequently the micelles aggregate to form a gel network. In contrast to ReGel technology, caprolactone present in InGell, stabilises the hydrogels allowing better control over drug releasing characteristics. The aliphatic modification further enhances the hydrophobicity of the triblock copolymer resulting in decreased burst effect, which is one of the challenges in controlled drug delivery applications (Petit et al. 2012).

Mebiol® gel

Mebiol gel is a copolymer consisting of thermoresponsive polymer PNIPAAm and hydrophilic polymer PEG (PNIPAAm-PEG) and is commercialised as a cell/tissue culture reagent (Kataoka and Huh 2010). Its unique sol-to-gel transition makes it ideal for cell/tissue culture. The thermoresponsive blocks are hydrophilic at low temperatures and are hydrophobic at 37°C. At high temperature in aqueous media, the hydrophobic interaction results in formation of a rigid 3D polymer network providing highly lipophilic environment that mimics physiological condition which is beneficial for cell growth and proliferation. Cells or tissues can be embedded in cooled Mebiol Gel solution and then cultured in a gel state at 37°C. Cultured cells can be conveniently recovered by cooling below the sol-gel transition temperature.

Conclusion

Increasing attention has been paid to hydrogels and their applications in drug delivery and tissue engineering due to their ease of preparation and handling. The specific porous structures permit loading of a wide range of drugs into the gel matrix and releasing drugs at a controlled and sustained rate to the target tissues. The 3D structure of the hydrogel mimics a physiological condition and provides the perfect environment for encapsulated cells to grow and differentiate into healthy tissues. Their excellent biocompatibility and biodegradability also make them competitive for *in vivo* biomedical applications. The major characteristic of thermosensitive hydrogels is their temperature sensitivity as they stay as a free flowing solution at room temperature but transform into gel after injection at body temperature. The sustained release of the loaded drugs can be achieved by modifying the physical, chemical and mechanical properties of thermosensitive copolymers. Considerable progress has been made in understanding the properties of thermosensitive hydrogels and their applications. New modification approaches and copolymers are still under investigation and the emerging thermosensitive hydrogels are expected to benefit the field of both tissue engineering and drug delivery science.

Reference

Alexander, A., Ajazuddin, J. Khan and S. Saraf. 2013. Poly(ethylene glycol)-poly(lactic-co-glycolic acid) based thermosensitive injectable hydrogels for biomedical applications. J. Control. Release 172(3): 715–729.

Alexandridis, P. and T.A. Hatton. 1995. Poly(ethylene oxide)-poly(propylene oxide)-poly(ethylene oxide) block copolymer surfactants in aqueous solutions and at interfaces: thermodynamics, structure, dynamics, and modeling. Colloids Surf. A 96(1): 1–46.

Ankareddi, I. and C.S. Brazel. 2007. Synthesis and characterization of grafted thermosensitive hydrogels for heating activated controlled release. Int. J. Pharm. 336(2): 241–247.

Arnott, S., A. Fulmer, W.E. Scott, I.C. Dea, R. Moorhouse and D.A. Rees. 1974. The agarose double helix and its function in agarose gel structure. J. Mol. Biol. 90(2): 269–284.

Balakrishnan, P., E.-K. Park, C.-K. Song, H.-J. Ko, T.-W. Hahn, K.-W. Song et al. 2015. Carbopol-incorporated thermoreversible gel for intranasal drug delivery. Molecules. 20(3): 4124.

Baloglu, E., S.Y. Karavana, Z.A. Senyigit and T. Guneri. 2011. Rheological and mechanical properties of poloxamer mixtures as a mucoadhesive gel base. Pharm. Dev. Technol. 16(6): 627–636.

Batrakova, E., S. Lee, S. Li, A. Venne, V. Alakhov and A. Kabanov. 1999. Fundamental relationships between the composition of pluronic block copolymers and their hypersensitization effect in mdr cancer cells. Pharm. Res. 16(9): 1373–1379.

Berger, J., M. Reist, J.M. Mayer, O. Felt, N.A. Peppas and R. Gurny. 2004. Structure and interactions in covalently and ionically crosslinked chitosan hydrogels for biomedical applications. Eur. J. Pharm. Biopharm. 57(1): 19–34.

Bhattarai, N., J. Gunn and M. Zhang. 2010. Chitosan-based hydrogels for controlled, localized drug delivery. Adv. Drug Deliv. Rev. 62(1): 83–99.

Bin Imran, A., K. Esaki, H. Gotoh, T. Seki, K. Ito, Y. Sakai et al. 2014. Extremely stretchable thermosensitive hydrogels by introducing slide-ring polyrotaxane cross-linkers and ionic groups into the polymer network. Nat. Commun. 5.

Boffito, M., P. Sirianni, A.M. Di Rienzo and V. Chiono. 2015. Thermosensitive block copolymer hydrogels based on poly(ε-caprolactone) and polyethylene glycol for biomedical applications: state of the art and future perspectives. J. Biomed. Mater. Res. A. 103(3): 1276–1290.

Bromberg, L.E. and E.S. Ron. 1998. Temperature-responsive gels and thermogelling polymer matrices for protein and peptide delivery. Adv. Drug Deliv. Rev. 31(3): 197–221.

Cabana, A., A. Aït-Kadi and J. Juhász. 1997. Study of the gelation process of polyethylene oxidea–polypropylene oxideb–polyethylene oxideacopolymer (poloxamer 407) aqueous solutions. J. Colloid. Interf. Sci. 190(2): 307–312.

Chang, G., T. Ci, L. Yu and J. Ding. 2011. Enhancement of the fraction of the active form of an antitumor drug topotecan via an injectable hydrogel. J. Control. Release. 156(1): 21–27.

Chang, J.Y., Y.-K. Oh, H.-g. Choi, Y.B. Kim and C.-K. Kim. 2002. Rheological evaluation of thermosensitive and mucoadhesive vaginal gels in physiological conditions. Int. J. Pharm. 241(1): 155–163.

ChangYang, G., Q. ZhiYong, L. CaiBing, H. MeiJuan, G. YingChun, W. YanJun et al. 2007. A thermosensitive hydrogel based on biodegradable amphiphilic poly(ethylene glycol)–polycaprolactone–poly(ethylene glycol) block copolymers. Smart Mater. Struct. 16(3): 927.

Chen, H. and M. Fan. 2008. Novel thermally sensitive pH-dependent chitosan/carboxymethyl cellulose hydrogels. J. Bioact. Compat. 23(1): 38–48.

Chen, J.-P. and T.-H. Cheng. 2006. Thermo-responsive chitosan-graft-poly(n-isopropylacrylamide) injectable hydrogel for cultivation of chondrocytes and meniscus cells. Macromol. Biosci. 6(12): 1026–1039.

Chen, J.-P. and W.-L. Lee. 2008. Collagen-grafted temperature-responsive nonwoven fabric for wound dressing. Appl. Surf. 255(2): 412–415.

Chen, J., R. Zhou, L. Li, B. Li, X. Zhang and J. Su. 2013. Mechanical, rheological and release behaviors of a poloxamer 407/poloxamer 188/carbopol 940 thermosensitive composite hydrogel. Molecules. 18(10): 12415.

Chenite, A., C. Chaput, D. Wang, C. Combes, M.D. Buschmann, C.D. Hoemann et al. 2000. Novel injectable neutral solutions of chitosan form biodegradable gels *in situ*. Biomaterials. 21(21): 2155–2161.

Cho, J.K., J.W. Park and S.C. Song. 2012. Injectable and biodegradable poly(organophosphazene) gel containing silibinin: its physicochemical properties and anticancer activity. J. Pharm. Sci. 101(7): 2382–2391.

Choi, S. and S.W. Kim. 2003. Controlled release of insulin from injectable biodegradable triblock copolymer depot in zdf rats. Pharm. Res. 20(12): 2008–2010.

Cilurzo, F., F. Selmin, P. Minghetti, M. Adami, E. Bertoni, S. Lauria et al. 2011. Injectability evaluation: an open issue. AAPS Pharm. Sci. Tech. 12(2): 604–609.

Danafar, H., K. Rostamizadeh, S. Davaran and M. Hamidi. 2014. PLA-PEG-PLA copolymer-based polymersomes as nanocarriers for delivery of hydrophilic and hydrophobic drugs: preparation and evaluation with atorvastatin and lisinopril. Drug Dev. Ind. Pharm. 40(10): 1411–1420.

Deasy, P.B. and K.J. Quigley. 1991. Rheological evaluation of deacetylated gellan gum (Gelrite) for pharmaceutical use. Int. J. Pharm. 73(2): 117–123.

Dessì, M., A. Borzacchiello, T.H.A. Mohamed, W.I. Abdel-Fattah and L. Ambrosio. 2013. Novel biomimetic thermosensitive β-tricalcium phosphate/chitosan-based hydrogels for bone tissue engineering. J. Biomed. Mater. Res. A. 101(10): 2984–2993.

Dumortier, G., J.L. Grossiord, F. Agnely and J.C. Chaumeil. 2006. A review of poloxamer 407 pharmaceutical and pharmacological characteristics. Pharm. Res. 23(12): 2709–2728.

Edsman, K., J. Carlfors and R. Petersson. 1998. Rheological evaluation of poloxamer as an *in situ* gel for ophthalmic use. Eur. J. Pharm. Sci. 6(2): 105–112.

Elstad, N.L. and K.D. Fowers. 2009. OncoGel (ReGel/paclitaxel)—Clinical applications for a novel paclitaxel delivery system. Adv. Drug Deliv. Rev. 61(10): 785–794.

Franz, G. 1986. Polysaccharides in Pharmacy. Springer Berlin Heidelberg.

Fu, S., G. Guo, C. Gong, S. Zeng, H. Liang, F. Luo et al. 2009. Injectable biodegradable thermosensitive hydrogel composite for orthopedic tissue engineering. 1. preparation and characterization of nanohydroxyapatite/poly(ethylene glycol)–poly(ε-caprolactone)–poly(ethylene glycol) hydrogel nanocomposites. J. Phys. Chem. B. 113(52): 16518–16525.

Fu, S., P. Ni, B. Wang, B. Chu, L. Zheng, F. Luo et al. 2012. Injectable and thermo-sensitive PEG-PCL-PEG copolymer/collagen/n-HA hydrogel composite for guided bone regeneration. Biomaterials. 33(19): 4801–4809.

Gai, H., J. Wu, C. Wu, X. Sun, F. Jia and Y. Yu. 2015. Synthesis and characterization of thermosensitive hydrogel with improved mechanical properties. J. Mater. Res. 30(16): 2400–2407.

Gandhi, A., A. Paul, S.O. Sen and K.K. Sen. 2015. Studies on thermoresponsive polymers: phase behaviour, drug delivery and biomedical applications. Asian J. Pharmacol. 10(2): 99–107.

Ganji, F., M.J. Abdekhodaie and A. Ramazani S.A. 2007. Gelation time and degradation rate of chitosan-based injectable hydrogel. J. Sol-Gel. Sci. Technol. 42(1): 47–53.

Gao, X., X. Deng, X. Wei, H. Shi, F. Wang, T. Ye et al. 2013. Novel thermosensitive hydrogel for preventing formation of abdominal adhesions. Int. J. Nanomedicine. 8: 2453–2463.

Gao, Y., Y. Sun, F. Ren and S. Gao. 2010. PLGA–PEG–PLGA hydrogel for ocular drug delivery of dexamethasone acetate. Drug Dev. Ind. Pharm. 36(10): 1131–1138.

Gibson, M.I. and R.K. O'Reilly. 2013. To aggregate, or not to aggregate? considerations in the design and application of polymeric thermally-responsive nanoparticles. Chem. Soc. Rev. 42(17): 7204–7213.

Gong, C., S. Shi, P. Dong, B. Kan, M. Gou, X. Wang et al. 2009a. Synthesis and characterization of PEG-PCL-PEG thermosensitive hydrogel. Int. J. Pharm. 365(1-2): 89–99.

Gong, C., T. Qi, X. Wei, Y. Qu, Q. Wu, F. Luo et al. 2013. Thermosensitive polymeric hydrogels as drug delivery systems. Curr. Med. Chem. 20(1): 79–94(16).

Hao, J., X. Wang, Y. Bi, Y. Teng, J. Wang, F. Li et al. 2014. Fabrication of a composite system combining solid lipid nanoparticles and thermosensitive hydrogel for challenging ophthalmic drug delivery. Colloids Surf, B. 114: 111–120.

Hatakeyama, H., A. Kikuchi, M. Yamato and T. Okano. 2006. Bio-functionalized thermoresponsive interfaces facilitating cell adhesion and proliferation. Biomaterials. 27(29): 5069–5078.

Hoare, T.R. and D.S. Kohane. 2008. Hydrogels in drug delivery: progress and challenges. Polymer. 49(8): 1993–2007.

Hrubý, M., S.K. Filippov and P. Štěpánek. 2015. Smart polymers in drug delivery systems on crossroads: which way deserves following? Eur. Polym. J. 65: 82–97.

Hsu, S.-H., W.-C. Kuo, Y.-T. Chen, C.-T. Yen, Y.-F. Chen, K.-S. Chen et al. 2013. New nerve regeneration strategy combining laminin-coated chitosan conduits and stem cell therapy. Acta Biomater. 9(5): 6606–6615.

Hurler, J., A. Engesland, B. Poorahmary Kermany and N. Škalko-Basnet. 2012. Improved texture analysis for hydrogel characterization: Gel cohesiveness, adhesiveness, and hardness. J. Appl. Polym. Sci. 125(1): 180–188.

Jeong, B., Y.H. Bae and S.W. Kim. 2000. Drug release from biodegradable injectable thermosensitive hydrogel of PEG–PLGA–PEG triblock copolymers. J. Control. Release. 63(1-2): 155–163.

Jeong, B., S.W. Kim and Y.H. Bae. 2012a. Thermosensitive sol–gel reversible hydrogels. Adv. Drug Deliv. Rev. 64: 154–162.

Jeong, B., S.W. Kim and Y.H. Bae. 2012b. Thermosensitive sol–gel reversible hydrogels. Adv. Drug Deliv. Rev. 54(1): 37–51.

Ji, Q.X., Q.S. Zhao, J. Deng and R. Lü. 2010. A novel injectable chlorhexidine thermosensitive hydrogel for periodontal application: preparation, antibacterial activity and toxicity evaluation. J. Mater. Sci. Mater. Med. 21(8): 2435–2442.

Jia, L., C. Guo, L. Yang, J. Xiang, Y. Tang, C. Liu et al. 2010. Mechanism of PEO–PPO–PEO micellization in aqueous solutions studied by two-dimensional correlation FTIR spectroscopy. J. Colloid. Interf. Sci. 345(2): 332–337.

Jiang, W.W., S.H. Su, R.C. Eberhart and L. Tang. 2007. Phagocyte responses to degradable polymers. J. Biomed. Mater. Res. A. 82(2): 492–497.

Jiang, Z., Y. You, X. Deng and J. Hao. 2007. Injectable hydrogels of poly(ε-caprolactone-co-glycolide)–poly(ethylene glycol)–poly(ε-caprolactone-co-glycolide) triblock copolymer aqueous solutions. Polymer. 48(16): 4786–4792.

Jin, R., L.S. Moreira Teixeira, P.J. Dijkstra, M. Karperien, C.A. van Blitterswijk, Z.Y. Zhong et al. 2009. Injectable chitosan-based hydrogels for cartilage tissue engineering. Biomaterials. 30(13): 2544–2551.

Jo, S., J. Kim and S.W. Kim. 2006. Reverse thermal gelation of aliphatically modified biodegradable triblock copolymers. Macromol. Biosci. 6(11): 923–928.

Jones, D.S., A.D. Woolfson and J. Djokic. 1996. Texture profile analysis of bioadhesive polymeric semisolids: mechanical characterization and investigation of interactions between formulation components. J. Appl. Polym. Sci. 61(12): 2229–2234.

Jones, D.S., A.D. Woolfson, A.F. Brown and M.J. O'Neill. 1997. Mucoadhesive, syringeable drug delivery systems for controlled application of metronidazole to the periodontal pocket: *in vitro* release kinetics, syringeability, mechanical and mucoadhesive properties. J. Control. Release. 49(1): 71–79.

Kataoka, K. and N. Huh. 2010. Application of a thermo-reversible gelation polymer, mebiol gel, for stem cell culture and regenerative medicine. J. Stem Cells Regen. Med. 6(1): 10–14.

Kim, M.S., K.S. Seo, G. Khang, H.C. Sun and B.L. Hai. 2004. Preparation of poly(ethylene glycol)-block -poly(caprolactone) copolymers and their applications as thermo-sensitive materials. J. Biomed. Mater. Res. A. 70(1): 154–158.

Kim, S., J.-H. Kim, O. Jeon, I.C. Kwon and K. Park. 2009. Engineered polymers for advanced drug delivery. Eur. J. Pharm. 71(3): 420–430.

Klouda, L. and A.G. Mikos. 2008. Thermoresponsive hydrogels in biomedical applications. Eur. J. Pharm. Biopharm. 68(1): 34–45.

Kumashiro, Y., M. Yamato and T. Okano. 2010. Cell attachment–detachment control on temperature-responsive thin surfaces for novel tissue engineering. Ann. Biomed. Eng. 38(6): 1977–1988.

Kuraitis, D., C. Giordano, M. Ruel, A. Musarò and E.J. Suuronen. 2012. Exploiting extracellular matrix-stem cell interactions: a review of natural materials for therapeutic muscle regeneration. Biomaterials. 33(2): 428–443.

Kwon, Y.M. and S.W. Kim. 2003. New biodegradable polymers for delivery of bioactive agents. Macromol. Symp. 201(1): 179–186.

Lai, P.-L., D.-W. Hong, K.-L. Ku, Z.-T. Lai and I.M. Chu. 2014. Novel thermosensitive hydrogels based on methoxy polyethylene glycol-co-poly(lactic acid-co-aromatic anhydride) for cefazolin delivery. Nanomedicine. 10(3): 553–560.

Langer, R. and J.P. Vacanti. 1993. Tissue engineering. Science (New York, N.Y.). 260(5110): 920–926.

Lee, J.W., F.-j. Hua and D.S. Lee. 2001. Thermoreversible gelation of biodegradable poly(ε-caprolactone) and poly(ethylene glycol) multiblock copolymers in aqueous solutions. J. Control. Release. 73(2-3): 315–327.

Legros, M., V. Dulong, L. Picton and D.L. Cerf. 2008. Self-organization of water soluble and amphiphile crosslinked carboxymethylpullulan. Polymer Journal. 40(12): 1132–1139.

Li, X., Y. Yu, Q. Ji and L. Qiu. 2015. Targeted delivery of anticancer drugs by aptamer AS1411 mediated Pluronic F127/cyclodextrin-linked polymer composite micelles. Nanomedicine 11(1): 175–184.

Li, Z. and J. Guan. 2011. Thermosensitive hydrogels for drug delivery. Expert Opin. Drug Deliv. 8(8): 991–1007.

Lin, G., L. Cosimbescu, N.J. Karin, A. Gutowska and B.J. Tarasevich. 2013. Injectable and thermogelling hydrogels of PCL-g-PEG: mechanisms, rheological and enzymatic degradation properties. J. Mater. Chem. B. 1(9): 1249–1255.

Liu, C., C. Gong, Y. Pan, Y. Zhang, J. Wang, M. Huang et al. 2007. Synthesis and characterization of a thermosensitive hydrogel based on biodegradable amphiphilic PCL-Pluronic (L35)-PCL block copolymers. Colloids Surf., A. 302(1-3): 430–438.

Liu, W., B. Zhang, W.W. Lu, X. Li, D. Zhu, K. De Yao et al. 2004. A rapid temperature-responsive sol–gel reversible poly(N-isopropylacrylamide)-g-methylcellulose copolymer hydrogel. Biomaterials. 25(15): 3005–3012.

Loh, X.J. and J. Li. 2007. Biodegradable thermosensitive copolymer hydrogels for drug delivery. Expert Opin. Ther. Pat. 17(8): 965–977.

Lutz, J.-F. and A. Hoth. 2006. Preparation of ideal PEG analogues with a tunable thermosensitivity by controlled radical copolymerization of 2-(2-methoxyethoxy) ethyl methacrylate and oligo (ethylene glycol) methacrylate. Macromolecules. 39(2): 893–896.

Lutz, J.F. 2008. Polymerization of oligo (ethylene glycol)(meth) acrylates: toward new generations of smart biocompatible materials. J. Polym. Sci. A Polym. Chem. 46(11): 3459–3470.

Madan, M., A. Bajaj, S. Lewis, N. Udupa and J.A. Baig. 2009. *In situ* forming polymeric drug delivery systems. Indian J. Pharm. Sci. 71(3): 242–251.

Matanović, M.R., J. Kristl and P.A. Grabnar. 2014. Thermoresponsive polymers: insights into decisive hydrogel characteristics, mechanisms of gelation, and promising biomedical applications. Int. J. Pharm. 472(1-2): 262–275.

Mattioli-Belmonte, M., A. Gigante, R.A. Muzzarelli, R. Politano, A. Benedittis, De, N. Specchia et al. 1999. N,N-dicarboxymethyl chitosan as delivery agent for bone morphogenetic protein in the repair of articular cartilage. Med. Biol. Eng. Comput. 37(1): 130–134.

Meeting, P.N.G., W. Burchard and S.B. Ross-Murphy. 1990. Physical networks: polymers and gels. Elsevier Applied Science.

Molinaro, G., J.C. Leroux, J. Damas and A. Adam. 2002. Biocompatibility of thermosensitive chitosanbased hydrogels: an *in vivo* experimental approach to injectable biomaterials. Biomaterials 23(13): 2717–2722.

Moreira, C.D.F., S.M. Carvalho, H.S. Mansur and M.M. Pereira. 2016. Thermogelling chitosan–collagen–bioactive glass nanoparticle hybrids as potential injectable systems for tissue engineering. Materials Science and Engineering: C. 58: 1207–1216.

Mu, Q. and Y.e. Fang. 2008. Preparation of thermosensitive chitosan with poly(N-isopropylacrylamide) side at hydroxyl group via O-maleoyl-N-phthaloyl-chitosan (MPCS). Carbohydr. Polym. 72(2): 308–314.

Muzzarelli, R.A.A. and C. Muzzarelli. 2005. Chitosan chemistry: Relevance to the biomedical sciences. Adv. Polym. Sci.

N. Sanoj, R., P.R. Sreerekha, K.P. Chennazhi, S.V. Nair and R. Jayakumar. 2011. Biocompatible, biodegradable and thermo-sensitive chitosan-g-poly N-isopropylacrylamide) nanocarrier for curcumin drug delivery. International Journal of Biological Macromolecules. 49(2): 161–172.

Ni, P.-Y., M. Fan, Z.-Y. Qian, J.-C. Luo, C.-Y. Gong, S.-Z. Fu et al. 2012. Synthesis and characterization of injectable, thermosensitive, and biocompatible acellular bone matrix/poly(ethylene glycol)-poly (ε-caprolactone)-poly(ethylene glycol) hydrogel composite. J. Biomed. Mater. Res. A. 100A(1): 171–179.

Ni, P., Q. Ding, M. Fan, J. Liao, Z. Qian, J. Luo et al. 2014. Injectable thermosensitive PEG–PCL–PEG hydrogel/acellular bone matrix composite for bone regeneration in cranial defects. Biomaterials. 35(1): 236–248.

Peppas, N., P. Bures, W. Leobandung and H. Ichikawa. 2000. Hydrogels in pharmaceutical formulations. Eur. J. Pharm. Biopharm. 50(1): 27–46.

Petit, A., B. Müller, P. Bruin, R. Meyboom, M. Piest, L.M.J. Kroon-Batenburg et al. 2012. Modulating rheological and degradation properties of temperature-responsive gelling systems composed of blends of PCLA–PEG–PCLA triblock copolymers and their fully hexanoyl-capped derivatives. Acta Biomater. 8(12): 4260–4267.

Petrusic, S., M. Lewandowski, S. Giraud, P. Jovancic, B. Bugarski, S. Ostojic et al. 2012. Development and characterization of thermosensitive hydrogels based on poly(N-isopropylacrylamide) and calcium alginate. J. Appl. Polym. Sci. 124(2): 890–903.

Piao, L., Z. Dai, M. Deng, X. Chen and X. Jing. 2003. Synthesis and characterization of PCL/PEG/PCL triblock copolymers by using calcium catalyst. Polymer. 44(7): 2025–2031.

Ramesh, C.R. and D.F. Kirk. 2008. ReGel Depot Technology. Modified-Release Drug Delivery Technology, Second Edition, CRC Press: 171–181.

Reed, J.A., A.E. Lucero, S. Hu, L.K. Ista, M.T. Bore, G.P. López et al. 2010. A low-cost, rapid deposition method for "smart" films: applications in mammalian cell release. ACS Appl. Mater. Interfaces. 2(4): 1048–1051.

Rees, D.A. and W.E. Jane. 1977. Secondary and tertiary structure of polysaccharides in solutions and gels. Angewandte Chemie International Edition. 16(4): 214–224.

Rozier, A., C. Mazuel, J. Grove and B. Plazonnet. 1989. Gelrite®: a novel, ion-activated, *in situ* gelling polymer for ophthalmic vehicles. Effect on bioavailability of timolol. Int. J. Pharm. 57(89): 163–168.

Ruel-Gariépy, E., G. Leclair, P. Hildgen, A. Gupta and J.C. Leroux. 2002. Thermosensitive chitosan-based hydrogel containing liposomes for the delivery of hydrophilic molecules. J. Control. Release. 82(2): 373–383.

Ruel-Gariépy, E. and J.-C. Leroux. 2004. *In situ*-forming hydrogels—review of temperature-sensitive systems. Eur. J. Pharm. Biopharm. 58(2): 409–426.

Ruel-Gariépy, E., M. Shive, A. Bichara, M. Berrada, D. Le Garrec, A. Chenite et al. 2004. A thermosensitive chitosan-based hydrogel for the local delivery of paclitaxel. Eur. J. Pharm. Biopharm. 57(1): 53–63.

Sang, C.L., W.C. Yong and K. Park. 2005. Control of thermogelation properties of hydrophobically-modified methylcellulose. J. Bioact. Compat. Polym. 20(1): 5–13.

Shiroya, T., N. Tamura, M. Yasui, K. Fujimoto and H. Kawaguchi. 1995. Enzyme immobilization on thermosensitive hydrogel microspheres. Colloids Surf. B. 4(5): 267–274.

Siemoneit, U., C.L.C. Schmitt, A. Luzardo, E.F. Otero, A. Concheiro and M.J. Blanco. 2006. Acrylic/cyclodextrin hydrogels with enhanced drug loading and sustained release capability. Int. J. Pharm. 312(1-2): 66–74.

Sinem Yaprak, K., R.b. Seda, e.i. Zeynep Ay and B.l. Esra. 2012. A new *in situ* gel formulation of itraconazole for vaginal administration. Pharmacol. Pharm. 3(4): 10.

Singh, K.P., G. Chhabra, V. Sharma and K. Pathak. 2014. Thermosensitive periodontal sol of ciprofloxacin hydrochloride and serratiopeptidase: Pharmaceutical and mechanical analysis. Int. J. Pharm. Investig. 4(1): 5–14.

Southall, N.T., K.A. Dill and A.D.J. Haymet. 2002. A view of the hydrophobic effect. J. Phys. Chem. B. 106(3): 521–533.

Stile, R.A. and K.E. Healy. 2001. Thermo-responsive peptide-modified hydrogels for tissue regeneration. Biomacromolecules. 2(1): 185–194.

Suk, K.M., S.K. Su, K. Gilson, C.S. Hang and L.H. Bang. 2004. Preparation of methoxy poly(ethylene glycol)/polyester diblock copolymers and examination of the gel-to-sol transition. J. Polym. Sci. A. Polym. Chem. 42(22): 5784–5793.

Sun, J. and H. Tan. 2013. Alginate-based biomaterials for regenerative medicine applications. Materials. 6(4): 1285.

Sun, S. and P. Wu. 2012. On the thermally reversible dynamic hydration behavior of oligo (ethylene glycol) methacrylate-based polymers in water. Macromolecules. 46(1): 236–246.

Tahrir, F.G., F. Ganji and T.M. Ahooyi. 2015. Injectable Thermosensitive chitosan/glycerophosphate-based hydrogels for tissue engineering and drug delivery applications: a review. Recent Pat. Drug Deliv. Formul. 9(2): 107–120.

Tan, H., C.M. Ramirez, N. Miljkovic, H. Li, J.P. Rubin and K.G. Marra. 2009. Thermosensitive injectable hyaluronic acid hydrogel for adipose tissue engineering. Biomaterials. 30(36): 6844–6853.

Tan, H. and K.G. Marra. 2010. Injectable, biodegradable hydrogels for tissue engineering applications. Materials. 3(3): 1746.

Tan, R., Z. She, M. Wang, Z. Fang, Y. Liu and Q. Feng. 2012. Thermo-sensitive alginate-based injectable hydrogel for tissue engineering. Carbohydr. Polym. 87(2): 1515–1521.

Teasdale, I. and O. Brüggemann. 2014. Polyphosphazenes for Medical Applications. Shrewsbury, Smithers Rapra.

Varghese, V., V. Raj, K. Sreenivasan and T.V. Kumary. 2010. In vitro cytocompatibility evaluation of a thermoresponsive NIPAAm-MMA copolymeric surface using L929 cells. J. Mater. Sci.: Mater. Med. 21(5): 1631–1639.

Velthoen, I.W. 2008. Thermo-responsive hydrogels based on branched block copolymers. University of Twente.

Vukelja, S.J., S.P. Anthony, J.C. Arseneau, B.S. Berman, C. Casey Cunningham, J.J. Nemunaitis et al. 2007. Phase 1 study of escalating-dose OncoGel® (ReGel®/paclitaxel) depot injection, a controlled-release formulation of paclitaxel, for local management of superficial solid tumor lesions. Anti-Cancer Drugs. 18(3): 283–289.

Wang, L. and J.P. Stegemann. 2010. Thermogelling chitosan and collagen composite hydrogels initiated with β-glycerophosphate for bone tissue engineering. Biomaterials. 31(14): 3976–3985.

Ward, M.A. and T.K. Georgiou. 2010. Thermoresponsive terpolymers based on methacrylate monomers: Effect of architecture and composition. J. Polym. Sci. A Polym. Chem. 48(4): 775–783.

Ward, M.A. and T.K. Georgiou. 2011. Thermoresponsive polymers for biomedical applications. Polymers. 3(3): 1215.

Wei, H., H. Yu, A.Y. Zhang, L.G. Sun and D. Hou. 2005. Synthesis and characterization of thermosensitive and supramolecular structured hydrogels. Macromolecules. 38(21): 8833–8839.

Wu, J., W. Wei, L.Y. Wang, Z.G. Su and G.H. Ma. 2007. A thermosensitive hydrogel based on quaternized chitosan and poly(ethylene glycol) for nasal drug delivery system. Biomaterials. 28(13): 2220–2232.

Wu, Q., N. Wang, T. He, J. Shang, L. Li, L. Song et al. 2015. Thermosensitive hydrogel containing dexamethasone micelles for preventing postsurgical adhesion in a repeated-injury model. Sci. Rep. 5: 13553.

Yang, Y., J. Wang, X. Zhang, W. Lu and Q. Zhang. 2009. A novel mixed micelle gel with thermo-sensitive property for the local delivery of docetaxel. J. Control. Release. 135(2): 175–182.

Yang, B., C. Gong, Z. Qian, X. Zhao, Z. Li, X. Qi et al. 2010. Prevention of post-surgical abdominal adhesions by a novel biodegradable thermosensitive PECE hydrogel. BMC Biotechnol. 10: 65.

Yang, H. and W. Kao. 2006. Thermoresponsive gelatin/monomethoxy poly(ethylene glycol)–poly(d,l-lactide) hydrogels: formulation, characterization, and antibacterial drug delivery. Pharm. Res. 23(1): 205–214.

Yang, Y., M. Liu, Y. Gu, S. Lin, F. Ding and X. Gu 2009. Effect of chitooligosaccharide on neuronal differentiation of PC-12 cells. Cell Biol. Int. 33(3): 352–356.

Yin, Y., Y.J. Yang and H. Xu. 2002. Hydrophobically modified hydrogels containing azoaromatic cross-links: swelling properties, degradation in vivo and application in drug delivery. Eur. Polym. J. 38(11): 2305–2311.

Yong, C.S., J.S. Choi, Q.-Z. Quan, J.-D. Rhee, C.-K. Kim, S.-J. Lim et al. 2001. Effect of sodium chloride on the gelation temperature, gel strength and bioadhesive force of poloxamer gels containing diclofenac sodium. Int. J. Pharm. 226(1-2): 195–205.

Yoshida, R., K. Sakai, T. Okano and Y. Sakurai. 1994. Modulating the phase transition temperature and thermosensitivity in N-isopropylacrylamide copolymer gels. J. Biomater. Sci. Polym. Ed. 6(6): 585–598.

Yuan, Y., Y. Cui, L. Zhang, H.-p. Zhu, Y.-S. Guo, B. Zhong et al. 2012. Thermosensitive and mucoadhesive in situ gel based on poloxamer as new carrier for rectal administration of nimesulide. Int. J. Pharm. 430(1-2): 114–119.

Zentner, G.M., R. Rathi, C. Shih, J.C. McRea, M.-H. Seo, H. Oh et al. 2001. Biodegradable block copolymers for delivery of proteins and water-insoluble drugs. J. Controlled Release. 72(1-3): 203–215.

Zhang, X.-Z., D.-Q. Wu and C.-C. Chu. 2004a. Synthesis, characterization and controlled drug release of thermosensitive IPN–PNIPAAm hydrogels. Biomaterials. 25(17): 3793–3805.

Zhang, X.Z., G.M. Sun, D.Q. Wu and C.C. Chu. 2004b. Synthesis and characterization of partially biodegradable and thermosensitive hydrogel. J. Mater. Sci. Mater. Med. 15(8): 865–875.

Zhang, Y., C. Gao, X. Li, C. Xu, Y. Zhang, Z. Sun et al. 2014. Thermosensitive methyl cellulose-based injectable hydrogels for post-operation anti-adhesion. Carbohydr. Polym. 101: 171–178.

Zhou, T., W. Wu and S. Zhou. 2010. Engineering oligo(ethylene glycol)-based thermosensitive microgels for drug delivery applications. Polymer. 51(17): 3926–3933.

CHAPTER 12

Silk Hydrogels for Drug and Cell Delivery

F. Philipp Seib

Introduction

Silk has fascinated humans since ancient times; silk fibres have been used in textiles for more than 5,000 years and for many centuries as a suturing material (Lubec et al. 1993; Omenetto and Kaplan 2010). The remarkable strength and toughness of silk stems from its evolution as a structural engineering material in nature (Vollrath and Porter 2009; Buehler 2013).

Silk is a sustainable and ecologically benign biopolymer that can be manufactured using green processes (Vollrath and Porter 2009). Over the past 25 years, we have seen a tremendous development of both bottom-up and top-down approaches for the generation of silk biopolymers. Specifically, reverse engineering of silk cocoons and the advent of recombinant technologies have been paramount for a better understanding of silks (Chung et al. 2012; Tokareva et al. 2014). For example, molecular simulation studies (Buehler 2013), coupled with dedicated mechanical testing of recombinant and natural silks (Vollrath and Porter 2009), have increased our appreciation of the critical importance of silk's hierarchal structure by which it serves its function (e.g., protects the developing moth in the silk cocoons and catches spider's prey in orb-webs) (Omenetto and Kaplan 2010). Thus, natural silk fibres can serve as blueprints for novel designer polymers.

Today, silk's remarkable physical properties have supported high-end applications, including its use in bulletproof vests (Gatesy et al. 2001), parachute cords (Kluge et al. 2008), composite materials for the aviation industry (Hardy and Scheibel 2009), photonics (Omenetto and Kaplan 2008) and electronics (Kim et al. 2010). The medical

Strathclyde Institute of Pharmacy and Biomedical Sciences, University of Strathclyde, 161 Cathedral Street, Glasgow, G4 0RE, UK.
E-mails: philipp.seib@strath.ac.uk or philipp.seib@SeibLab.com

use of silk dates back to its use as a suture material; here the unique physical properties, handling and biocompatibility of silk fibres have been critical for its continued success, as well as for its approval by the Food and Drug Administration (FDA) as a biopolymer for use in humans. However, the medical applications of silk that have emerged over the past decade go beyond its traditional load-bearing applications (Altman et al. 2003; Omenetto and Kaplan 2010). In this chapter, we examine the role of silk in drug and cell delivery applications, with specific reference to silk hydrogels, and we highlight emerging trends, opportunities and challenges, as well as provide a sound background on silk biopolymers for the silk novice.

Silk Structure-Function Relationships

For the purpose of this chapter, we use the term silk to refer to protein-based fibre-forming materials spun by living organisms. Spiders and silkworms are the most prominent organisms associated with silk production, although silks are made by many arthropod taxa (Vollrath and Porter 2009; Porter et al. 2013). Furthermore, spiders make more than one type of silk. For example, the common European garden spider, *Araneus diadematus,* and the golden silk spider, *Nephila clavipes,* spin seven different silks from seven sets of different silk glands (Vollrath 1992); these silks are often used in combination simultaneously to fine tune the overall fibre composition and subsequent performance. Nonetheless, the silks used for drug delivery applications are typically those produced by the silkworm, *Bombyx mori,* or recombinant versions of spider silks (Yucel et al. 2014). Where appropriate, we distinguish between silkworm silk (fibroin) from the cocoons of *B. mori* and spider silks. We also differentiate silk materials that are reverse engineered native proteins from those generated in heterologous hosts via genetic engineering. When not specifically stated, we refer to silkworm silk because *B. mori* silk is most commonly used due to its abundance (Seib and Kaplan 2013). The hierarchal structure of silk enables this biopolymer to serve specific functions (Fig. 1a,b), including tailored drug release and payload protection. The following section details silk structure with specific reference to drug delivery.

Bombyx mori Silk

The *B. mori* silk heavy chain consists predominantly of five amino acids: 45.9% glycine (G), 30.3% alanine (A), 12.1% serine (S), 5.3% tyrosine (Y), and 1.8% valine (V) and only 4.6% of the other 15 amino acid types (Zhou et al. 2001). *B. mori* silk is a very large (2.3 MDa) protein that is made up of a heavy chain (approximately 350 kDa) (Zhou et al. 2000) and a light chain (approximately 26 kDa) (Yamaguchi et al. 1989) that are held together by a single disulphide bond at the C terminus (Tanaka et al. 1999) (Fig. 1b); this disulphide linkage is critically important for the successful secretion of silk from the silk gland. The 2.3 MDa elementary silk unit is composed of six sets of disulphide-linked heavy and light chain heterodimers that assemble and are physically complexed by one molecule of fibrohexamerin (P25, approximately 25 kDa). Fibrohexamerin has *N*-linked high mannose type oligosaccharide chains that facilitate the physical interaction with the silk heavy chain (Inoue et al. 2000; Inoue et al. 2004). The 6:6:1 molar ratio of heavy chain, light chain and fibrohexamerin that makes up

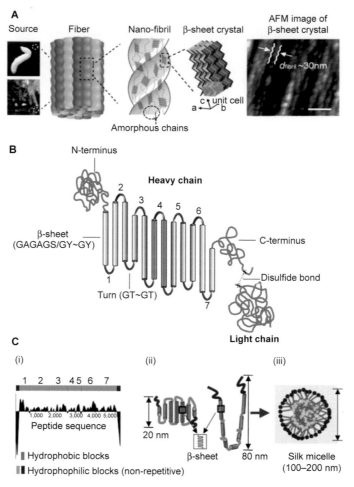

Fig. 1. Overview of the different scales and hierarchical structure of silkworm and spider dragline silk fibres. (A) Both spider and silkworm silks are similar and are composed of numerous interlocking nano-fibrils. The β-sheet crystals stabilise the silk fibril and provides strength while and the amorphous segments within these nano-fibrils endow silk with elasticity. Each β-sheet crystal is composed of stacked sheets that are stabilised by hydrogen bonding between each sheet. The yellow box indicates the unit cell of a single β-sheet crystal. Atomic force microscopy image of the nano-fibrillar structure in *B. mori* silk (scale bar 100 nm). (B) 2 dimensional schematic of *B. mori* silk. Numbers are aligned with the hydrophobicity pattern. (C) Model of *B. mori* heavy chain folding and micelle formation. (i) Hydrophobicity pattern of the heavy chain with (ii) possible chain folding and (iii) micelle assembly of silk in water. Micelle formation is based on the block copolymer configuration of silk with internal smaller hydrophilic domains to promote solubility in water and larger chain terminal hydrophilic blocks in contact with the continuous water phase. (Panel A reproduced with permission from (Xu et al. 2014), panel B from (Ha et al. 2005) and panel C modified from (Jin and Kaplan 2003)).

the silk elementary unit ensures solubility during transport, both intracellularly and in the silk gland (Zhou et al. 2001). However, the heavy chain is of particular importance for the overall physical performance of silk and is believed to have a critical influence on the ability of silk to serve as a biopolymer for drug delivery as well as to assume various forms, including hydrogels (Seib and Kaplan 2013).

The primary sequence of *B. mori* silk heavy chain resembles that of an amphiphilic block co-polymer, with hydrophobic blocks alternating with hydrophilic ones (Ha et al. 2005; Yucel et al. 2014) (Fig. 1c). This block co-polymer is flanked by hydrophilic C- and N-termini composed of completely non-repeating amino acid residues. Specifically, the heavy chain has 12 long hydrophobic, "crystallisable" blocks that are interspaced by 11 nearly identical, less repetitive and more hydrophilic "amorphous" blocks that have an anionic character; the result is an overall silk isoelectric point of approximately 4 (Fig. 1b). The crystallisable blocks are made up of GX repeats and account for 94% of the silk heavy chain sequence (Zhou et al. 2001) (Fig. 1c). The hexa-amino acid sequence, GAGAGS, is the main component of the typical silk β-sheet crystal and is interspersed with small, irregular GAAS tetrapeptides and 60 residues containing GY (GY~GY) sequences (Ha et al. 2005). These GAGAGS/GY~GY crystalline building blocks are usually composed of glycine (G), alanine (A), serine (S), and tyrosine (Y), while valine (V), threonine (T), isoleucine (I) and phenylalanine (F) are not major residue types but sometimes appear in GAGAGS/GY~GY blocks (Ha et al. 2005).

One silk heavy chain has 12 intramolecular antiparallel β-strands and 11 amorphous regions. The amorphous regions typically consist of 31 amino acid with sequence irregularity (GT~GT), but always contain proline residues that can act as major factors for changing the backbone direction (Fig. 1b). The crystalline and amorphous blocks in the silk heavy chain contribute significantly to the fibre's physical properties (Ha et al. 2005). In particular, sequence motifs, such as poly alanine-glycine (polyAG) and polyalanine (polyA) (β sheet–forming), GXX (31-helix), GXG (stiffness), and GPGXX (β spiral), are key components, and their relative positioning and arrangement are intimately tied to the overall material properties (Omenetto and Kaplan 2010).

Manipulation of the crystal form and content allow fine-tuning of the physical properties of silk and subsequently affect its performance as a drug delivery system (Yucel et al. 2014). In aqueous solutions, the crystallisable domains of silk form β-strands and 3-stranded β-sheets, which are stabilised through hydrogen bonding; the increasing interaction of the hydrophobic blocks drives β-sheet formation through lateral and facial packing (Ha et al. 2005; Yucel et al. 2014). The hydrophobic, crystallisable blocks are interspaced by hydrophilic blocks and capped by N- and C-terminal sequences; this block copolymer arrangement drives the formation of 100–200 nm sized spherical micellar structures that contain a hydrophobic core of crystalline/amorphous domains, and a hydrophilic shell of the terminal domains (Jin and Kaplan 2003) (Fig. 1c). These micelles remain loosely assembled, and the assembly process is reversible (Lu et al. 2012).

Under aqueous conditions that mimic the *B. mori* silk gland microenvironment, these nanometre-sized micelles assemble into larger microscale globules (0.8–15 μm) and gel-like states, while maintaining solubility (Werner and Meinel 2015). However, a number of external triggers, such as stretching, shearing, electromagnetic fields, solution concentration, pH and ionic strength cause irreversible physical intermicellar and inter globular crosslinking (Werner and Meinel 2015). The resulting silk networks have an increased β-sheet content and are formed though the self-assembly process detailed above, thereby eliminating the need for use of any harsh chemicals or crosslinkers. The self-assembly of silk into these globular micelles is exploited when generating silk nanoparticles (Werner and Meinel 2015); for example, the addition of an aqueous silk solution to a miscible organic solvent (e.g., acetone) results in nanoprecipitation and formation of nanoparticles (Seib et al. 2013) that are characterised by high crystallinity in the densely packed core (reviewed in (Zhao et al. 2015)).

The silk heavy chain shows crystalline polymorphism with three predominant forms, namely silk I, II and III (Marsh et al. 1955; Valluzzi et al. 1999; Asakura et al. 2013). Silk I is the metastable silk form present in silk solutions (Asakura et al. 2013); it is characterised by intra- and intermolecular bonding repeats of type II and a β-turn structure that result in a more compact silk conformation than seen with silk II (Asakura et al. 2013). Silk II represents the antiparallel β-sheets of crystallised silk that are found in spun silk fibres (Marsh et al. 1955; Asakura et al. 2013); silk III forms a 3-fold extended helix at a water-air interface (Valluzzi et al. 1999). Silk-based drug delivery devices are typically made up of a mixture of β-sheets, β-turns, helices and random coils, although the extent of each can be fined tuned, and this is known to influence drug release (Seib and Kaplan 2013; Yucel et al. 2014).

Spider silks

To date, *B. mori* silk cocoons are the most commonly used silk source for the development of drug delivery systems because *B. mori* silk can be readily mass-produced using sericultures (Seib and Kaplan 2013). In contrast, spiders cannot be farmed; therefore, spider silks are typically obtained by expression using a heterologous host via genetic engineering (Chung et al. 2012). Dragline spider silk is the most commonly studied spider silk because this silk is used to build the frames and radii of orb webs, as well as serving as the spider's safety line (Vollrath and Porter 2009; Porter et al. 2013). This silk is thus endowed with an exceptionally high tensile strength and elasticity to serve its function. Dragline silk is composed of two major proteins: the major ampullate spidroin 1 and 2 (MaSp1 and MaSp2) in silk from the Gold Orb weaver spider (*Nephila clavipes*) and Araneus diadematus fibroin 3 and 4 (ADF-3 and -4) in silk from the common European garden spider (Scheibel 2004). The small peptide motifs of spider silks can be grouped into four major categories: (i) crystalline β-sheet rich poly(A)/poly(GA) motifs (ii) helix forming GGX repeats, (iii) an elastic β-turn-like proline-rich region, composed of multiple GPGXX motifs (where P is proline and X is mostly glutamine) and (iv) a spacer region with currently unknown functions (Tokareva et al. 2014).

Across all araneid, the dragline spider silks have a very high molecular weight (reviewed in (Scheibel 2004)). For example, MaSP 1 and 2 silk proteins possess similar motifs and are approximately 3,500 amino acids long, resulting in a protein with a molecular mass of 250–350 kDa (Sponner et al. 2005; Ayoub et al. 2007). As is the case with *B. mori* silk, spider silks contain long repetitive sequences that are rich in glycine and alanine and are flanked at the C and N termini by non-repeating amino acid sequences approximately 100 amino acids in length (Ayoub et al. 2007); these non-repeating sequences are thought to orchestrate the self-assembly process during spinning (Jin and Kaplan 2003; Exler et al. 2007; Askarieh et al. 2010; Hagn et al. 2010). Analogous to the situation with *B. mori* silk, the polyalanine residues give high tensile strength to the silk fibre. These hydrophobic polyalanine blocks are typically made up of six to nine alanines and several polyalanine chains are required to form the crystalline β-sheet stacks. The glycine-rich motifs, such as GGX or GPGXX, adopt flexible helical structures and act as molecular springs interspersed among the crystalline regions to provide elasticity to the silk thread (Chung et al. 2012; Tokareva et al. 2014).

Unlike *B. mori,* which can be raised as sericultures, spiders are more challenging to raise for silk production and are rarely used as a primary silk source. The large size of naturally occurring spider silks and the highly repetitive nature of these proteins also pose challenges during expression in heterologous hosts, in part due to the limits of the glycyl-tRNA pools in the expression host (Seib and Kaplan 2013). This has recently been overcome by the use of metabolically engineered *E. coli,* where recombinantly expressed silk matched the protein made by spiders with respect to its molecular weight and mechanical properties (Xia et al. 2010). However, most studies that have explored spider silks for drug delivery applications have used the ADF-4 and MaSp1 sequences to generate spider silk-inspired biopolymers that are tens of kDa in size. For example, eADF4-(C16) consists of 16 repeats of module C (GSSAAAAAAAASGPGGYG PENQGPSGPGGYGPGGP), which mimics the repetitive core sequence of ADF4 of the European garden spider and yields a biopolymer 48 kDa in size. This eADF4-(C16) biopolymer has been explored for various drug delivery applications, including silk nanoparticle (Lammel et al. 2011) and hydrogels (Schacht et al. 2015) for drug delivery. Recombinant silks have been the foundation for a number of spin out companies, including eADF4-(C16) which is central to AMSilk's commercial portfolio which now includes silk-based fibres, coatings and cosmetics.

In addition to ADF4, the *Nephila clavipes* MaSp1 silk consensus repeat SGRGGLGGQGAGAAAAAGGAGQGGYGGLGSQGT has been widely studied for the generation of silk (nano)particles, fibres, hydrogels and hybrid materials for both tissue engineering applications and drug delivery (Tokareva et al. 2014). The isolation of spider silk from the expression host will not be reviewed here (see excellent reviews; for example (Scheibel 2004; Chung et al. 2012; Ebrahimi et al. 2015)). However, the extraction procedure used to isolate silk from cocoons has a significant impact on the final biopolymer properties, so this will be briefly reviewed.

Reverse Engineering Silk Cocoons

Silkworm fibres consist of two types of proteins: silk fibroin (commonly referred to as silk) and sericins. Sericin is used by the worm during the spinning process to "glue" silk fibres together. Sericins are commonly removed when processing *B. mori* cocoons, as they are thought to induce an inflammatory response, especially in combination with silk (reviewed in (Altman et al. 2003)). Typical strategies for sericin removal include boiling (i.e., degumming) the cocoons in an aqueous alkaline solution (e.g., sodium carbonate) (Rockwood et al. 2011). While most studies report degumming times ranging from 20 to 60 minutes, a short 5 minute degumming process is usually sufficient to remove the sericin and minimise degradation of the silk. Silk is degraded into smaller fragments during prolonged boiling, which particularly affects the silk light chain, the disulphide bond between the light and heavy chain, and the amorphous regions in the silk heavy chain (Wray et al. 2011). After degumming, the extracted silk fibres can be used to generate yarns, sutures or woven fabrics. However, the generation of new silk material formats, such as silk hydrogels, typically requires that the extracted silk fibre be reverse engineered into an aqueous silk solution that resembles the silk dope found the silk worm's gland. Therefore, the silk fibre is dismantled with the use of chaotropic agents at elevated temperatures (e.g., 9.3 M LiBr at 60°C for up to 4 hours) to disrupt hydrogen bonding and unfold the silk crystalline domains.

The resulting silk solution is dialysed extensively against water to yield an aqueous silk solution of typically 6% w/v. A more concentrated silk solution can be readily obtained by dialysing silk against a 10% w/v polyethylene glycol solution, which withdraws water from the silk preparation. The aqueous silk solution can be processed into various material formats, such as films, fibres, scaffolds, micro- and nanoparticles, as well as hydrogels (Rockwood et al. 2011) (Fig. 2). Irrespective of the silk format, the material needs to be suited for its intended use. In the following section, we will examine the rationale for using the silk biopolymer for drug and cell delivery.

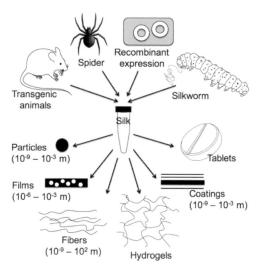

Fig. 2. Diagram of silk sources and silk formats. Numbers in parentheses refer to the approximate sizes of these materials; diameters or thicknesses in the case of particles and films/coatings, respectively (reproduced with permission from (Seib and Kaplan 2013)).

Rationale for Using Silk for Drug and Cell Delivery

A number of important attributes are typically cited in support of using silk for cell and drug delivery, including (i) biocompatibility, (ii) biodegradability, (iii) mild processing conditions, (iv) protection of the payload and (v) approved use in humans. Silk fibres are United States of America Food and Drug Administration (FDA) and European Medicines Authority (EMA) approved biomaterials for use in humans as medical sutures; silk-based surgical meshes have also received FDA/EMA approval. These meshes have been developed by Serica Technologies, Inc. Medford MA,

USA (subsequently acquired in 2010 by Allergan, Inc.) using technology originally developed by David Kaplan and co-workers at Tufts University, MA, USA. Data from two clinical trials with these surgical meshes have been encouraging, with high levels of investigator and patient satisfaction scores and no adverse reactions due to the silk mesh (De Vita et al. 2014; Fine et al. 2015). Early phase trials are currently ongoing to test BioShield-S1 silk coatings of silicone breast implants to improve host–tissue responses [based on eADF4(C16) spider silks manufactured by AMSilk, Munich, Germany]; these clinical studies were preceded by successful *in vivo* studies that showed no acute systemic toxicity and immunogenicity with eADF4(C16), as well as a significant reduction in capsule formation with the silk-coated silicon implants (Zeplin et al. 2014). In particular, the successful track record of silk sutures for use in humans has served as the launching platform for the development of silk-based materials for biomedical applications, including cell and drug delivery.

Biocompatibility

Nonetheless, the generic use of the term "biocompatibility" to describe silks is potentially misleading. In particular, the notion that any natural material automatically qualifies as biocompatible is widespread but misleading, with potentially disastrous consequences. For example, some of the most toxic compounds known to man are of natural origin (e.g., botulinum toxin). When used clinically and for aesthetic purposes, both the dose and route of administration are critical for safe use. Therefore, all (bio)materials need careful assessment prior to their *in vivo* use. The biocompatibility definition by David Williams "refers to the ability to perform as a substrate that will support the appropriate cellular activity, including the facilitation of molecular and mechanical signalling systems, in order to optimise tissue regeneration, without eliciting any undesirable local or systemic responses in the eventual host" (Williams 2008). Although silk has a proven track record in humans as a suture material, context specific biocompatibility assessment is still required when silk is being used beyond its licensed applications. For example, silk has been proposed for various vascular tissue engineering applications, but without first undergoing rigorous haematocompatibility assessment. We have assessed the blood compatibility of silk and were able to demonstrate a low haemostasis activity but an inflammatory response that was in part dependent on the processing history of the silk (Seib et al. 2012; Seib et al. 2014).

Silk biocompatibility

In vivo studies in rats indicated that silk films implanted intramuscularly induced a mild inflammatory response, appearing in the form of fibroblasts, few new blood vessels and macrophages at the implant-host interface. This type of tissue response was more noticeable for polylactide and collagen films at 6 weeks post implantation than for silk films (Meinel et al. 2005). The silk scaffolds also showed different *in vivo* degradation behaviour depending on whether they were generated by water- or solvent-based processing. For example, water-based silk scaffolds with large pore sizes (850–1,000 μm) were completely degraded and resorbed within 6 months, while solvent-based silk scaffolds with a similar pore size showed significantly less degradation over the same time course, with residual material still present one year after implantation. Throughout the study, the animals showed no visible signs of any adverse response. The low host immune response towards the implant was inferred by comparing mRNA expression of various markers, including interferon-γ, tumour necrosis factor-α and interleukins, from the retrieved scaffolds and control tissues (Wang et al. 2008). The results indicated that the macrophages recruited towards the silk were the main contributors to silk degradation, because only scaffolds that allowed cell infiltration showed any substantial degradation over the study period (Wang et al. 2008). Silk has been reported to induce a transient and mild foreign body response that activates the complement system, but this response typically subsides within 14 days and does not progress to a chronic inflammatory response (Thurber et al. 2015).

All biomaterials derived from a non-autologous source will elicit a foreign body response following implantation *in vivo*, albeit to varying degrees (Altman et al. 2003). Historically, adverse reactions reported for silk sutures can be largely attributed to the use of virgin silk fibres that contained contaminating sericin, as this causes an allergic reaction, or to the use of braided silk fibres that were coated with waxes (commonly referred to as black braided silk) (Altman et al. 2003). Silk fibroin elicits a foreign body response following implantation *in vivo* (Thurber et al. 2015), but this response is comparable to that elicited by the most popular synthetic materials in use today as biomaterials [e.g., poly(lactic-co-glycolic acid), polycaprolactone, polylactic acid].

The intensity of the biological response also depends on the implantation site and the model used for investigation. For example, silk scaffolds, films and hydrogels are commonly implanted subcutaneously (Thurber et al. 2015) and are expected to result in different biological responses when compared to that triggered by their placement into immune privileged sites such as the back of the eye (e.g., vitreous, retina), the testicles and, to some extent, the articular cartilage. A different biological response would be expected yet again following the administration of silk directly into tissues of the immune system, such as the spleen, lymph nodes or liver.

Information is currently limited regarding the tissue response towards silk hydrogels, but the available data are encouraging (Etienne et al. 2009; Critchfield et al. 2014; Hamilton et al. 2015). For example, injection of sonication-induced silk hydrogels into the cervix of pregnant rats (gestational day 13) as a potential therapeutic approach to preterm birth (Critchfield et al. 2014; Brown et al. 2016) resulted in a mild foreign body response similar to that observed with polyglycolic acid and poly(ethylene terephthalate) sutures (Critchfield et al. 2014). These *in vivo* studies assessed the biological response at 4 days post treatment, and they were supplemented by *in vitro* studies with human cervical cells, which showed no up-regulation of inflammatory markers. However, the longer-term effects, such as longitudinal inflammatory responses, biodegradation or impacts on pregnancy (e.g., a shift to a post-term pregnancy), are currently unknown (Critchfield et al. 2014).

One longer-term study compared silk hydrogels to collagen type I hydrogels both *in vitro* and *in vivo* (Etienne et al. 2009). Nude mice, at one and two weeks post implantation of silk hydrogels, showed signs of inflammation in the tissues surrounding the silk hydrogels, as indicated by the presence of eosinophils, neutrophils and macrophages around the hydrogel periphery, but showed no infiltration of these cells within the hydrogel network. However, this silk-induced inflammatory response was less intense than that observed for collagen hydrogels, which attracted numerous neutrophils, eosinophils and macrophages that infiltrated the material and subsequently degraded the hydrogel completely within 4 weeks. At week 4, the inflammation around the silk hydrogel was greatly reduced and the hydrogel had cracks that were populated by spindle shaped cells; at 3 months, no inflammatory cells could be detected in or around the silk hydrogels, but vascularisation was apparent and the interstitial spaces were populated by stromal cells. Corroborating these observations are results from subcutaneously implanted 8% w/v silk hydrogels in rats, where significant hydrogel remodelling was initiated at 15 weeks post implantation, resulting in vascularisation, loss of hydrogel shape and degradation (Hamilton et al. 2015).

Silk Biodegradation

Most studies reporting the *in vivo* biodegradation of silk have assessed films and scaffolds; only a few studies have characterized silk hydrogels. One study used sonication-induced sol-gels that were preformed *ex vivo* and subsequently surgically implanted in mice. Cylindrically shaped 8 × 6 mm silk hydrogels generated from a 4% w/v silk solution were subcutaneously implanted in nude mice and the biological response assessed over 12 weeks (Etienne et al. 2009). At the endpoint of this study, fragmentation of the silk hydrogel was reported, although the hydrogel maintained its shape and showed signs of vascularisation (Etienne et al. 2009). However, the exact extent of silk hydrogel degradation was not assessed as well as the process of vascularisation.

Silk is biodegradable due to its susceptibility to proteases and enzyme-catalysed hydrolysis reactions. In particular, the disulphide bond between the light and heavy chains, as well as the amorphous silk sequences, are highly susceptible to degradation. In contrast, the crystalline regions are most resistant to proteolytic degradation due to reduced chain flexibility and access. Therefore, the β-sheet content has a protective effect on silk degradation both *in vitro* (Li et al. 2003; Horan et al. 2005; Meinel et al. 2005; Numata et al. 2010; Brown et al. 2015) and *in vivo* (Meinel et al. 2005; Wang et al. 2008). However, differences in packing geometries exist within the crystalline regions, ranging from tight to looser chain packing. This, in turn, results in differences in degradation behaviour; the tightly packed crystalline regions are made up of highly ordered β-sheets while the looser packing contains less ordered β-sheets as well as turn-and random-coil structures (Numata et al. 2010). In particular, the more loosely packed crystalline regions are susceptible to degradation and are degraded first.

Protease XIV is a useful proteolytic model enzyme for uncovering some of the fundamentals of silk degradation over short study intervals (e.g., hours to days). For example, protease XIV studies showed that digestion of the more loosely packed β-sheets yielded nanofibrils around 4 nm thick and 80–100 nm wide that persisted over the course of the *in vitro* degradation study (24 h), as well as soluble silk fragments. Cytotoxicity studies indicated that these protease XIV digested silk samples reduced cell viability (IC_{50} 75 µg/ml), whereas disease-associated β-sheets of amyloid β-peptide fibrils (IC_{50} 20 µg/ml) were more cytotoxic (Numata et al. 2010).

At first sight, these observations might seem alarming, but a number of points need to be considered. First, no similar observations were made with silk that was degraded using α-chymotrypsin to yield insoluble silk crystals and soluble hydrophilic domains; these showed no cytotoxicity at the maximum tested concentration ($IC_{50} > 225$ μg/ml), in sharp contrast to protease XIV degradation that generated soluble fragments with β-sheet structures (Numata et al. 2010). Second, protease XIV is a non-mammalian enzyme; therefore, its degradation products are not necessarily encountered *in vivo*. Third, the degradation products generated by chymotrypsin, a mammalian enzyme, showed no cytotoxicity. Fourth, *in vivo* studies, and indeed observations in human clinical trials and during routine use of silk sutures, have not shown any overt adverse effects due to inadequate biodegradation. The US Pharmacopeia classifies silk sutures as non-resorbable. However, this is based on the definition that the material "loses most of its tensile strength within 60 days" post-implantation *in vivo*. Silk sutures significantly degrade within 1 year, and they are completely resorbed within 2 years (Altman et al. 2003).

In vitro studies and mapping of the silk primary sequence to a known protease cleavage site indicated that serine proteases (e.g., α-chymotrypsin, collagenase) and matrix metalloproteinases (MMPs) (MMP-1, interstitial collagenase, and MMP-2, gelatinase A) are particularly active in silk degradation (Brown et al. 2015). Our current understanding of silk degradation (Brown et al. 2015) and emerging evidence suggest that the amorphous regions of silk hydrogels are degraded first. Thus, at an equivalent silk and β-sheet content, silk in hydrogel form is likely to be degraded fastest due to the open hydrogel frame structure, followed by porous scaffolds and films, where the monolithic structure restricts water ingress and thus hinders access of enzymes to the amorphous silk segments.

Silk Hydrogel Manufacture

Silk hydrogels can be broadly classified into physically (Ayub et al. 1993) and chemically crosslinked systems (Min et al. 1998).

Physically crosslinked silk hydrogels

A number of strategies have been explored to generate physically crosslinked silk hydrogels, including (i) ultrasound (Wang et al. 2008), (ii) vortexing (Yucel et al. 2009), (iii) CO_2 acidification (Floren et al. 2012), (iv) non-solvent induced phase separation (Kasoju et al. 2016), (v) electrical fields (Leisk et al. 2010; Lu et al. 2011), (vi) temperature (Kim et al. 2004), (vii) osmotic stress (Kim et al. 2004; Ribeiro et al. 2014) and (viii) pH (Ayoub et al. 2007). The underlying basis of all these systems is the self-assembling behaviour of silk, which forms hydrogels due to the physical entanglements and hydrogen bonding between hydrophobic domains of the silk block copolymer. Under aqueous conditions, this self-assembly into micelles is a thermodynamic process, whose kinetics depend on molecular mobility, charge, hydrophilic interactions and concentration (Lu et al. 2012). Therefore, any changes in these parameters due to the chosen processing technique will directly affect the final format of the silk.

Emerging evidence suggests that the silk I format is promoted by a high silk solution concentration (20% w/v) that causes the silk micelles to assemble initially into nanofilamentous structures. These silk I structures are metastable and do not involve changes in secondary structure, but they undergo weak hydrogen bonding as well as hydrophobic and electrostatic interactions (Matsumoto et al. 2006; Lu et al. 2012). This initial stage is followed by changes to the secondary structure, including the formation of β-sheets (Matsumoto et al. 2006), which give rise to strong intermolecular interactions and stabilise the silk hydrogel network, making the hydrogel structure essentially irreversible (Matsumoto et al. 2006). In contrast, low silk concentrations (1% w/v) promote the formation of silk micelles that transition directly into micellar aggregates (Lu et al. 2012).

Shearing of silk aqueous solutions (i.e., by vortexing, sonication, etc.) speeds up the self-assembling kinetics and results in the formation of silk hydrogels within minutes to hours. These hydrogels transition from a random coil conformation to a β-sheet that contains some inter-chain physical crosslinks. In time, large numbers of inter-chain β-sheet crosslinks form and stabilise the overall structure (Wang et al. 2008). The kinetics of this process can be further expedited by increasing the silk concentration, solution temperature, concentration of K^+ ions, acidity (i.e., low pH) and energy input. However, excessive sonication leads to fragmentation of the silk fibres and negatively impacts hydrogel formation (Samal et al. 2013).

The hydrogels that are produced by reducing the solution pH to a value close to the silk isoelectric point (pH 4.2) are characterized by extensive β-sheets (Ayub et al. 1993). The responsiveness of silk to pH is governed by its amphiphilic nature, due to the presence of large hydrophobic blocks interspersed with hydrophilic amorphous regions, and due to its hydrophilic C- and N-termini. The N-terminus of the silk heavy chain is acidic (isoelectric point 4.6) and the C-terminus is basic (isoelectric point 10.5) whereas the C-terminus of the light chain is acidic (isoelectric point 5.1) (Kapoor and Kundu 2016). The acidic groups become protonated at low pH, leading to a reduced charge-charge repulsion that subsequently allows silk to adopt a more ordered state, with the formation of β-sheets that exclude water (He et al. 2012).

The use of high pressure CO_2 during silk hydrogel manufacture acidifies the silk solution while changing the hydration shell and increasing the propensity for reduced volume states of silk. At high pressure, CO_2 generates carbonic acid and, according to Henry's law, this process is directly proportional to the applied pressure. Experimental and theoretical calculations have shown the occurrence of robust gelation within 2 hours, yielding silk hydrogels that were at least 2 fold more robust mechanically than hydrogels generated using traditional pH approaches (Floren et al. 2012).

Water exclusion and subsequent β-sheet formation have been proposed for silk hydrogels formed under osmotic stress, pH, increased temperature (Matsumoto et al. 2006) and non-solvent induced phase separation (Kasoju et al. 2016). However, silk hydrogels generated using low electrical DC fields differ markedly from those formed by these other processes, as they are formed through electrogelation (and are therefore referred to as e-gels). They deposit on the positive electrode and their formation is completed within minutes (Leisk et al. 2010).

The electrogelation process is based on local pH changes that occur due to water electrolysis. The local pH drops at the positive electrode to a value below the

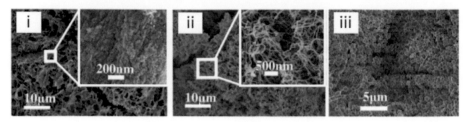

Fig. 3. Silk e-gel processing, characterisation and structure. Scanning electron micrographs of different hydrogel morphologies derived from silk solution (i) of low and (ii) high concentration and (iii) silk e-gel. Reproduced with permission from (Lu et al. 2012).

isoelectric point of silk, thereby enabling silk deposition on the electrode (Lu et al. 2011; Kojic et al. 2012). The formation of the silk hydrogel can be predicted by ion electrodiffusion (Kojic et al. 2012).

Analysis of the secondary structure of the silk in e-gels indicated a transition from a random coil conformation to a helical conformation, but no changes in β-sheet content (as typically seen for sonicated or vortexed silk hydrogels). Reversal of the electric field led to a dissociation of the silk hydrogel and subsequent formation at the new positive electrode; this process could undergo many repeat cycles (Leisk et al. 2010). High resolution imaging showed that these hydrogels were formed from nanometre sized silk micelles that were metastable (Lu et al. 2011). In the presence of a weak electric field, these silk micelles formed larger spherical structures that ranged from nanometres to several micrometres in size. These particles were able to assemble into hydrogels because the negative surface charge of the silk particles was screened by the low pH in the vicinity of the positive electrode (Lu et al. 2011). Overall, silk e-gels have been proposed for a range of biomedical applications due to their ability to control silk hydrogel assembly and to trigger the release of silk particles upon charge reversal, and because of the excellent adhesive properties of these hydrogels (Leisk et al. 2010; Lu et al. 2011; Kojic et al. 2012).

Physically crosslinked silk hydrogels are particularly promising for drug delivery and biomedical applications because their formation does not rely on chemical crosslinking and therefore avoids the use of potentially harmful agents such as organic solvents, chemical initiators or UV irradiation. Residual chemicals can leach from chemically crosslinked hydrogels, while UV-based polymerisation techniques are incompatible with cell viability. Silk hydrogels formed by sonication and vortexing are particularly well suited for drug and cell delivery because the payload can be added after the silk treatment but prior to the onset of gelation (Seib and Kaplan 2013). However, physically crosslinked silk hydrogels show limited elastic behaviour and plastic deformation occurs typically at strains greater than 10%.

Most physically crosslinked silk hydrogels rely on β-sheet crystals to stabilise the hydrogel network, which results in brittleness that prevents long range displacements and culminates in low elastic behaviour. The e-gels are notable exceptions, as they have outstanding elastic properties and can withstand strains of up to 2,500%. Nevertheless, they require the use of an electric current to generate the low pH; an approach that is not compatible with cells. Therefore, alternative silk hydrogels are being developed that show better elastic behaviour.

Chemically crosslinked silk hydrogels

Chemically crosslinked silk hydrogels have been synthesised using a range of chemistries (Kapoor and Kundu 2016). For example, horseradish peroxidase has been used to crosslink the phenol groups in the tyrosine amino acids in the silk protein (Partlow et al. 2014). This generated elastic silk hydrogels that could withstand a shear strain of 100% and a compressive strain greater than 70%. The stiffness of these silk hydrogels could be fine tuned to range from 200 to 10,000 Pa by adjusting the silk degumming times between 60 and 10 minutes, respectively. These crosslinked silk hydrogels are optically clear over the visible wavelength spectrum (Partlow et al. 2014), making them different from physically crosslinked gels that typically contain nanocrystalline regions that scatter light. Horseradish peroxidase crosslinked silk hydrogels have subsequently been exposed to low-energy ultrafast laser pulses to generate complex 3D patterns within the hydrogels that could subsequently be populated with cells (Applegate et al. 2015). Riboflavin, a photoactive crosslinker, has recently been used to generate *in situ* crosslinked silk corneal prostheses with the aim of improving visual acuity (Applegate et al. 2016).

Examples of Silk Hydrogels for Cell and Drug Delivery

Silk hydrogels have been studied for a broad range of biomedical applications, including cell and drug delivery. For example, self-assembling silk hydrogels were developed for breast cancer focal therapy (Seib et al. 2013). Sonication-induced hydrogels were drug loaded prior to the onset of gelation and drug release was subsequently assessed *in vitro*. Drug release was not affected by the silk degumming time, but doxorubicin release from these hydrogels was significantly affected by the weight percentage of the silk. Hydrogels with the lowest silk content released the drug fastest (27% cumulative drug release over 30 days), whereas the hydrogels with the highest amount of silk had the slowest drug release (17% cumulative drug release over 30 days) (Seib et al. 2013). Injection of drug loaded silk hydrogels in close proximity to well-established orthotopic breast tumours, followed by *in vivo* monitoring and necropsy, showed that these hydrogels were well tolerated in biological systems. Complete tumour regression was observed in two of five animals investigated, and breast cancer metastasis was reduced when compared to animals administered an equivalent amount of doxorubicin by bolus intravenous injection (Seib et al. 2013).

Sonication-induced silk hydrogels have also been used for ocular drug delivery of an antivascular endothelial growth factor (bevacizumab) (Lovett et al. 2015). *In vitro* drug release from 2% w/v silk hydrogels loaded with 5.0 mg of bevacizumab revealed a controlled drug release over 90 days for both doses. By contrast, the control

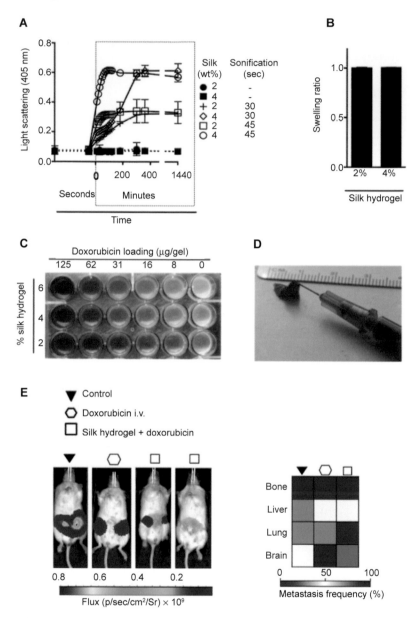

Fig. 4. Self-assembling silk hydrogels for focal breast cancer focal therapy. (A) Impact of processing parameters on the sol-gel kinetics of silk. (B) Silk hydrogels show no swelling post sol-gel transition. (C) Silk hydrogels can be readily loaded with drug; here, doxorubicin was added prior to the onset of gelation. (D) Injectability of drug loaded silk hydrogels. (E) Response of human breast cancer xenografts to treatment. Bioluminescence imaging of primary breast tumours at the end of the study and extent of metastasis (Reproduced with permission from (Seib et al. 2013)).

drug formulation, Avastin, was eliminated form the test system within 30 days. The hydrogels showed an initial burst release (up to day 10) and a similar release profile to Avastin between days 11 and 20, but then showed a sustained zero order drug release over the remaining 60 days of the study. By contrast, drug release was exhausted for the Avastin control group by day 30. Pharmacokinetic assessment of the bevacizumab loaded silk hydrogels revealed an increase of two to three fold in the terminal elimination half-life in the vitreous and aqueous humour. *In vivo* biocompatibility studies indicated no overt adverse reactions due to the silk hydrogels over the course of the study, as verified by gross examination of the hydrogels, ophthalmic examination and fundus imaging. The silk hydrogels showed some signs of degradation from day 30 onwards, although the hydrogels (50 µl volume) were still present at the end of the study (day 90) (Lovett et al. 2015).

Physically crosslinked silk hydrogels show shear thinning, making them well suited for injection. Silk also has a remarkable ability to stabilise therapeutic proteins, largely due to the nanocrystalline regions that perform several functions, including providing a buffering capacity, tailoring water content at the nanoscale level and providing physical protection (reviewed in (Pritchard et al. 2012)). Therefore, silk hydrogels serve as a delivery vehicle but they also provide active support for the payload.

The excellent material properties of silk have supported the development of various hydrogel systems for soft and hard tissue engineering applications (Omenetto and Kaplan 2010). More recently, silk hydrogels have been assessed as a potential delivery system for pancreatic islet transplantation (Hamilton et al. 2015). Vortex induced silk hydrogels were generated and pancreatic islets were added prior to the onset of gelation and compared *in vivo* to pancreatic islet transplantations in the absence of silk. A third treatment group included silk hydrogel transplants that contained pancreatic islets and mesenchymal stem cells (MSCs). Diabetic mice regained glycaemic control, with the best control observed with the pancreatic islets and MSC silk hydrogels. However, histological assessment indicated that the MSCs had not only supported the graft but had also differentiated into bone and cartilage; an outcome that was not intended. Therefore, silk hydrogels not only served as a delivery vehicle but also mimicked the extracellular matrix (ECM) that stem cells sense and respond to (Hamilton et al. 2015). The viscoelastic properties of physically crosslinked silk hydrogels have received little attention to date, although emerging evidence indicates that rapid stress relaxation of viscoelastic hydrogels supports osteogenesis of MSCs (Chaudhuri et al. 2015). Indeed, ECMs found *in vivo* are viscoelastic; therefore, physically crosslinked silk hydrogels are well placed to serve as ECM mimetics. However, these silk hydrogels are brittle, so alternatives to chemical crosslinking need to be explored. In this context, the inclusion of silk fibres has emerged as a valuable strategy (Yodmuang et al. 2015), and silk fibre reinforced silk hydrogels have now been successfully used for the culture of chondrocytes. At day 40, these tissue engineered cartilage constructs closely resembled native tissue in both composition and physical performance (Yodmuang et al. 2015).

The spectrum of use of silk hydrogels goes beyond typical cell and drug delivery applications. For example, as part of the 3R initiative (i.e., replacement, refinement and reduction of animal experiments), silk-based brain dummies made from silk scaffolds and collagen type I hydrogels have been developed to study traumatic brain injury (Tang-Schomer et al. 2014). These constructs faithfully recapitulate the brain's biophysical properties (Tang-Schomer et al. 2014) and, in future studies, could be used as a model system to study neurophysiology. Print technologies have been used to process both chemically modified *B. mori* silk solution (Suntivich et al. 2014) and recombinant spider silks (Schacht et al. 2015). The spider silks were used as aqueous solutions to encapsulate cells and were then allowed to undergo gelation. This mixture was subsequently extruded by application of pressure through an electromagnetically controlled valve. The resulting 3D constructs could be readily manufactured to a 500 μm resolution, and they supported cell viability.

Summary and Outlook

This chapter summarises recent developments in the production and use of silk-based hydrogels for cell and drug delivery. We have primarily focused on silk hydrogels, but have used other silk formats for reference purposes, as a substantial body of work is available regarding silk particles, films and scaffolds for drug and cell delivery (Kasoju and Bora 2012; Seib and Kaplan 2013; Yucel et al. 2014; Zhao et al. 2015). This chapter has also omitted the development of silk "alloys" (e.g., recombinantly engineered silk elastins, reviewed in (Rnjak-Kovacina and Kaplan 2013; Price et al. 2014)) due to space constraints. Overall, silk is a truly remarkable biopolymer that will continue to amaze us. Clearly, at the time of this writing, silk is poised to change the way we deliver cells and drugs in the clinical setting.

Acknowledgement

The author would like to thank Thidarat Wongpinyochit for feedback on the manuscript and Dr. Jelena Rnjak-Kovacina, University of New South Wales, Sydney, Australia for insightful discussion and advice. This research was supported in part by a Marie Curie FP7 Career Integration Grant 334134 within the 7th European Union Framework Program and an EPSRC First Grant EP/N03127X/1.

References

Altman, G.H., F. Diaz, C. Jakuba, T. Calabro, R.L. Horan, J. Chen et al. 2003. Silk-based biomaterials. Biomaterials. 24: 401–416.

Applegate, M.B., J. Coburn, B.P. Partlow, J.E. Moreau, J.P. Mondia, B. Marelli et al. 2015. Laser-based three-dimensional multiscale micropatterning of biocompatible hydrogels for customized tissue engineering scaffolds. Proc. Natl. Acad. Sci. USA. 112: 12052–12057.

Applegate, M.B., B.P. Partlow, J. Coburn, B. Marelli, C. Pirie, R. Pineda et al. 2016. Photocrosslinking of silk fibroin using riboflavin for ocular prostheses. Adv. Mater.

Asakura, T., Y. Suzuki, Y. Nakazawa, G.P. Holland and J.L. Yarger. 2013. Elucidating silk structure using solid-state NMR. Soft Matter. 9: 11440–11450.

Askarieh, G., M. Hedhammar, K. Nordling, A. Saenz, C. Casals, A. Rising et al. 2010. Self-assembly of spider silk proteins is controlled by a pH-sensitive relay. Nature. 465: 236–238.

Ayoub, N.A., J.E. Garb, R.M. Tinghitella, M.A. Collin and C.Y. Hayashi. 2007. Blueprint for a high-performance biomaterial: full-length spider dragline silk genes. PLoS One. 2: e514.

Ayub, Z.H., M. Arai and K. Hirabayashi. 1993. Mechanism of the gelation of fibroin solution. Biosci. Biotech. Biochem. 57: 1910–1912.

Brown, J., C.L. Lu, J. Coburn and D.L. Kaplan. 2015. Impact of silk biomaterial structure on proteolysis. Acta Biomater. 11: 212–221.

Brown, J.E., B.P. Partlow, A.M. Berman, M.D. House and D.L. Kaplan. 2016. Injectable silk-based biomaterials for cervical tissue augmentation: an *in vitro* study. Am. J. Obstet. Gynecol. 214: 118 e111–119.

Buehler, M.J. 2013. Materials by design-a perspective from atoms to structures. MRS Bull. 38: 169–176.

Chaudhuri, O., L. Gu, D. Klumpers, M. Darnell, S.A. Bencherif, J.C. Weaver et al. 2015. Hydrogels with tunable stress relaxation regulate stem cell fate and activity. Nat. Mater.

Chung, H., T.Y. Kim and S.Y. Lee. 2012. Recent advances in production of recombinant spider silk proteins. Curr. Opin. Biotechnol. 23: 957–964.

Critchfield, A.S., R. McCabe, N. Klebanov, L. Richey, S. Socrate, E.R. Norwitz et al. 2014. Biocompatibility of a sonicated silk gel for cervical injection during pregnancy: *in vivo* and *in vitro* study. Reprod. Sci. 21: 1266–1273.

De Vita, R., E.M. Buccheri, M. Pozzi and G. Zoccali. 2014. Direct to implant breast reconstruction by using SERI, preliminary report. J. Exp. Clin. Cancer Res. 33: 78.

Ebrahimi, D., O. Tokareva, N.G. Rim, J.Y. Wong, D.L. Kaplan and M.J. Buehler. 2015. Silk—its mysteries, how it is made, and how it is used. ACS Biomater. Sci. Eng. 1: 864–876.

Etienne, O., A. Schneider, J.A. Kluge, C. Bellemin-Laponnaz, C. Polidori, G.G. Leisk et al. 2009. Soft tissue augmentation using silk gels: an *in vitro* and *in vivo* study. J. Periodontol. 80: 1852–1858.

Exler, J.H., D. Hummerich and T. Scheibel. 2007. The amphiphilic properties of spider silks are important for spinning. Angew. Chem. Int. Ed. Engl. 46: 3559–3562.

Fine, N.A., M. Lehfeldt, J.E. Gross, S. Downey, G.M. Kind, G. Duda et al. 2015. SERI surgical scaffold, prospective clinical trial of a silk-derived biological scaffold in two-stage breast reconstruction: 1-year data. Plast. Reconstr. Surg. 135: 339–351.

Floren, M.L., S. Spilimbergo, A. Motta and C. Migliaresi. 2012. Carbon dioxide induced silk protein gelation for biomedical applications. Biomacromolecules. 13: 2060–2072.

Gatesy, J., C. Hayashi, D. Motriuk, J. Woods and R. Lewis. 2001. Extreme diversity, conservation, and convergence of spider silk fibroin sequences. Science. 291: 2603–2605.

Ha, S.W., H.S. Gracz, A.E. Tonelli and S.M. Hudson. 2005. Structural study of irregular amino acid sequences in the heavy chain of Bombyx mori silk fibroin. Biomacromolecules. 6: 2563–2569.

Hagn, F., L. Eisoldt, J.G. Hardy, C. Vendrely, M. Coles, T. Scheibel et al. 2010. A conserved spider silk domain acts as a molecular switch that controls fibre assembly. Nature. 465: 239–242.

Hamilton, D.C., H.H. Shih, R.A. Schubert, S.A. Michie, P.N. Staats, D.L. Kaplan et al. 2015. A silk-based encapsulation platform for pancreatic islet transplantation improves islet function *in vivo*. J. Tissue Eng. Regen. Med.

Hardy, J.G. and T.R. Scheibel. 2009. Silk-inspired polymers and proteins. Biochem. Soc. Trans. 37: 677–681.

He, Y.X., N.N. Zhang, W.F. Li, N. Jia, B.Y. Chen, K. Zhou et al. 2012. N-Terminal domain of *Bombyx mori* fibroin mediates the assembly of silk in response to pH decrease. J. Mol. Biol. 418: 197–207.

Horan, R.L., K. Antle, A.L. Collette, Y. Wang, J. Huang, J.E. Moreau et al. 2005. *In vitro* degradation of silk fibroin. Biomaterials. 26: 3385–3393.

Inoue, S., K. Tanaka, F. Arisaka, S. Kimura, K. Ohtomo and S. Mizuno. 2000. Silk fibroin of *Bombyx mori* is secreted, assembling a high molecular mass elementary unit consisting of H-chain, L-chain, and P25, with a 6:6:1 molar ratio. J. Biol. Chem. 275: 40517–40528.

Inoue, S., K. Tanaka, H. Tanaka, K. Ohtomo, T. Kanda, M. Imamura et al. 2004. Assembly of the silk fibroin elementary unit in endoplasmic reticulum and a role of L-chain for protection of α1,2-mannose residues in N-linked oligosaccharide chains of fibrohexamerin/P25. Eur. J. Biochem. 27: 356–366.

Jin, H.J. and D.L. Kaplan. 2003. Mechanism of silk processing in insects and spiders. Nature. 424: 1057–1061.

Kapoor, S. and S.C. Kundu. 2016. Silk protein-based hydrogels: promising advanced materials for biomedical applications. Acta Biomater. 31: 17–32.

Kasoju, N. and U. Bora. 2012. Silk fibroin in tissue engineering. Adv. Healthc. Mater. 1: 393–412.

Kasoju, N., N. Hawkins, O. Pop-Georgievski, D. Kubies and F. Vollrath. 2016. Silk fibroin gelation via non-solvent induced phase separation. Biomater. Sci.

Kim, D.H., J. Viventi, J.J. Amsden, J. Xiao, L. Vigeland, Y.S. Kim et al. 2010. Dissolvable films of silk fibroin for ultrathin conformal bio-integrated electronics. Nat. Mater. 9: 511–517.

Kim, U.J., J. Park, C. Li, H.J. Jin, R. Valluzzi and D.L. Kaplan. 2004. Structure and properties of silk hydrogels. Biomacromolecules. 5: 786–792.

Kluge, J.A., O. Rabotyagova, G.G. Leisk and D.L. Kaplan. 2008. Spider silks and their applications. Trends Biotechnol. 26: 244–251.

Kojic, N., M.J. Panzer, G.G. Leisk, W.K. Raja, M. Kojicd and D.L. Kaplan. 2012. Ion electrodiffusion governs silk electrogelation. Soft Matter. 8: 6897–6905.

Lammel, A., M. Schwab, M. Hofer, G. Winter and T. Scheibel. 2011. Recombinant spider silk particles as drug delivery vehicles. Biomaterials. 32: 2233–2240.

Leisk, G.G., T.J. Lo, T. Yucel, Q. Lu and D.L. Kaplan. 2010. Electrogelation for protein adhesives. Adv. Mater. 22: 711–715.

Li, M., M. Ogiso and N. Minoura. 2003. Enzymatic degradation behavior of porous silk fibroin sheets. Biomaterials. 24: 357–365.

Lovett, M.L., X. Wang, T. Yucel, L. York, M. Keirstead, L. Haggerty et al. 2015. Silk hydrogels for sustained ocular delivery of anti-vascular endothelial growth factor (anti-VEGF) therapeutics. Eur. J. Pharm. Biopharm. 95: 271–278.

Lu, Q., Y. Huang, M. Li, B. Zuo, S. Lu, J. Wang et al. 2011. Silk fibroin electrogelation mechanisms. Acta Biomater. 7: 2394–2400.

Lu, Q., H. Zhu, C. Zhang, F. Zhang, B. Zhang and D.L. Kaplan. 2012. Silk self-assembly mechanisms and control from thermodynamics to kinetics. Biomacromolecules. 13: 826–832.

Lubec, G., J. Holbaubek, C. Feidl, B. Lucec and E. Strouhal. 1993. Use of silk in acient Egypt. Nature. 362: 25.

Marsh, R.E., R.B. Corey and L. Pauling. 1955. An investigation of the structure of silk fibroin. Biochem. Biophys. Acta. 16: 1–34.

Matsumoto, A., J. Chen, A.L. Collette, U.J. Kim, G.H. Altman, P. Cebe et al. 2006. Mechanisms of silk fibroin sol-gel transitions. J. Phys. Chem. B. 110: 21630–21638.

Meinel, L., S. Hofmann, V. Karageorgiou, C. Kirker-Head, J. McCool, G. Gronowicz et al. 2005. The inflammatory responses to silk films *in vitro* and *in vivo*. Biomaterials. 26: 147–155.

Min, S., T. Nakamura, A. Teramoto and K. Abe. 1998. Preparation and characterization of crosslinked porous silk fibroin gel. Fiber. 54: 85–92.

Numata, K., P. Cebe and D.L. Kaplan. 2010. Mechanism of enzymatic degradation of beta-sheet crystals. Biomaterials. 31: 2926–2933.

Omenetto, F.G. and D.L. Kaplan. 2008. A new route for silk. Nat. Photonics. 2: 641–643.

Omenetto, F.G. and D.L. Kaplan. 2010. New opportunities for an ancient material. Science. 329: 528–531.

Partlow, B.P., C.W. Hanna, J. Rnjak-Kovacina, J.E. Moreau, M.B. Applegate, K.A. Burke et al. 2014. Highly tunable elastomeric silk biomaterials. Adv. Funct. Mater. 24: 4615–4624.

Porter, D., J. Guan and F. Vollrath. 2013. Spider silk: super material or thin fibre? Adv. Mater. 25: 1275–1279.

Price, R., A. Poursaid and H. Ghandehari. 2014. Controlled release from recombinant polymers. J. Control. Release. 190: 304–313.

Pritchard, E.M., P.B. Dennis, F.G. Omenetto, R.R. Naik and D.L. Kaplan. 2012. Physical and chemical aspects of stabilization of compounds in silk. Biopolymers. 97: 479–498.

Ribeiro, M., M.A. de Moraes, M.M. Beppu, F.J. Monteiro and M.P. Ferraz. 2014. The role of dialysis and freezing on structural conformation, thermal properties and morphology of silk fibroin hydrogels. Biomatter. 4: e28536.

Rnjak-Kovacina, J. and D.L. Kaplan. 2013. Multifunctional silk-tropoelastin biomaterial systems. Israel J. Chem. 53: 777–786.

Rockwood, D.N., R.C. Preda, T. Yucel, X. Wang, M.L. Lovett and D.L. Kaplan. 2011. Materials fabrication from Bombyx mori silk fibroin. Nat. Protoc. 6: 1612–1631.

Samal, S.K., D.L. Kaplan and E. Chiellini. 2013. Ultrasound sonication effects on silk fibroin protein. Macromol. Mater. Eng. 298: 1201–1208.

Schacht, K., T. Jungst, M. Schweinlin, A. Ewald, J. Groll and T. Scheibel. 2015. Biofabrication of cell-loaded 3D spider silk constructs. Angew. Chem. Int. Ed. Engl. 54: 2816–2820.

Scheibel, T. 2004. Spider silks: recombinant synthesis, assembly, spinning, and engineering of synthetic proteins. Microb. Cell Fact. 3: 14.

Seib, F.P., M.F. Maitz, X. Hu, C. Werner and D.L. Kaplan. 2012. Impact of processing parameters on the haemocompatibility of Bombyx mori silk films. Biomaterials. 33: 1017–1023.

Seib, F.P. and D.L. Kaplan. 2013. Silk for drug delivery applications: opportunities and challenges. Israel J. Chem. 53: 756–766.

Seib, F.P., E.M. Pritchard and D.L. Kaplan. 2013. Self-assembling doxorubicin silk hydrogels for the focal treatment of primary breast cancer. Adv. Funct. Mater. 23: 58–65.

Seib, F.P., G.T. Jones, J. Rnjak-Kovacina, Y. Lin and D.L. Kaplan. 2013. pH-dependent anticancer drug release from silk nanoparticles. Adv. Healthc. Mater. 2: 1606–1611.

Seib, F.P., M. Herklotz, K.A. Burke, M.F. Maitz, C. Werner and D.L. Kaplan. 2014. Multifunctional silk-heparin biomaterials for vascular tissue engineering applications. Biomaterials. 35: 83–91.

Sponner, A., B. Schlott, F. Vollrath, E. Unger, F. Grosse and K. Weisshart. 2005. Characterization of the protein components of Nephila clavipes dragline silk. Biochemistry. 44: 4727–4736.

Suntivich, R., I. Drachuk, R. Calabrese, D.L. Kaplan and V.V. Tsukruk. 2014. Inkjet printing of silk nest arrays for cell hosting. Biomacromolecules. 15: 1428–1435.

Tanaka, K., N. Kajiyama, K. Ishikura, S. Waga, A. Kikuchi, K. Ohtomo et al. 1999. Determination of the site of disulfide linkage between heavy and light chains of silk fibroin produced by Bombyx mori. Biochim. Biophys. Acta. 1432: 92–103.

Tang-Schomer, M.D., J.D. White, L.W. Tien, L.I. Schmitt, T.M. Valentin, D.J. Graziano et al. 2014. Bioengineered functional brain-like cortical tissue. Proc. Natl. Acad. Sci. USA. 111: 13811–13816.

Thurber, A.E., F.G. Omenetto and D.L. Kaplan. 2015. *In vivo* bioresponses to silk proteins. Biomaterials. 71: 145–157.

Tokareva, O., M. Jacobsen, M. Buehler, J. Wong and D.L. Kaplan. 2014. Structure-function-property-design interplay in biopolymers: spider silk. Acta Biomater. 10: 1612–1626.

Valluzzi, R., S.P. Gido, W. Muller and D.L. Kaplan. 1999. Orientation of silk III at the air-water interface. Int. J. Biol. Macromol. 24: 237–242.

Vollrath, F. 1992. Spider webs and silks. Scientific American. 266: 70–76.

Vollrath, F. and D. Porter. 2009. Silks as ancient models for modern polymers. Polymer. 50: 5623–5632.

Wang, X., J.A. Kluge, G.G. Leisk and D.L. Kaplan. 2008. Sonication-induced gelation of silk fibroin for cell encapsulation. Biomaterials. 29: 1054–1064.

Wang, Y., D.D. Rudym, A. Walsh, L. Abrahamsen, H.J. Kim, H.S. Kim et al. 2008. *In vivo* degradation of three-dimensional silk fibroin scaffolds. Biomaterials. 29: 3415–3428.

Werner, V. and L. Meinel. 2015. From silk spinning in insects and spiders to advanced silk fibroin drug delivery systems. Eur. J. Pharm. Biopharm. 97: 392–399.

Williams, D.F. 2008. On the mechanisms of biocompatibility. Biomaterials. 29: 2941–2953.

Wray, L.S., X. Hu, J. Gallego, I. Georgakoudi, F.G. Omenetto, D. Schmidt et al. 2011. Effect of processing on silk-based biomaterials: reproducibility and biocompatibility. J. Biomed. Mater. Res. B Appl. Biomater. 99: 89–101.

Xia, X.X., Z.G. Qian, C.S. Ki, Y.H. Park, D.L. Kaplan and S.Y. Lee. 2010. Native-sized recombinant spider silk protein produced in metabolically engineered *Escherichia coli* results in a strong fiber. Proc. Natl. Acad. Sci. USA. 107: 14059–14063.

Xu, G., L. Gong, Z. Yang and X.Y. Liu. 2014. What makes spider silk fibers so strong? From molecular-crystallite network to hierarchical network structures. Soft Matter. 10: 2116–2123.

Yamaguchi, K., Y. Kikuchi, T. Takagi, A. Kikuchi, F. Oyama, K. Shimura et al. 1989. Primary structure of the silk fibroin light chain determined by cDNA sequencing and peptide analysis. J. Mol. Biol. 210: 127–139.

Yodmuang, S., S.L. McNamara, A.B. Nover, B.B. Mandal, M. Agarwal, T.A. Kelly et al. 2015. Silk microfiber-reinforced silk hydrogel composites for functional cartilage tissue repair. Acta Biomater. 11: 27–36.

Yucel, T., P. Cebe and D.L. Kaplan. 2009. Vortex-induced injectable silk fibroin hydrogels. Biophys. J. 97: 2044–2050.

Yucel, T., M.L. Lovett and D.L. Kaplan. 2014. Silk-based biomaterials for sustained drug delivery. J. Control. Release. 190: 381–397.

Zeplin, P.H., N.C. Maksimovikj, M.C. Jordan, J. Nickel, G. Lang, A.H. Leimer et al. 2014. Spider silk coatings as a bioshield to reduce periprosthetic fibrous capsule formation. Adv. Funct. Mater. 24: 2658–2666.

Zhao, Z., Y. Li and M.B. Xie. 2015. Silk fibroin-based nanoparticles for drug delivery. Int. J. Mol. Sci. 16: 4880–4903.

Zhou, C.Z., F. Confalonieri, N. Medina, Y. Zivanovic, C. Esnault, T. Yang et al. 2000. Fine organization of Bombyx mori fibroin heavy chain gene. Nucleic Acids Res. 28: 2413–2419.

Zhou, C.Z., F. Confalonieri, M. Jacquet, R. Perasso, Z.G. Li and J. Janin. 2001. Silk fibroin: structural implications of a remarkable amino acid sequence. Proteins. 44: 119–122.

CHAPTER 13

In Situ Forming Phase–Inversion Injectable Hydrogels for Controlled Drug Release

Thakur Raghu Raj Singh,[1,*] *Hannah L. McMillan,*[1]
Ravi Sheshala,[2] *Ismaiel Abdo Tekko,*[1,3]
Farhan Alshammari[1] *and Prashant Kesharwani*[4]

Introduction

Drugs that require recurrent administration often result in poor patient compliance, especially if the method of administration is painful or difficult. To overcome these problems, controlled release systems emerged, which allowed a reduction in the frequency of administration. Subcutaneous and intramuscular controlled release depot implants were developed as an attractive alternative to instant release preparations. These depots and pre-formed implants were attractive due to their uniform release profiles, improved patient compliance in terms of dosing and obviously longer-term release. They do however have inherent drawbacks. Minor surgery is required if pre-formed controlled release implants are used. But for non-biodegradable pre-formed

[1] School of Pharmacy, Medical Biology Centre Queen's University Belfast, 97 Lisburn Road, Belfast BT9 7BL, United Kingdom.
[2] Department of Pharmaceutics, Faculty of Pharmacy, Universiti Teknologi MARA (UiTM), Puncak Alam Campus, Selangor, 42300, Malaysia.
   E-mail: ravisheshala@uitm.edu.my
[3] Department of Pharmaceutics and Pharmaceutical Technology, Faculty of Pharmacy, Aleppo University, Aleppo, Syria.
[4] Department of Pharmaceutical Sciences, Eugene Applebaum College of Pharmacy and Health Sciences, Wayne State University, Detroit, Michigan 48201, USA.
* Corresponding author: r.thakur@qub.ac.uk

implants, a second surgery is essential once the drug supply has been exhausted (Kapoor et al. 2012).

Of the many controlled drug release technologies, *in situ* forming (ISF) implant systems have risen in their popularity for a range of biomedical applications such as tissue repair, cell encapsulation, microfluidics, bioengineering and drug delivery (Lendlein and Shastri 2010). The widespread interest in ISF systems can be attributed to a range of advantages which include site-specific action due to localized delivery, easy and less invasive application, extended delivery times, reduction in side effects associated with systemic delivery and also improved patient compliance and comfort (Hatefi and Amsden 2002; Chitkara et al. 2006). Depending upon their mechanism of implant formation, the ISF systems can be categorised into different types such as phase separation systems (e.g., thermoresponsive, solvent exchange and pH), crosslinked systems (e.g., photo-initiated, chemical and physical) and solidifying organogels (e.g., solubility change) (Abashzadeh et al. 2011; Gil and Hudson 2004). The most commonly used ISF systems are the thermoresponsive, pH, ions, photocrosslinked and solvent induced phase inversion (SPI) hydrogel implants. Importantly, administration by this method allows the injection of a relatively low viscosity material into the body which then solidifies to form a semi-solid depot that controls the drug delivery to provide long-term therapeutic action (Chitkara et al. 2006).

The Southern Research Institute carried some of the earliest work in the 1980s, which focused on the development of injectable depot systems for the treatment of periodontal disease with chemotherapeutics. The polymeric system allowed localised delivery of chemotherapeutic drugs, such as antimicrobials, directly into the infected gingival tissue instead of into the periodontal pocket between the infected tissue and tooth. The patents note the potential use of microspheres, microcapsules, nanoparticles, liposomes, fibres, spheres, films or rods made preferentially from biodegradable polymers, as removal would not be required after the chemotherapeutic agent was exhausted. The advantage cited for these systems is that the local delivery into the gingival tissue overcame the loss of active agent from the periodontal pocket due to the outward flow of the crevicular fluid. The liquid systems also allowed relatively simple administration to the required site and retention by the gingival tissue ensuring effective concentrations of the antimicrobial to kill the bacteria involved in peridontitis (Dunn et al. 1990; Dunn et al. 1997).

There are numerous methods by which implants may form *in situ*. This process a free flowing system solidify once introduced into the physiological environment. Depending upon their mechanism of implant formation the ISF can be categorised into different types such as phase separation systems.

The *in situ* formation of polymeric drug delivery systems can be attributed to a single or combination of different stimuli (Abashzadeh et al. 2011). Stimuli-sensitive polymers are often referred to as 'smart' polymers as their properties and characteristics are modified once they are exposed to stimuli. The ability of stimuli sensitive gels to swell or shrink is dependant on change of environmental conditions. A large number of possible stimuli and polymers have been investigated to determine their suitability and feasibility in relation to drug delivery and release. Both physical and chemical triggers have been applied to induce changes in systems. Chemical stimuli include ions, pH changes and chemical agents (Gil and Hudson 2004). Physical stimuli include electrical fields, temperature, solvent changes, light, pressure, magnetic fields and pressure.

A stimuli responsive system has a number of distinct advantages over conventional polymeric delivery systems, depending on the type of polymer. Those systems that once exposed to a stimuli experience a sharp rise in viscosity are initially of low viscosity and therefore allow easy administration through a syringe. A system that gels, or is triggered to release drug particles, once exposed to a change in pH can result in targeted drug delivery. As well as in drug delivery, stimuli responsive polymers are being utilized in a number of different fields such as aerospace, textiles, sensors, microfluidics, bioengineering, packaging and actuators (Lendlein and Shastri 2010).

In Situ Forming SPI Hydrogel Implants

This aims to discuss the SPI-based ISF hydrogel implant technology, which has attracted significant attention among pharmaceutical/drug delivery companies, leading to the development of commercial therapeutic products for a wide range of clinical applications. Importantly, SPI mode of ISF implants has a number of advantages over its counterparts, e.g., need for critical temperature (for thermoresponsive ISF implants), presence of ions (for charge sensitive ISF implants), and change in pH (for pH sensitive ISF implants) is not required to trigger implant formation. Therefore, considering the growing interest in SPI type ISF drug delivery systems, this work critically assessed the literature available in relation to SPI hydrogel implant technology.

SPI is known by a number of different terms throughout published literature, namely, non-solvent induced phase separation (NIPS) (Wang et al. 2004), solvent exchange (Ruel-Gariépy and Leroux 2004), solvent/non-solvent exchange (Kranz and Bodmeier 2008), solvent removal (Hatefi and Amsden 2002; Chitkara et al. 2006), liquid-liquid phase separation (Brodbeck et al. 1999a), solvent-removal precipitation (Dong et al. 2011), polymer precipitation (Packhaeuser et al. 2004; Körber and Bodmeier 2008) and phase-sensitive ISFIs (Yu and Singh 2008). This method of implant formation *in situ* has numerous benefits compared to its counterparts mentioned above. For example, control of temperature is not an issue, which is in contrast to those systems that require a critical temperature for gelation to take place. Also the application of an external energy source, such as a UV light, is not required (Hatefi and Amsden 2002). These systems first came into existence through the work of Richard Dunn and colleagues at the Southern Research Institute in the 1990s (Dunn et al. 1990).

SPI hydrogel systems are comprised of a water insoluble polymer that is dissolved in an organic, water-miscible, biocompatible solvent, into which a drug is incorporated. Once this system is introduced into aqueous environment, the organic solvent dissipates out of the system and water ingress via diffusion (Graham et al. 1999). This exchange of solvents results in sol-to-gel transformation causing polymer precipitation that leads to hydrogel implant formation, which in turn controls the rate of drug release.

Effect of polymer type

The body of knowledge relating to phase inversion is vast and this has led to the investigation of a number of polymers for their potential to form ISFI (Brodbeck et al. 2000). When there was a move towards sustained release systems natural polymers were considered for their production such as albumin, gelatin, collagen and alginate but the favour for these polymers has waned over the years due to batch inconsistency and a contamination hazard due to prions (Matschke et al. 2002). With the emergence of *in situ* forming systems, synthetic polymers were considered for use. The most commonly employed polymers for ISFI are of a synthetic nature (Abashzadeh et al. 2011; Astaneh et al. 2009) and as previously mentioned are usually biodegradable and biocompatible (Hatefi and Amsden 2002; Luan and Bodmeier 2006). These polymers are hydrophobic and insoluble in water and it is this characteristic that allows for the solid implant to form after polymer precipitation takes place (Hatefi and Amsden 2002; Brodbeck et al. 1999; Liu et al. 2010). Polymer selection for industrial production also involves consideration of both chemical and physical stability therefore careful selection of polymers is required (Matschke et al. 2002).

Biodegradable polymers have risen in popularity as they have a distinct advantage over those that are non-biodegradable. Non-biodegradable systems require surgery to implant the system and once the drug supply has been spent, invasive surgery is necessary to remove the implant from its site of injection (Lee et al. 2010; DesNoyer and McHugh 2001). Regarding the use of non-biodegradable polymers in the treatment of vitreo-retinal diseases, this invasive surgery has been linked with a number of serious side effects such as vitreous haemorrhage, cataract formation and retinal detachment (Kiernan and Mieler 2009; Yasukawa et al. 2001; Mohammad et al. 2007). With biodegradable polymers, invasive surgery is avoided as the implant degrades to form non-toxic by products (Luan and Bodmeier 2006), which are removed by the tricarboxylic acid cycle (Krebs cycle) that yields carbon dioxide and water as metabolic end products (Schoenhammer et al. 2010).

Biodegradable polymers that are commonly used in SPI systems are from polyhydroxyacid, polyanhydride and polyorthoester families. Aliphatic esters from the poly-α-hydroxyacid family such as poly(glycolic acid) (PGA), poly(lactic acid) (PLA) and PLGA which is a co-polymer of PGA and PLA, are extremely popular (Brannon-Peppas 1995; Lee et al. 2010). Poly-ε-caprolactone (PCL) (Bae et al. 2006), poly(lactide-co-caprolactone) copolymer, poly(acrylic acid) (PAA) and its derivatives (Haglund et al. 1996) such as poly(methacrylic acid) (PMA)—poly(ethylene glycol) (PEG) have also being investigated as potential SPI polymers (Ismail et al. 2000). These polyesters degrade by random chain scissions of ester bonds that result in a steady reduction in molecular weight but a delayed loss of weight, known as bulk hydrolysis.

PLA and PLGA have been the most popular polymers in SPI formulation (Table 1). PLGA has a long history of use in biomedical applications and was described in the earliest work completed by Dunn et al. 1990. It has been approved for parenteral use (Eliaz and Kost 2000; Fredenberg et al. 2011) by US Food and Drug Administration (US-FDA), which is prepared by polymerisation of lactic acid and glycolic acid monomers (Merkli et al. 1998). The glass transition temperature (T_g) of PLGA copolymers are above physiological temperature of 37°C, which imparts a moderately rigid chain configuration and therefore the mechanical strength at ambient temperatures. Jamshidi et al. 1988 observed a decrease in T_g when the ratio of lactic acid monomers also decreased. Availability of PLGA in different commercial grades such as lactide to glycolide ratio and molecular weight is also raised its popularity, as

Table 1. Recent publications in PLA and PLGA based SPI.

Molecule	Polymer	Solvent	Approximate Release time (Reference)
Sodium fluorescein (model drug)	PLGA	NMP	*In vivo:* 7 d (Luis and Exner 2015)
Fenretinide	PLGA	NMP	30 d (Wischke et al. 2010)
Doxorubicin HCl	PLGA	NMP	7 d (Li et al. 2015)
Betamethasone	PLGA	NMP	Up to 90 d (Rafienia et al. 2009)
Thymosin-1-alpha	PLGA	NMP/with & without triacetin	28 d (Fredenberg et al. 2011)
Asenapine	PLGA	NMP	21 d (Avachat and Kapure 2014)
Ivermectine	PLA	NMP, 2-pyrrolidone, triacetin or benzyl benzoate	96 d (Camargo et al. 2013)
Tinidazole	PLA	NMP	7 d (Qin et al. 2012)
HIV-fusion inhibitor	PLGA	DMSO/TA	2 d (Kapoor et al. 2012)
Haloperidol	PLGA	NMP	*In vivo:* up to 1 mon (Ahmed et al. 2012)
Granisetron HCl	PLGA	Dimethylsulphoxide/ prophylenecarbonate	21 d (Yapar et al. 2014)
Risperidone	PLGA	Benzyl alcohol/benzyl benzoate	Prolonged MRT: 32.6 hr (Dong et al. 2011)
Insulin	PLGA	Benzyl alcohol/benzyl benzoate	*In vivo:* Up to 15 d (Sanju et al. 2010)
Plasmid DNA	PLGA	glycofurol	70 d (Jeon et al. 2011)
Cucurbitacin	PLGA	NMP/DMSO	28 d (Guo et al. 2015)
Metronidazole	PLGA	NMP/benzyl alcohol	10 d (Kilicarslan et al. 2014)

this can allow researchers to obtain different drug release profiles (Eliaz and Kost 2000; Fredenberg et al. 2011; Merkli et al. 1998). SPI-based implants, containing PLGA, has been used to deliver a wide range of molecules ranging from small hydrophilic and/or hydrophobic to large protein/peptide molecules such as bupivacaine (Ruel-Gariepy and Leroux 2004), diltiazem (Kranz and Bodmeier 2007), leuprolide acetate (Zare et al. 2008), human growth hormone, buserelin acetate (Kranz and Bodmeier 2007), aspirin (Tang and Singh 2008), naltrexone (Bakhshi et al. 2006), fenretinide (Wischke et al. 2010), thymosin alpha-1 (Fredenberg et al. 2011) and risperidone (Dong et al. 2011). Poly(caprolactone) (PCL) is another widely studied polymer but its popularity wane due to the rise in interest of PLGA and related polymers. PCL is a semi-crystalline polymer with a T_g of around –60°C and a low melting point of 59–64°C. The rate of PCL degradation is markedly slower than that of PLA, with the homopolymer taking up to 2 to 3 yr to degrade (Middleton and Tipton 2000). Its use for extremely prolonged release implants is therefore ideal. This polymer is widely accepted as being non-toxic and so biocompatibility is no issue (Gunatillake and Adhikari 2003). Recently, Zhang et al. 2015 studied the feasibility of using (ε-caprolactone-co-DL-lactide) as a biodegradable polymer for ISP system. The investigations proved that sustained *in situ* testosterone undeconate delivery could be obtained from (ε-caprolactone-co-DL-lactide). In addition, Ueda et al. 2007 investigated the use of the linear, polyester polymer poly(propylene-fumarate) (PPF) (an alternative to poly-α-hydroxyacid family) in SPI systems. PPF was used to study *in vitro* release of fluocinolone acetonide (FA) intended for ocular drug delivery applications. A release period of up to 62 wk was observed for the implants with an overall conclusion being drawn that PPF shows promise as a biocompatible polymer for use in SPI in ocular drug delivery (Ueda et al. 2007).

However, PLGA, PLA, and PLA-PEG causes accumulation of acidic degradation products generated during the hydrolysis and show a non-linear release profiles, which is especially challenging for delivery of hydrophilic macromolecules (i.e., peptides and proteins). To overcome this issues a collaborative research between Philipps-University of Marburg and Novartis Pharma AG led to the use of poly(ethylene carbonate) (PEC) polymer in SPI systems. PEC degrades through surface erosion, providing linear release profile. PEC containing SPI system has shown selective reduction in burst release of bovine serum albumin, which was depended upon solvent type chosen (Liu et al. 2010).

A biodegradable copolymer based on ε-caprolactone (CL) and D,L-lactide (LA), i.e. ([poly(ε-caprolactone)-random-poly(D,L-lactide)]-*block*-poly(ethyleneglycol)-*block*-[poly(ε-caprolactone)-random-poly(D,L-lactide)]), known as PLEC, was investigated as SPI-based implants. Introduction of PEG in this copolymer was to overcome the low hydrophilicity of LA and CL copolymers. Combining PLEC with tetrahydrofurfuryl alcohol (GF), a biocompatible solvent that has been used to deliver drugs such as phenytoin and diazepam as well as proteins by injection (Cornacchione et al. 2012; Renette et al. 2012), results in a SPI depot. This group concluded that this material was a successful candidate for further investigations relating to the development of ISF (Nasongkla et al. 2012).

Effect of solvent on SPI hydrogels

In order for an *in situ* forming polymer system to be feasible, the selected polymers must possess a good solubility in the solvent, with biocompatibility being a very important characteristic. A SPI hydrogel system uses solvents that are water miscible, biocompatible and organic in nature. Importantly, solvents should efficiently dissolve the polymer, be miscible with water and bodily fluids. Polarity of the solvent should be such that at least 10% should be soluble in water (Dunn et al. 2004) (Table 2). Solvent viscosity also plays an important role in SPI implant formation. For example, highly viscous solvents, combined with around 30% of polymer as well as drug, could pose difficulty when injecting via conventional needles. Therefore overall viscosity should be within the range that is syringeable. Formulations with a rate index of below one are those, which exhibit shear-thinning behaviour. This would therefore be beneficial as the application of force to inject the polymer formulation would exert a shear stress

Table 2. Properties of commonly used solvents in the preparation of SPI formulations. Information obtained from Sigma-Aldrich.

Solvent	Type	Physical characteristics	Water solubility	Melting Point (°C)	Boiling Point (°C)
NMP	HP	Colourless liquid	Completely miscible	−24	202
DMSO (Dimethyl sulfoxide)	HP	Colourless liquid	Completely miscible	16–19	189
Triacetin	HO	Colourless liquid	61.2 g/L at 20°C	3	258–260
Ethyl benzoate	HO	Colourless liquid	Limited solubility	−34	212
Benzyl benzoate (BB)	HO	Colourless liquid	15.4 mg/L at 20°C	17–20	323–324
Benzyl alcohol (BA)	HP	Colourless liquid	33 g/L at 20°C	−16–13	203–205
PEG500DME	HP	Light brown liquid	Completely miscible	−23	>250

HP: Hydrophilic; HO: Hydrophobic

and therefore cause thinning of the material (Kapoor et al. 2012). Solvent strength and its affinity for water direct the nature of phase inversion and implant formation. For example, solvent that have a high water affinity exhibit fast hydrogel forming phase inversion (fPI) such as NMP (Bakhshi et al. 2006; Malik et al. 2010; Wang et al. 2012) and DMSO (Kranz and Bodmeier 2007; 2008; Wang et al. 2012). Hydrophobic solvents exhibit slow forming phase inversion (sPI) such as triacetin (Brodbeck et al. 1999; Kranz and Bodmeier 2007; Malik et al. 2010) and ethylbenzoate (McHugh 2005; Brodbeck et al. 1999), this is further discussed in Section 4. Solvents that possess a water solubility of below 7% w/w have been shown to result in slower drug release due to a reduction in water uptake (Brodbeck et al. 2000). Solvents with high water miscibility exhibit higher rate of drug release relative to low water miscible solvents following order NMP > 2-pyrrolidone > triacetin > benzyl benzoate (Camargo et al. 2013).

A number of other solvents have also been detailed in the literature such as glycofurol (Eliaz and Kost 2000; Eliaz et al. 2000) and tetrahydrofuran (Hatefi and Amsden 2002) but studies on these solvent are limited. The mixture of BA and BB can also be used to obtain desired release profile (Kang and Singh 2005; Dong et al. 2011). However, SPI systems most commonly use DMSO and NMP solvents preferentially due to their pharmaceutical precedence over other solvents (Dunn et al. 1997). Schoenhammer et al. 2009a,b have described the use of poly(ethylene glycol) 500 dimethylether (PEG500DME) and also poly(ethylene glycol) dialkylether (PEG-DAE) as novel solvents for use in SPI systems. PEG500DME shown to stabilize the PLGA containing SPI systems and resulted in rapid phase inversion as the solvent has a high affinity for water (Schoenhammer et al. 2009a). The use of PEG-DAE also showed stability of injectable SPI systems for up to two months (Schoenhammer et al.

2009b). Limited number of studies also showed use of glycerol formal and triacetin in SPI systems, these solvents has earlier history of using in veterinary formulations (Bleiberg et al. 1993).

The search for novel solvents for use in SPI systems is an on-going process with a number of factors such as polymer solubility, toxicity, system stability, biocompatibility and the potential for a single unit formulation posing barriers to this development. Although the regulatory authorities approve the 'gold-standard' solvents such as NMP and DMSO, evidence relating to toxicity and suitability is conflicting and sometimes contradictory therefore there is a need for further research and improvement. Movement towards the use of solvent mixtures can be observed through literature in order to obtain the most suitable 'solvent strength' to enable predictable and modifiable controlled release. For example, Zingermann and Chern patented a combination of glycerol formal (hydrophilic) and triacetin (hydrophobic) solvent that showed the blood levels of fipronil (flea adulticide) for 12 mon after subcutaneous injection (Chern and Zingerman 2004).

2.3 Method of SPI hydrogel implant formation

Two different forms of phase inversion have been identified and recorded in previous literature, according to their rate of phase inversion as detailed below. For example, rapid injection of the SPI hydrogel formulations results in rod-like implants whereas slower injection yields more spherical implants (Schoenhammer et al. 2009a).

2.3.1 Fast Phase Inversion (fPI)

These systems undergo phase inversion at a rapid rate (from seconds to minutes) resulting in formation of a thin membrane with a porous implant structure (Graham et al. 1999; Packhaeuser et al. 2004) (Fig. 1). This change is a result of solvents that are 'strong' and 'hydrophilic' in nature (McHugh 2005). As the affinity of the solvent for the non-solvent increases, the rate of sol-to-gel phase inversion also increases. fPI systems are of a lower viscosity and, therefore, require lower force of injection. fPI have improved biocompatibility hydrophilic nature of the solvent (Raman and McHugh 2005). Mashak et al. 2011 investigated the addition of aliphatic esters, namely ethyl heptanoate, methyl heptanoate and ethyl nonanoate, to a PLGA in NMP solution. Here rapid NMP removal resulted in implant formation, which is due to increased interaction between PLGA and the esters and also by a reduction of the affinity between PLGA/ester and NMP. Additives resulted in highly porous matrix compared control PLGA/NMP system. Most rapid phase inversion was seen in the systems containing ethyl heptanoate.

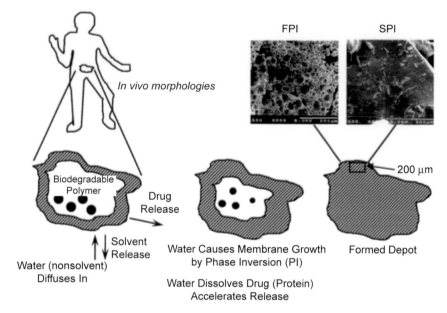

Fig. 1. Schematic illustration of membrane formation/drug release in an injectable system. Morphologies in upper right show fast phase inversion (FPI) and slow phase inversion (SPI) hardened membrane structures (McHugh 2005).

2.3.2 Slow Phase Inversion (sPI)

These systems undergo phase inversion at a slow rate (from hours to days) (McHugh 2005). Solvents used in sPI are weaker and are hydrophobic in nature. Therefore gelation/implant formation occurs at a slow rate. In contrast to the fPI, the implant conformation can be described as being uniformly dense with a limited number of pores (McHugh 2005; Raman and McHugh 2005; Chitkara et al. 2006) (Fig. 1). The limited pores resulted in slower drug release from these implants than that from fPI implants but burst release is highly reduced. The extended period of time for solidification of implant formation is not ideal. The viscosities of sPI solutions are usually of an order that makes injection difficult unless the system is pre-emulsified or preheated to 37°C (Raman and McHugh 2005). These systems have an inherent disadvantage in relation to drug delivery as the hydrophobicity of the solvent can result in foreign protein adhesion to the implant surface and therefore inhibition of drug release (McHugh 2005).

3. Drug Release from SPI Hydrogel Implants

Depending on the solubility of a drug, it can either be dissolved or dispersed in the polymer solution therefore this method of delivery via injection is appealing for a wide variety of drugs. Drug is entrapment within the polymer matrix occurs when the phase inversion takes place to form a solid implant, allowing release to be controlled

(Royals et al. 1999). Graham et al. determined that the release rate of protein is directly influenced by the rate of phase inversion and morphology of the formed implant (Graham et al. 1999).

Once injected into an aqueous environment SPI system forms a polymeric implant that controls drug release over defined time period (Royals et al. 1999). A number of publications and patents over the last few decades have indicated that release can be modified so that SPI hydrogel implants can deliver drugs over 2-week to 6-month period. Fredenberg et al. 2011 identified three basic ways in which drugs could be released from PLGA-based matrices as (i) transport through water-filled channels, (ii) transport through the polymer, and (iii) due to dissolution of the encapsulating polymer. They deduced that the mechanism of release of encapsulated biopharmaceuticals, proteins and peptides, was through water-filled pores as these molecules are large and hydrophilic therefore transport through the polymer phase would be limited (Fredenberg et al. 2011).

An ideal prolonged drug release profile would conform to zero-order release kinetics. Typically the drug release profile from SPI hydrogel implants can be described as triphasic (Fig. 2); (i) a sudden burst release of drug that is attributed to a lag period before the implant forms after injection, where drug is released from the surface of the system through pores, (ii) a slow diffusion facilitated release of non-entailment drug molecules in the matrix, and (iii) degradation of polymer matrix in which once the molecular weight of the polymer reaches a lower threshold, erosion results in a second rapid phase of release in the profile (Zare et al. 2008; Astaneh et al. 2008; Ahmed et al. 2012). The rate of drug release can be attributed to a number of parameters such as molecular weight of polymer, concentration of polymer solution, solvent/solution hydrophilicity and system additives. Modification of theses parameters can allow tailoring the drug delivery. Following sections details the effect of each parameter on drug release from SPI hydrogel implants.

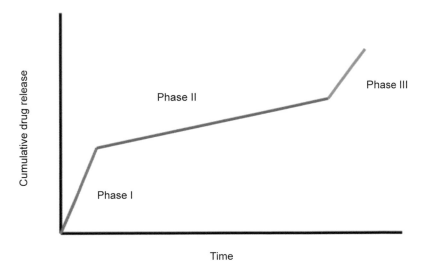

Fig. 2. Schematic representation of general drug release profile from solvent-induced ISFI.

Unfortunately, these systems are subject to burst release, which is the amount of drug released in the first 24 hours after formation (Wang et al. 2004). This is due to time taken for complete implant formation (Hatefi and Amsden 2002), during which the surface layer of the implant quickly inverts (Graham et al. 1999) resulting in a relatively large bolus amount of drug released before the release rate reaches a stable profile. A number of studies have explained the process of burst release both experimentally and theoretically. Commonly, it is observed with drugs of low molecular weight due to the small molecular size and osmotic pressures that heighten the gradient of concentration (Huang and Brazel 2001). It stands to sense that small molecular weight drugs have the ability to pass easily through porous structures of implants and those drugs that are hydrophilic are therefore soluble in aqueous environment that promotes drug release. Depending on the intended use, burst release can either have positive or negative effects. It is however seen as being detrimental due to large amounts of drug being released in a short period that potentially result in concentrations outside of therapeutic levels, leading to adverse effects (Shively et al. 1995). Potent drugs with narrow therapeutic windows, such as chemotherapeutics and human growth hormones may therefore be problematic (Wang et al. 2004). High burst release also reduce the effective lifetime of the implant (Huang and Brazel 2001; Patel et al. 2010), as potential for local or systemic toxicity, a shortened half-life of drugs *in vivo*, the drug is wasted in both an economically and therapeutic manner and also the total drug release profile is shortened therefore more frequent dosing is required (Huang and Brazel 2001). Furthermore, *in vivo* environment could have a significant impact on the burst release. For example, sodium fluorescein implant formed *in vivo* has remarkably higher burst release relative to implant formed *in vitro* (Luis and Exner 2015). Burst release has however been utilized to deliver drugs at high release rates to achieve an initial loading dose, such as antibiotics (Setterstrom et al. 1984). Huang and Brazel 2001, recorded the instances where burst release may be advantageous such as in wound treatment, for encapsulating flavours, to target delivery via triggered burst release and the ability of pulsatile release. Even in the instances that burst release is desired, the drug release profile is unpredictable, variable amounts of drug are released and it is difficult to control the amount of drug released during the period (Patel et al. 2010).

Numerous studies have been carried out in relation to the modification of burst release. The majority of studies have investigated methods to alter this initial, extensive drug release and prevent it from occurring to produce a better control release system, typical zero-order release kinetics. A number of different formulation parameters have been investigate for their ability to reduce the extent of burst release.

3.1 Rate modifying agents

The most extensive body of work has focused on the addition of rate modifying agents that aim to reduce the rate at which phase inversion takes place and therefore the extent of burst release. These agents are added into the polymeric formulation with the aim of altering the release profiles of solvent-induced ISFI. Table 3 gives a broad list of rate modifying additives that have been investigated in literature with varying levels of success.

Table 3. Effect of rate modifying agents on the burst release from SPI hydrogel implants.

Type of Additive	Polymer/Solvent system	Drug	Amount of additive	Mean burst release (no additive)	Mean burst release (with additive)	Ref.
Triacetin	PLGA/NMP	Aspirin	NA	36.9%	65%	Tang and Singh 2008
PVP	PLGA/NMP	Chicken egg lysozyme	3%	NA	8 fold increase	Graham et al. 1999
Ethyl benzoate	PLGA/NMP	Leuprolide acetate	12.8%	14.50%	5.53%	Astaneh et al. 2008
PEG 400	PLGA/NMP	Aspirin	20%	36.9%	30%	Tang and Singh 2008
Glycerol	PLGA/NMP	Naltrexone HCl	1% 3% 5%	67%	62% 61% 60%	Bakhshi et al. 2006
Ethyl heptanoate	PLGA/NMP	Naltrexone HCl	1% 3% 5%	67%	62% 50% 44%	Bakhshi et al. 2006
PEG 4000	PLLA/NMP PLLGA/NMP	Heparin	5%	40% 20%	5% NA	Tan et al. 2004
Glyceryl monosterate	PLGA/BB and BA	Risperidone	2%	32.2%	4.7%	Dong et al. 2011
Steric Acid	PLGA/BB and BA	Risperidone	2%	32.2%	23.4%	Dong et al. 2011
Zinc complexation	PLGA/NMP, triacetin, ethyl benzoate, BB	Human growth hormone	30 mM	ND	Reduction in all cases	Brodbeck et al. 1999
Pluronic L101	PDLA/NMP	Lysozyme	5.4%	25%	18%	DesNoyer and McHugh 2003
Pluronic L121	PDLA/NMP	Lysozyme	5.4%	25%	10%	DesNoyer and McHugh 2003
DiI	PLGA/NMP	Sodium fluorescein	4%	28.8%	6.9%	Solorio et al. 2010
Water	PLGA/NMP	Sodium fluorescein	10% of the solvent	28.8%	15.1%	Solorio et al. 2010

ND: No details, DiI: 1, 1'-dioctadecyl-3,3,3'3,3,tetramethylindocarbocyanine perchlorate

3.2 Polymer molecular weight

Altering the molecular weight (MW) of the polymer used in the system can have a profound effect on release profile. Polymer MW is an exceptionally important property that can alter a number of physicochemical and mechanical properties such as solubility, diffusivity, viscosity, glass transition temperature and modulus (Omelczuk and McGinity 1992). Published literature has stated that an increase in MW will reduce the drug release from a system. By utilising this parameter and the wide availability of different MW of polymers means that release profiles can be modified without the addition of another agent. Astaneh et al. deduced that a solvent-induced ISFI system prepared using a high Mw of PLGA resulted in a significant reduction in leuprolide acetate burst release compared to a system using a lower Mw of PLGA (Astaneh et al. 2009). Although burst release is reduced in this case, the higher Mw means an increase in viscosity and therefore an increase in the work of syringeability, which will be problematic for administration reasons. A lower bioavailability may also be observed with increasing Mw, as the incorporated drug my not show 100% release from the implants. Liu and colleagues concluded that the use of a low MW PLGA aiding delivery as the formulation was less viscous, however thymosin alpha 1 (Tα1) burst release was increased due to a faster rate of phase inversion (Liu et al. 2010).

3.3 Polymer concentration

By increasing the polymer concentration, the rate of phase inversion is reduced, therefore reducing the extent of burst release. A slowing of the rate of water ingress into the system alters the internal morphology of the implant resulting in a more dense structure (Graham et al. 1999). A reduction in the release of FITC-bovine serum albumin (Lambert and Peck 1995) and Tα1 (Liu et al. 2010) was seen with increasing concentrations of PLGA, with both studies conforming that the reduced rate of phase inversion was the reason. Likewise, Ahmed et al. 2014 accredited drop in montelukast release with increase in the concentration of PLGA increased from 20 to 40%. As with increasing polymer MW, increasing the polymer concentration has a number of effects such as altering viscosity and therefore syringeability, reduced diffusivity and increased system hydrophobicity, some of which can be detrimental (Graham et al. 1999; Liu et al. 2010).

3.4 Polymer end-capping

Studies conducted by Wang et al. showed that the alteration of the acidic end group of PLGA to a lauryl ester group reduced the release of sirolimus from a multi-layered PLGA stent (Wang et al. 2006). A similar result was also seen when investigating the release of leuprolide from a PLGA microparticulate system. A reduced release rate was observed when the carboxylic end groups were esterified (Luan and Bodmeier 2006). This reduced in release can be attributed to the polymer being rendered more hydrophobic and therefore requiring less hydrophilic solvents to allow dissolution (Chhabra et al. 2007).

3.5 Monomer ratios

PLGA is a copolymer of lactic acid and glycolic acid monomers and is available for purchase in a variety of monomer ratios. The number of lactic acid monomers is inextricably linked to the hydrophobicity of the polymer. An increase in the number of lactic acid monomers results in a reduced water uptake into the system. The bulky, hydrophobic methyl side groups of the lactic acid monomers reduce water uptake and therefore dampen the rate of phase inversion (Göpferich 1996b).

3.6 Polymer crystallinity

There is a growing body of work investigating the effect of t polymer crystallinity on drug release. A model injectable implant system that employs a crystallisable polymer should initially be amorphous to permit easy injection but should then crystallise swiftly after injection (DesNoyer and McHugh 2001). Systems with limited crystallinity result in more uniformly, dense morphologies, which lack micropores. This is a result of mild liquid–liquid demixing and therefore slower release rates of drugs. Conversely, a more crystalline system will result in more rapid release due to porous morphologies forming through phase inversion after the lag period during which crystallisation occurs. Two distinct regions are apparent in the release profiles of systems based on crystallisable polymers. Firstly a lag phase followed by burst release. Knowledge about this important polymer parameter therefore permits tailoring of drug release profiles by altering the semi-crystalline: amorphous polymer ratios (DesNoyer and McHugh 2001; Miyajima et al. 1997).

4. Biodegradation of SPI Hydrogel Implants

Biodegradation of injectable implants is essential so as to accommodate a follow on injection. Ideally, degradation should take place in parallel to drug release so that the implant is reabsorbed upon complete drug release. This will avoid any surgical intervention for implant extraction or issues with follow on administration. Thankfully, most of polymeric implants are utilized in SPI-based systems are biodegradable—through hydrolysis or oxidation mechanism. The degradation by hydrolysis is rather a fast process that can be influenced by a number of factors such as pH, type of chemical bond, copolymer composition, drug type, and water uptake (Gopferich 1996a). The degradation by oxidation is intrinsically very slow processes (Acemoglu 2004). It is also important to take into consideration polymers physical and physico-mechanical properties (e.g., molecular weight, polydispersity, melting point), as well as morphology of the formed implant. Overall, biodegradation of SPI implants is dependent upon the polymer type, molecular weight, co-polymer ratio, polydispersity and drug type and concentration. It is also dependent upon the site of administration, as the locally available micronutrients and enzymes further effect the overall biodegradation. Table 4 provides degradation characteristics of polymers that have been commonly used in SPI systems.

Table 4. Biodegradation characteristics of commonly used polymers in SPI formulations. Adapted from Gunatillake and Adhikari 2003.

Polymer	Melting Point (°C)	Glass Transition (°C)	Approximate degradation time (in months)	Mode of Degradation and degraded products
PGA	225–230	35–40	6–12	Hydrolysis & GA
PLA	173–178	60–65	>24	Hydrolysis & l-LA
Poly(d,l-lactic acid)	Amorphous	55–60	12–16	Hydrolysis & d,l-LA
PLGA (85/15)	Amorphous	45–55	1–6	Hydrolysis & d,l-LA & GA
PCL	58–63	–65–60	>24	Hydrolysis & Caproic acid
PPF	Amorphous	31.9 for infinite MW	Several months	Hydrolysis & Fumaric acid, propylene glycol
PLEC	No details	No details	Weeks to months	Hydrolysis & CL & d,l-LA
PEC	No details	No details	Weeks to months	Oxidation & Ethylene carbonate

5. Currently Marketed SPI Systems

Even though this *in situ* forming technology shows great promise in the field of drug delivery, currently there are only a small number of devices that are marketed and approved for use by the FDA. Initial work using this technology completed by Dunn and co-workers surfaced in the 1990s with Atridox® being the first system to be released onto the market after FDA approval in late 1998, marketed by Tolmar Inc. in the United States. The system consists of poly DL-lactide, NMP and doxycycline and the MHRA granted a marketing authorisation to Atrix Laboratories Limited in the United Kingdom on 1st March 2003 for Atridox® (MHRA 2003). Atridox® is licensed for the treatment of chronic periodontal disease and it utilises the initially liquid state of the polymer solution to allow injection of the antibiotic and polymer formulation into the periodontal pocket before the controlled release implant is formed. This system has been reported to allow the release of doxycycline over 21 days (Stoller et al. 1998). Advantages of this product detailed by the company in relation to marketing draw on the advantages of *in situ* forming devices. Atridox® allows local treatment of the periodontal disease via direct application of the antibiotic and also that removal is not required as the system of bioabsorbable.

A number of clinical studies were conducted to determine the benefits of this treatment compared to previously licensed treatment modalities. Garrett, Johnson and Drisko in 1999 conducted two multicenter studies comparing locally delivered doxycycline to oral hygiene measures, scaling and root planning and also a placebo measure. They determined that the local delivery of doxycycline resulted in a gain in clinical attachment and also a reduction in probing depths. A similar study comparing the local delivery of doxycycline in a controlled release manner in comparison to scaling and root planning indicated that the local delivery resulted in a reduction in bleeding on probing (Garrett et al. 1999).

Tolmar also market Atrisorb® FreeFlow™ which was granted FDA approval on 21st March 2006 (US Food and Drug Administration 2012). This product utilises the *in situ* gelation of a polymer and solvent formulation (PLA and NMP) to produce a Guided Tissue Regeneration (GTR) barrier for use after periodontal surgery. The formation of the gel at the site of surgery encourages the growth of tissue via custom-fitted barrier. Due to its bioabsorbable properties, like Atridox®, it does not need further surgery for removal. A study of this formulation by Coonts et al. (1998) determined that the integrity of the barrier structure remained intact for approximately six months, with complete bioabsorption within nine to twelve months (Coonts et al. 1998). An advancement of this product involves the introduction of 4% doxycycline into the formulation to inhibit local bacterial growth as healing takes place. This system is marketed as Atrisorb-D® FreeFlow™ and it was granted FDA approval in September 2000. Currently the Atrisorb® FreeFlow™ products are not licensed for use in the United Kingdom.

Eligard™ is a sustained release delivery system marketed by Sanofi-Aventis, that employs a similar polymeric delivery system (PLGA and NMP) utilised by Atridox® to deliver leuprolide acetate, a gonadotropin releasing hormone (GnRH) agonist (Sartor 2003). It is licensed for the management of advanced prostate cancer and allows flexible dosing regimes of every 1, 3, 4 or 6 months due to variation of polymer molecular weight and solvent concentrations. This system requires the mixing of the leuprolide acetate with polymer/solvent combination immediately prior to injection via a 20-gauge needle into subcutaneous tissue. The drug is then released in a controlled manner and the solid implant that forms does not need surgery for removal as the degradation products are removed by body processes.

Clinical trials conducted by Chu et al. indicated that both the 1-month and 3-month formulations were effective in reducing the levels of testosterone in patients below castration levels previously stated by the FDA of 50 ng/dL but also those levels advocated by the NCCN for LHRH agonist monotherapy (≤20 ng/dL) (Chu et al. 2002; Sartor 2003). The U.S. Food and Drug Administration (FDA) released a safety announcement on 5th May 2003 regarding the use Gonadotropin-Releasing Hormone (GnRH) Agonists in the treatment of prostate cancer. It is evaluating whether GnRH agonists may increase the risk of diabetes and certain cardiovascular diseases males receiving these medications for the treatment of prostate cancer. This safety alert is still active and therefore medical professionals are advised to exercise diligence when considering the use of these treatments to treat advanced prostate cancer (US Food and Drug Administration 2011).

Lupron Depot™ is a prolonged release formulation of leuprolide acetate, composed of PLGA and NMP like Eligard, and was initially approved in the United States in 1995 for the palliative treatment of advanced prostate cancer. Three different formulations are available which allow a variety of dosing intervals for prostate cancer. The 22.5 mg formulation releases drug over a 3-month period therefore a single intramuscular injection is required every 12 weeks. The 30 mg formulation releases over 4 months and so dosing is needed every 16 weeks and the 45 mg formulation requires dosing every 24 weeks as it has the ability to release controlled amounts of leuprolide over 6 months (US Food and Drug Adminsitration 2011). A further development included the development of 3.75 mg and 11.25 mg depot formulations for the treatment of endometriosis and fibroids. As with Eligard, the Safety Alert issued in relation to GnRH agonists applies to Lupron Depot™ therefore prescribers are advised to exercise caution. A further formulation development has resulted in the production of Lupron Depot-Ped™ 7.5 mg, 11.25 mg and 15 mg for 1-month and 11.25 mg and 30 mg for 3-month administration for the treatment of children with central precocious puberty (CPP).

Sandostatin LAR is a prolonged-release Octreotide formulation consisting of PLGA and NMP. Octreotide is a synthetic analogue of somatostatin that is used to treat agromegaly by controlling the levels of growth hormone (GH) and IGF-1, which reduces the size of turmors and regulates symptoms. It is also used in the treatment of gastroenteropancreatic neuroendocrine tumors (GEP NETs) by controlling gastrointestinal hormone secretion. FDA approval of the LAR formulations was granted to Novartis Pharmaceuticals Corporation on 25th November 1998, with Novartis Pharmaceuticals UK Limited trading as Sandoz Pharmaceuticals granted marketing authorizations by the MHRA for 10, 20 and 30 mg formulations in June 2007 (Novartis Pharmaceuticals UK Ltd. 2011). This product is injected intramuscularly and the prolonged release nature of the formulation allows for monthly dosing, regardless of dose.

Modlin et al. in 2010 reviewed a number of articles that focused on the use of Sandostatin LAR in the treatment of GEP NETs, as well as other SST analogues. The review consisted of examining 15 previously published studies, which included 481 patients. They determined that the use of Sandostatin LAR accomplished symptomatic relief in 74.2%, biochemical response in 51.4% and tumour response in 69.8% (Modlin et al. 2010). A multicenter study conducted which was published in 2002, compared patient outcomes in relation to GH levels, IGF-1 levels and tumor size after treatment of acromegaly with the subcutaneous or long acting octreotide formulations. Before treatment, the mean GH level was 30 mU/litre but with the initial 24 weeks of subcutaneous treatment, GH levels were reduced to less than 5 mU/litre in 9 patients, with IGF-1 levels being reduced to normal in 8 patients. A tumor size decline of 49% was seen in those patients with microadenomas and a 43% reduction in those with macroadenomas. Upon completion of the study, 79% of patients showed a mean serum GH level of less than 5 mU/litre, 53% had normalized IGF-1 levels and a 23% reduction in tumor volume was reported in 73% of patients (James et al. 2002).

Current Issues with Solvent-Induced SPI

Although SPI are an attractive alternative to other currently used methods of drug delivery, they do however face a number of problematic issues. The first to consider is the susceptibility to burst release. As shown, this can be extensive within the first 24 hours after injection. A large initial release may result in drug levels that are above the therapeutic window and could be toxic. This is obviously is more problematic for those drugs that have narrow therapeutic window. As this review has shown, many groups have investigated a range of methods to modify this burst release, but to date no product with an altered release profile has made it to market.

Secondly, due to the issue of the stability of PLGA in NMP, the Atridox® system is only available as a two component system that must be mixed prior to use by a trained individual. This can be a lengthy process and is obviously not ideal. A two-component system could therefore be detrimental in terms of progress towards a patient self-administered formulation. Some work has been completed to combat the issue of PLGA instability in the form of alternative solvents. It has been shown that PLGA stability is increased when formulated in end-capped PEGs and the resultant solvents (PEG500DME and PEG-DAE) have shown favorable release and toxicity profiles (Schoenhammer et al. 2009a; Schoenhammer et al. 2009b).

Due to conflicting data relating to the toxicity of these ISFI, this area is still of concern to research groups and may be limiting their use in practice. The main concern relates to the use of organic solvents. The consideration of other solvents has resulted in ethyl benzoate and low molecular weight PEGs being shown to be compatible (Kranz et al. 2001). As stated previously, Schoenhammer et al. have shown the promise that lies with end-capped PEGs for use in these systems (Schoenhammer et al. 2009a; Schoenhammer et al. 2009b). Currently, there are no marketed or near to market systems that fulfill the criteria of an ideal ISFI but this is an area that is rapidly moving and research is growing.

Conclusion

In situ forming systems are gaining significant interest among pharmaceutical and biotechnology industries to formulate control drug delivery applications—particularly, due to enhanced patient compliance and simple administration procedure. *In situ* forming SPI implants has unique advantages over other forms of ISFI as sustained release systems such as thermo, pH, and ion responsive systems. These systems have many inherent advantages such as ease of production, biocompatibility of components, controlled release profiles and also the accommodation of both hydrophilic and hydrophobic drugs for delivery. However, as mentioned previously, solvent-induced ISFIs are not without their drawbacks. These implants are currently susceptible to burst release meaning that levels of drug above the therapeutic range may be released in the first 24 hours after implantation, possibly resulting in toxicity-related adverse effects. Also, there is conflicting information relating to the use to organic solvents and their toxicity within the body therefore there is a pressing need for alternative, non-toxic solvents for use in these systems. Issues relating to stability of polymers, such as PLGA, in organic solvents have resulted in those systems currently available on the market being produced as two-component systems that require extensive mixing prior to use. This may cause problems if mixing instructions are not stringently adhered to resulting in a non-homogenously mixed system that is injected. Due to the issues underlined, as of yet, there are a limited number of products on the market utilizing this promising technology therefore efforts must be made to produce commercial products that will benefit patients worldwide.

References

Abashzadeh, S., R. Dinarvand, M. Sharifzadeh, G. Hassanzadeh, M. Amini and F. Atyabi. 2011. Formulation and evaluation of an *in situ* gel forming system for controlled delivery of triptorelin acetate. Eur. J. Pharm. Sci. 4: 514–521.

Acemoglu, M. 2004. Chemistry of polymer biodegradation and implications on parenteral drug delivery. Int. J. Pharma. 277: 133–139.

Ahmed, T., H. Ibrahim, F. Ibrahim, A.M. Samy, A. Kaseem, M.T. Nutan et al. 2012. Development of biodegradable *in situ* implant and microparticle injectable formulations for sustained delivery of haloperidol. J. Pharma. Sci. 101: 3753–3762.

Ahmed, T.A., H.M. Ibrahim, A.M. Samy, A. Kaseem, M.T. Nutan and M.D. Hussain. 2014. Biodegradable injectable in situ implants and microparticles for sustained release of montelukast: *in vitro* release, pharmacokinetics, and stability. AAPS PharmSciTech. 15(3): 772–80.

Astaneh, R., M. Erfan, J. Barzin and H. Mobedi. 2008. Effects of ethyl benzoate on performance, morphology, and erosion of plga implants formed *in situ*. Adv. Polym. Techno. 27: 17–26.

Astaneh, R., M. Erfan, H. Moghimi and H. Mobedi. 2009. Changes in morphology of *in situ* forming PLGA implant prepared by different polymer molecular weight and its effect on release behavior. J. Pharm. Sci. 98: 135–145.

Atrisorb® FreeFlow™, Zila Inc., US Food and Drug Administration, Devices@FDA. 2012.

Avachat, A.M. and S.S. Kapure. 2014. Asenapine maleate *in situ* forming biodegradable implant: an approach to enhance bioavailability. Int. J. Pharm. 477: 64–72.

Bae, S.J., M.K. Joo, Y. Jeong, S.W. Kim, W.K. Lee, Y.S. Sohn et al. 2006. Gelation behavior of poly(ethylene glycol) and polycaprolactone triblock and multiblock copolymer aqueous solutions. Macromol. 39: 4873–4879.

Bakhshi, R., E. Vasheghani-farahani, H. Mobedi, A. Jamshidi and M. Khakpour. 2006. The effect of additives on naltrexone hydrochloride release and solvent removal rate from an injectable *in situ* forming PLGA implant release profiles. Polym. Adv. Tech. 17: 354–359.

Bleiberg, B., T. Beers, M. Persson and J. Miles. 1993. Metabolism of triacetin-derived acetate in dogs. Am. J. Clin. Nutr. 58: 908–911.

Brannon-Peppas, L. 1995. Recent advances on the use of biodegradable microparticles and nanoparticles in controlled drug delivery. Int. J. Pharm. 116: 1–9.

Brodbeck, K.J., S. Pushpala and A.J. McHugh. 1999a. Sustained release of human growth hormone from PLGA solution depots. Pharm. Res. 16: 1825–1829.

Brodbeck, K.J.J., J.R.R. Desnoyer and A.J.J. McHugh. 1999b. Phase inversion dynamics of PLGA solutions related to drug delivery. Part II. The role of solution thermodynamics and bath-side mass transfer. J. Control. Release. 62: 333–344.

Brodbeck, K.J., A.T. Gaynor-Duarte and T. Shen. 2000. Gel Composition and Methods. U.S. Patent # 6,130,200.

Camargo, J.A., A. Sapin, C. Nouvel and P. Maincent. 2013. Injectable PLA-based *in situ* forming implants for controlled release of Ivermectin a BCS Class II drug: solvent selection based on physico-chemical characterization. Drug Dev. Ind. Pharm. 39: 146–155.

Chern, R.T. and J.R. Zingerman. 2004. Liquid Polymeric Compositions for Controlled Release of Bioactive Substances. U.S. Patent # 6,733,767 B2.

Chhabra, S., V. Sachdeva and S. Singh. 2007. Influence of end groups on *in vitro* release and biological activity of lysozyme from a phase-sensitive smart polymer-based *in situ* gel forming controlled release drug delivery system. Int. J. Pharm. 342: 72–77.

Chitkara, D., A. Shikanov, N. Kumar and A.J. Domb. 2006. Biodegradable injectable *in situ* depot-forming drug delivery systems. Macromol. Biosci. 6: 977–990.

Chu, F.M., M. Jayson, M.K. Dineen, R. Perez, R. Harkaway and R.C. Tyler. 2002. A clinical study of 22.5 mg. La-2550: a new subcutaneous depot delivery system for leuprolide acetate for the treatment of prostate cancer. J. Urology. 168: 1199–1203.

Coonts, B.A., S.L. Whitman, M. O'Donnell, A.M. Polson, G. Bogle, S. Garrett et al. 1998. Biodegradation and biocompatibility of a guided tissue regeneration barrier membrane formed from a liquid polymer material. J. Biomed. Mater. Res. 42: 303–311.

DesNoyer, J. and A. McHugh. 2003. The effect of pluronic on the protein release kinetics of an injectable drug delivery system. J. Control. Rel. 86: 15–24.

DesNoyer, J.R. and A.J. McHugh. 2001. Role of crystallization in the phase inversion dynamics and protein release kinetics of injectable drug delivery systems. J. Control. Release. 70: 285–294.

Dong, S., S. Wang, C. Zheng, W. Liang and Y. Huang. 2011. An *in situ*-forming, solid lipid/PLGA hybrid implant for long-acting antipsychotics. Soft Matter. 7: 5873–5878.

Dunn, R.L., J.P. English, D.R. Cowsar and D.P. Vanderbilt. 1990. Biodegradable *In-situ* Forming Implants and Methods of Producing the Same. US Patent 4,938,763.

Dunn, R.L., A.J. Tipton, G.L. Southard and J.A. Rogers. 1997. Biodegradable Polymer Composition. U.S. Patent # 5,599,552.

Dunn, R.L., J.P. English, D.R. Cowsar and D.D. Vanderbilt. 2004. Biodegradable *In-situ* Forming Implants and Methods of Producing the Same. U.S. Patent # 5,278,202.

Eliaz, R., D. Wallach and J. Kost. 2000. Delivery of soluble tumor necrosis factor receptor from *in-situ* forming plga implants: *in-vivo.* Pharm. Res. 17: 1546–1550.

Eliaz, R.E. and J. Kost. 2000. Characterization of a polymeric PLGA-injectable implant delivery system for the controlled release of proteins. Journal of Biomedical Materials Research. 50(3): 388–96.

Fredenberg, S., M. Wahlgren, M. Reslow and A. Axelsson. 2011. The mechanisms of drug release in poly(lactic-co-glycolic acid)-based drug delivery systems-A review. Int. J. Pharma. 415: 34–55.

Garrett, S., L. Johnson, C.H. Drisko, D.F. Adams, C. Bandt, B. Beiswanger et al. 1999. Two multi-center studies evaluating locally delivered doxycycline hyclate, placebo control, oral hygiene, and scaling and root planing in the treatment of periodontitis. J. Periodont. 70: 490–503.

Gil, E. and S. Hudson. 2004. Stimuli-reponsive polymers and their bioconjugates. Prog. Polym. Sci. 29: 1173–1222.

Göpferich, A. 1996a. Mechanisms of polymer degradation and erosion. Biomater. 17: 103–114.

Göpferich, A. 1996b. Polymer degradation and erosion: mechanisms and applications. Eur. J. Pharm. Biopharm. 42: 1–11.

Graham, P.D.D., K.J.J. Brodbeck and A.J.J. McHugh. 1999. Phase inversion dynamics of PLGA solutions related to drug delivery. J. Control. Release. 58: 233–245.

Gunatillake, P.a. and R. Adhikari. 2003. Biodegradable synthetic polymers for tissue engineering. European Cells & Materials. 5: 1–16; discussion 16.

Guo, J., J. Wang, C. Cai, J. Xu, H. Yu, H. Xu et al. 2015. The anti-melanoma efficiency of the intratumoral injection of cucurbitacin-loaded sustained release carriers: *in situ*-forming implants. AAPS Pharm. Sci. Tech. 16: 973–985.

Haglund, B.O., R. Joshi and K.J. Himmelstein. 1996. An *in situ* gelling system for parenteral delivery. J. Control. Release. 41: 229–235.

Hatefi, A. and B. Amsden. 2002. Biodegradable injectable *in situ* forming drug delivery systems. J. Control. Release. 80: 9–28.

Huang, X. and C.S. Brazel. 2001. On the importance and mechanisms of burst release in matrix-controlled drug delivery systems. J. Control. Release. 73: 121–136.

Ismail, F.A., J. Napaporn, J.A. Hughes and G.A. Brazeau. 2000. *In situ* gel formulations for gene delivery: release and myotoxicity studies. Pharm. Dev. Technol. 5: 391–397.

James, R.A., M.M.C. Connell, G.A. Roberts, M.F. Scanlon, P.M. Stewart, E. Teasdale et al. 2002. Primary medical therapy for acromegaly: An open, prospective, multicenter study of the effects of subcutaneous and intramuscular slow-release octreotide on growth hormone, insulin-like growth factor-I, and tumor size. J. Clinic Endocrinol. Metabol. 87: 4554–4563.

Jamshidi, K., S.H. Hyon and Y. Ikada. 1988. Thermal characterization of polylactides. Polymer. 29: 2229–2234.

Jeon, O., M. Krebs and E. Alsberg. 2011. Controlled and sustained gene delivery from injectable, porous PLGA scaffolds. J. Biomed. Mater. Res. A. 98: 72–79.

Kang, F. and J. Singh. 2005. *In vitro* release of insulin and biocompatibility of in situ forming gel systems. Int. J. Pharm. 304: 83–90.

Kapoor, D.N., O.P. Katare and S. Dhawan. 2012. *In situ* forming implant for controlled delivery of an anti-HIV fusion inhibitor. Int. J. Pharm. 426: 132–143.

Kiernan, D.F. and W.F. Mieler. 2009. The use of intraocular corticosteroids. Expert Opin. Pharmacother. 10: 2511–2525.

Kilicarslan, M., M. Korber and R. Bodmeier. 2014. *In situ* forming implants for the delivery of metronidazole to periodontal pockets: formulation and drug release studies. Drug Dev. Ind. Pharm. 40: 619–624.

Körber, M. and R. Bodmeier. 2008. Development of an *in situ* forming PLGA drug delivery system I. Characterization of a non-aqueous protein precipitation. Eur. J. Pharma. Sci. 35: 283–292.

Kranz, H., G.A. Brazeau, J. Napaporn, R.L. Martin, W. Millard and R. Bodmeier. 2001. Myotoxicity studies of injectable biodegradable in-situ forming drug delivery systems, Int.J..Pharm. 212: 11–18.

Kranz, H. and R. Bodmeier. 2007. A novel *in situ* forming drug delivery system for controlled parenteral drug delivery. Int. J. Pharma. 332: 107–114.

Kranz, H. and R. Bodmeier. 2008. Structure formation and characterization of injectable drug loaded biodegradable devices: *in situ* implants versus *in situ* microparticles. Eur. J. Pharma. Sci. 34: 164–172.

Lambert, W.J. and K.D. Peck. 1995. Development of an *in situ* forming biodegradable poly-lactide-coglycolide system for the controlled release of proteins. J. Control. Rel. 33: 189–195.

Lee, S.S., P. Hughes, A.D. Ross and M.R. Robinson. 2010. Biodegradable implants for sustained drug release in the eye. Pharm. Res. 27: 2043–2053.

Lendlein, A. and V.P. Shastri. 2010. Stimuli-sensitive polymers. Adv. Mater. 22: 3344–3347.

Liu, Q., H. Zhang, G. Zhou, S. Xie, H. Zou, Y. Yu et al. 2010. *In vitro* and *in vivo* study of thymosin alpha1 biodegradable *in situ* forming poly(lactide-co-glycolide) implants. Int. J. Pharma. 397: 122–129.

Liu, Y., A. Kemmer, K. Keim, C. Curdy, H. Petersen and T. Kissel. 2010. Poly(ethylene carbonate) as a surface-eroding biomaterial for *in situ* forming parenteral drug delivery systems: a feasibility study. Eur. J. Pharm. Biopharm. 76: 222–229.

Luan, X. and R. Bodmeier. 2006. Influence of the poly(lactide-co-glycolide) type on the leuprolide release from *in situ* forming microparticle systems. J. Control. Release. 110: 266–272.

Luis, S. and A.A. Exner. 2015. Effect of the subcutaneous environment on phase-sensitive *in situ*-forming implant drug release, degradation, and microstructure. J. Pharm. Sci. 104: 4322–4328.

Malik, K., I. Singh, M. Nagpal and S. Arora. 2010. Atrigel: a potential parenteral controlled drug delivery system. Der Pharmacia Sinica. 1: 74–81.

Mashak, A., H. Mobedi, F. Ziaee and M. Nekoomanesh. 2011. The effect of aliphatic esters on the formation and degradation behavior of PLGA-based *in situ* forming system. Polym. Bull. 66: 1063–1073.

Matschke, C., U. Isele, P. Van Hoogevest and A. Fahr. 2002. Sustained-release injectables formed *in situ* and their potential use for veterinary products. J. Control. Release. 85: 1–15.

McHugh, A.J. 2005. The role of polymer membrane formation in sustained release drug delivery systems. J. Control. Release. 109: 211–221.

Merkli, A., C. Tabatabay, R. Gurny and J. Heller. 1998. Biodegradable polymers for the controlled release of ocular drugs. Prog. Polym. Sci. 23: 563–580.

Middleton, J.C. and A.J. Tipton. 2000. Synthetic biodegradable polymers as orthopedic devices. Biomater. 21: 2335–2346.

Miyajima, M., A. Koshika, J. Okada, M. Ikeda and K. Nishimura. 1997. Effect of polymer crystallinity on papaverine release from poly(L-lactic acid) matrix. J. Control. Release. 49: 207–215.

Modlin, I.M., M. Pavel, M. Kidd and B.I. Gustafsson. 2010. Review article: somatostatin analogues in the treatment of gastroenteropancreatic neuroendocrine (carcinoid) tumours. Aliment Pharmacol. Therapeut. 31: 169–188.

Mohammad, D.A., B.V. Sweet and S.G. Elner. 2007. Retisert: is the new advance in treatment of uveitis a good one? Ann. Pharmacother. 41: 449–454.

Nasongkla, N., A. Boongird, S. Hongeng, C. Manaspon and N. Larbcharoensub. 2012. Preparation and biocompatibility study of *in situ* forming polymer implants in rat brains. J. Mater. Sci. Mater. Medi. 23: 497–505.

Novartis Pharmaceuticals UK Ltd., Summary of Product Characteristics of Sandostatin LAR (2011).

Omelczuk, M.O. and J.W. McGinity. 1992. The influence of polymer glass transition temperature and molecular weight on drug release from tablets containing poly(DL-lactic acid). Pharm. Res. 9: 26–32.

Packhaeuser, C.B., J. Schnieders, C.G. Oster and T. Kissel. 2004. *In situ* forming parenteral drug delivery systems: an overview. Eur. J. Pharm. Biopharm. 58: 445–455.

Patel, R.B., A.N. Carlson, L. Solorio and A.A. Exner. 2010. Characterization of formulation parameters affecting low molecular weight drug release from *in situ* forming drug delivery systems. J. Biomed. Mater. Res. Part A. 94: 476–484.

Qin, Y., M. Yuan, L. Li. and J. Xue. 2012. Formulation and evaluation of *in situ* forming PLA implant containing tinidazole for the treatment of periodontitis. J. Biomed. Mater. Res. B Appl. Biomater. 100: 2197–2202.

Rafienia, M., S.H. Emami, H. Mirzadeh and S. Karbasi. 2009. Influence of poly (lactide-co-glycolide) type and gamma irradiation on the betamethasone acetate release from the *in situ* forming systems. Curr. Drug Deliv. 6: 184–191.

Raman, C. and A.J. McHugh. 2005. A model for drug release from fast phase inverting injectable solutions. J. Control. Release. 102: 145–157.

Royals, M.A., S.M. Fujita, G.L. Yewey, J. Rodriguez, P.C. Schultheiss and R.L. Dunn. 1999. Biocompatibility of a biodegradable *in situ* forming implant system in rhesus monkeys. J. Biomed. Mater. Res. 45: 231–239.

Ruel-Gariépy, E. and J.C. Leroux. 2004. *In situ*-forming hydrogels—review of temperature-sensitive systems. Eur. J. Pharma. Biopharma. 58: 409–426.

Sanju, D., R. Kapil and D.N. Kapoor. 2010. Development and evaluation of *in situ* gel-forming system for sustained delivery of insulin. J. Biomater. App. 25: 699–720.

Sartor, O. 2003. Eligard: leuprolide acetate in a novel sustained-release delivery system. Urology. 61: 25–31.

Schoenhammer, K., H. Petersen, F. Guethlein and A. Goepferich. 2009a. Poly(ethyleneglycol) 500 dimethylether as novel solvent for injectable *in situ* forming depots. Pharm. Res. 26: 2568–2577.

Schoenhammer, K., H. Petersen, F. Guethlein and A. Goepferich. 2009b. Injectable *in situ* forming depot systems: PEG-DAE as novel solvent for improved PLGA storage stability. Int. J. Pharma. 371: 33–39.

Schoenhammer, K., J. Boisclair, H. Schuetz, H. Petersen and A. Goepferich. 2010. Biocompatibility of an injectable *in situ* forming depot for peptide delivery. J. Pharma. Sci. 99: 4390–4399.

Setterstrom, J.A., T.R. Tice, W.E. Meyers and J. Vincent. 1984. Development of encapsulated antibiotics for topical administration to wounds. In: Second World Congress on Biomaterials 10th Annual Meeting of the Society for Biomaterials, Washington. p. 4.

Shively, M.L., B.A. Coonts, W.D. Renner, J.L. Southard and A.T. Bennett. 1995. Physico-chemical characterization of a polymeric injectable implant delivery system. J. Control. Rel. 33: 237–243.

Solorio, L., B.M. Babin, R.B. Patel, J. Mach, N. Azar and A.A. Exner. 2010. Noninvasive characterization of *in situ* forming implants using diagnostic ultrasound. J. Control. Release. 143: 183–190.

Stoller, N.H., L.R. Johnson, S. Trapnell, C.Q. Harrold and S. Garrett. 1998. The pharmacokinetic profile of a biodegradable controlled-release delivery system containing doxycycline compared to systemically delivered doxycycline in gingival crevicular fluid, saliva, and serum. J. Periodont. 69: 1085–1091.

Tan, L.P., S.S. Venkatraman, P.F. Sung and X.T. Wang. 2004. Effect of plasticization on heparin release from biodegradable matrices. Int. J. Pharma. 283: 89–96.

Tang, Y. and J. Singh. 2008. Controlled delivery of aspirin: effect of aspirin on polymer degradation and *in vitro* release from PLGA based phase sensitive systems. Int. J. Pharma. 357: 119–125.

Ueda, H., M.C. Hacker, A. Haesslein, S. Jo, D.M. Ammon, R.N. Borazjani et al. 2007. Injectable, *in situ* forming poly(propylene fumarate)-based ocular drug delivery systems. J. Biomed. Mater. Res. Part A. 83: 656–666.

US Food and Drug Adminsitration, Highlights of Prescribing Information, (2011).

Wang, L., S. Venkatraman and L. Kleiner. 2004. Drug release from injectable depots: two different *in vitro* mechanisms. J. Control. Release. 99: 207–216.

Wang, L., A. Wang, X. Zhao, X. Liu, D. Wang, F. Sun et al. 2012. Design of a long-term antipsychotic *in situ* forming implant and its release control method and mechanism. Int. J. Pharma. 427: 284–292.

Wang, X., S.S. Venkatraman, F.Y.C. Boey, J.S.C. Loo and L.P. Tan. 2006. Controlled release of sirolimus from a multilayered PLGA stent matrix. Biomater. 27: 5588–5595.

Wischke, C., Y. Zhang, S. Mittal and S.P. Schwendeman. 2010. Development of PLGA-based injectable delivery systems for hydrophobic fenretinide. Pharm. Res. 27: 2063–2074.

Yapar, E.A., N.D. Ari and T. Baykara. 2014. Evaluation of *in vitro* and *in vivo* performance of granisetron *in situ* forming implants: effect of sterilization, storage condition and degradation. Trop. J. Pharm. Res. 13: 319–325.

Yasukawa, T., H. Kimura, Y. Tabata and Y. Ogura. 2001. Biodegradable scleral plugs for vitreoretinal drug delivery. Adv. Drug Deliv. Rev. 52: 25–36.

Yu, T. and J. Singh. 2008. Controlled delivery of aspirin: effect of aspirin on polymer degradation and *in vitro* release from PLGA based phase sensitive systems. Int. J. Pharm. 357: 119–125.

Zare, M., H. Mobedi, J. Barzin, H. Mivehchi, A. Jamshidi and R. Mashayekhi. 2008. Effect of additives on release profile of leuprolide acetate in an *in situ* forming controlled-release system: *in vitro* study. J. App. Polym. Sci. 107: 3781–3787.

Zhang, X., C. Zhang, W. Zhang, S. Meng, D. Liu, P. Wang et al. 2015. Feasibility of Poly (ε-caprolactone-co-DL-lactide) as a biodegradable material for *in situ* forming implants: evaluation of drug release and *in vivo* degradation. Drug Dev. Ind. Pharm. 41: 342–352.

CHAPTER 14

Transdermal Applications of Hydrogels

Helen L. Quinn and *Ryan F. Donnelly**

Introduction

A hydrogel is a three-dimensional polymeric network, which has the ability to swell and retain water, yet remains insoluble. The water-absorbing capacity of the gel arises from the preponderance of hydrophilic functional groups on the polymeric backbone, while the insolubility occurs as a result of the cross-linked structure (Peppas et al. 2000). This cross-linking is essential for maintaining the elastic hydrogel structure and can be physical or chemical in nature, depending on the nature of the associations. The unique properties of hydrogels have led to their application in a variety of drug delivery systems, from implantable devices to topical formulations (Hoare and Kohane 2008). The porous structure creates a carrier matrix for drug loading, with the option of controlling release by modification of the hydrogel properties. The drug release from a hydrogel proceeds at a rate dependent on the diffusion coefficient of the drug through the polymeric network, which in turn is largely dependent upon the structure and pore size of the hydrogel, in addition to the properties of the drug itself (Thakur et al. 2009). These hydrogel characteristics can easily be tuned by adjustment of the cross-link density, with the tangible outcome of controlling the swelling behaviour of the hydrogel in a given solvent. The two most important characteristics of hydrogels in controlled release applications are, therefore, the intrinsically linked properties of network permeability and swelling behaviour. Understanding and manipulating these hydrogel characteristics will aid in modeling solute release from candidate hydrogel-based controlled drug-delivery systems. As researchers seek to optimise drug delivery processes, the use of novel routes for drug administration is of great interest, with transdermal delivery the focus of much research. Having found many applications

School of Pharmacy, Queen's University, Belfast, 97 Lisburn Road, Belfast, BT9 7BL, UK.
* Corresponding author: r.donnelly@qub.ac.uk

in advanced drug delivery systems, hydrogels have inevitably played a role in the innovative transdermal formulations investigated.

Transdermal Drug Delivery

The delivery of drugs via the transdermal route offers many advantages in terms of both patient comfort and, also, the action of the drug. The primary attraction with such a system is considered to be the convenient and non-invasive nature, which can lead to increased patient adherence and satisfaction, particularly in comparison to delivery methods associated with pain and discomfort, such as injections (Jenkins 2014). By circumventing the gastrointestinal tract, the risk of degradation of the active is removed and variables which may cause unpredictable drug absorption are minimised, such as pH, enzymatic activity and drug-food interactions (Morrow et al. 2007). Hepatic first-pass metabolism is also avoided, proffering the possibility for improved bioavailability of the drug. Drug transport across the skin typically progresses at a relatively slow rate, facilitating sustained delivery of drug and achieving a steady-state effect instead of the typical peak-trough profile. The maintenance of drug levels within the therapeutic window for extended durations of time with the same transdermal patch is therefore possible. The relatively constant plasma concentrations can also reduce the occurrence of adverse effects. For compounds with a short biological half-life, this can lead to a reduced dosing frequency. Termination of therapy in the event of a serious adverse effect or toxicity is also easily achieved, as a straightforward removal of the patch should cease drug delivery.

The number of drugs able to passively diffuse across the skin barrier is inherently limited in terms of the molecular requirements. A number of physicochemical drug properties have been identified as important for transdermal permeation, including a molecular mass less than 600 Da, an octanol-water partition coefficient between 1 and 3 and reasonably high potency (Prausnitz and Langer 2008). Since the FDA approval of the first transdermal product in 1979 (scopolamine), the market for conventional transdermal patches has not consistently expanded, as the number of drugs that can be formulated for passive permeation through the skin has dwindled. To enable the delivery of a wider range of drug compounds and overcome the permeability barrier of the skin anatomy, methods of permeation enhancement are required.

Hydrogels offer attractive transdermal materials because of their high water content, providing a comfortable feeling on the patient's skin, which may lead to better adherence to therapy (Mazzitelli et al. 2013). On the converse, however, transdermal drug delivery can be challenging, due to the hydrophilic nature of the gels (Rehman and Zulfakar 2014). In terms of application to the skin, hydrogels have found their greatest use to date in wound healing and dressing, with a number of successful marketed products using this type of polymeric scaffold for wound protection and facilitation of healing. Hydrogels are ideal for maintaining suitable moist environmental conditions for wound healing, promoting granulation, epithelialization, and autolytic debridement (Ghobril and Grinstaff 2015). In some cases, a hydrogel can be simultaneously used for controlled local drug delivery in addition to providing a wound dressing. To this end, hydrogels have been extensively investigated for topical delivery of antimicrobials, such as silver sulfadiazine (Jodar et al. 2015), anti-inflammatory agents, such as curcumin (Gong et al. 2013) and local anaesthetics, for example, lidocaine (Negi et al. 2014). Distinct from these examples, there are also numerous reports of hydrogels being applied transdermally for the purposes of systemic delivery. For example, chitosan hydrogels have been used for delivery of glimepiride (Ammar et al. 2008) the active S-enantiomer of racemic propranolol (Suedee et al. 2008). Liu et al. (2014) designed a hydrogel formulation of tolterodine for the treatment of overactive bladder, achieving sustained release over 24 h and greater bioavailability than oral administration of tablets in rats. Considering marketed products, IONSYS®, a fentanyl iontophoretic transdermal system, has recently been re-launched, indicated for the short-term management of acute postoperative pain in hospital settings (Scott 2016). The fentanyl in this patch is contained within a hydrogel reservoir, the electrical current essential for driving the fentanyl across the skin upon activation of the system. However, despite the examples discussed, the use of a hydrogel formulation alone is generally not sufficient to guarantee transdermal penetration of the active ingredient. The technologies showing the greatest promise in transdermal delivery are those that are designed to temporarily manipulate the skin barrier, increasing permeation by disruption of the outermost layer of skin, the *stratum corneum* (Prausnitz and Langer 2008). Microneedles are an example of this, mechanically creating pores in the *stratum corneum* and physically bypassing the principal skin barrier. A microneedle array is a collection of numerous micron-sized projections (50–900 μm), amassed on a baseplate (Fig. 1). When applied to the skin, the tiny needles puncture the *stratum corneum*, forming aqueous conduits for diffusion to the dermal microcirculation. Microneedle drug delivery can occur via a variety of mechanisms including drug-coated microneedles, soluble microneedles with drug incorporated or infusion through hollow microneedles (Tuan-Mahmood et

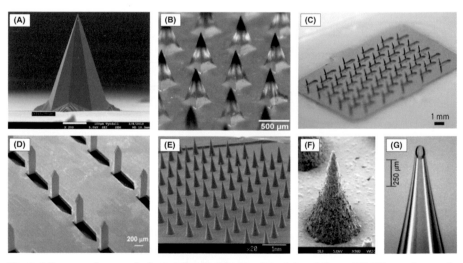

Fig. 1. Microscope images of microneedles used for transdermal drug delivery. (A) Silicon microneedle of height 400 μm (O'Mahony 2014). (B) Dissolving microneedles prepared from sucrose and PVA (Edens et al. 2015). (C) Array of 100 stainless steel microneedles of height 750 μm (Norman et al. 2014). (D) Out-of-plane stainless steel microneedles of height 700 μm (Gill and Prausnitz 2007). (E) Dissolving microneedle array (needle height 800 μm) prepared from poly(vinyl pyrrolidone) (Wang et al. 2015). (F) Single polymeric microneedle of height 600 μm (Donnelly et al. 2010). (G) Hollow glass microneedle (Martanto et al. 2006).

al. 2013). Alternatively, a drug reservoir can be applied following skin piercing with a microneedle array. Solid microneedles prepared from materials such as silicon and metal have been combined with hydrogel patches in this 'poke and patch' approach, for systemic delivery of the active. For example, silicon microneedles have been used in tandem with a hydrogel patch formulation, loaded with hepatitis B surface antigen, and cholera toxin B as an adjuvant (Guo et al. 2013). Female Balb/c mice were pretreated with the microneedle array, followed by application of a carbomer hydrogel patch, producing a longer duration of stable IgG titres compared with an intramuscular control group. However, the cumbersome two-step process, alongside concerns about breakage or debris of these materials in the skin and high production costs, has led to interest in the use of FDA-approved polymeric substances for microneedle manufacture. These materials are often inexpensive and widely available, amenable for microneedle manufacture without the use of harsh processing conditions, e.g., elevated temperatures. The majority of polymeric microneedles are designed to dissolve, releasing the drug loading by dissolution of the microneedles. In one novel approach of this type, hydrogel microparticles were incorporated into biodegradable poly-lactic-co-glycolic acid (PLGA) microneedles, in an attempt to achieve sustained delivery of both hydrophobic and hydrophilic drugs (Kim et al. 2012). Upon insertion of the microneedle array into the skin, the encapsulated hydrogel particles rapidly absorbed water and expanded, causing cracking of the microneedle structures, due to the difference in volume expansion between the needle matrix polymer and the hydrogel particles. Total breakdown of the microneedles then occurred, depositing the tips and loaded drug into the skin. This method, however, similar to other dissolving microneedle delivery strategies, may lead to the deposition of polymer in the skin. Likely of little concern for occasional use such as vaccination, it would be preferable to minimize polymer delivery into the skin when considering long-term microneedle use (Donnelly and Woolfson 2014). The use of hydrogels, which remain intact after absorption of aqueous fluid, for microneedle manufacture has, therefore, been investigated.

Hydrogel-Forming Microneedles

Hydrogel-forming microneedles are a relatively new concept, first described by Donnelly et al. (2012). They reported a novel strategy, involving an integrated system, consisting of drug-free microneedles prepared from a hydrogel-forming polymer and a separate drug reservoir attached to the supporting baseplate. Hard in the dry state and, hence, able to be reliably inserted, these microneedles swell upon application to the skin, due to the uptake of interstitial fluid from the tissue. This triggers diffusion of the drug from the attached reservoir, through the swollen micro-projections, which act as conduits, into the dermal layers of the skin for uptake by the microcirculation, as illustrated in Fig. 2. Another strategy, described by Yang et al. (2012), has the drug incorporated directly into the needle tip hydrogel matrix, for diffusion outwards upon insertion and contact with the interstitial fluid. In both scenarios, regardless of the initial location of the drug, the rate of drug diffusion into the lower skin layers is controlled by the degree of swelling of the cross-linked polymer, which forms the hydrogel matrix. Altering the polymer cross-link density can, therefore, control the

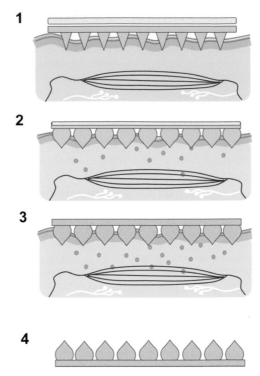

Fig. 2. Schematic illustration of the mechanism of action of hydrogel-forming microneedles.

rate of microneedle swelling, thus conferring the ability to govern drug release rate, which can be tailored for specific drugs. As with other microneedles, hydrogel-forming microneedles are painless and blood-free upon application, with the additional benefit of being removed intact from the skin following use, thereby depositing no measurable residual polymer. Importantly, however, the microneedles are suitably softened by the interstitial fluid, preventing reinsertion of the array, thereby reducing the risk of infection transmission that may arise from needle reuse.

Materials and manufacture

The first hydrogel-forming microneedles were manufactured using aqueous blends of specific polymeric materials, namely poly(methyl vinyl ether-co-maleic acid) (PMVE/MA), cross-linked with poly(ethylene glycol) (PEG) (Donnelly et al. 2012). Upon heating, these two polymers undergo an esterification reaction (Fig. 3) to produce a cross-linked material, confirmed using attenuated total reflectance (ATR)-Fourier transform infra-red (FTIR) spectroscopy and the observation of a carbonyl peak shift from 1708 to 1731 cm^{-1}, due to formation of an ester carbonyl (Luppi et al. 2003; Thakur et al. 2009). The swelling and network parameters of the hydrogels formed by the cross-linking of PMVE/MA with PEG have been extensively characterized, investigating the effect of PEG molecular weight, as well as differing ratios of the two components (Thakur et al. 2009). Using a high molecular weight PEG (1,000–10,000

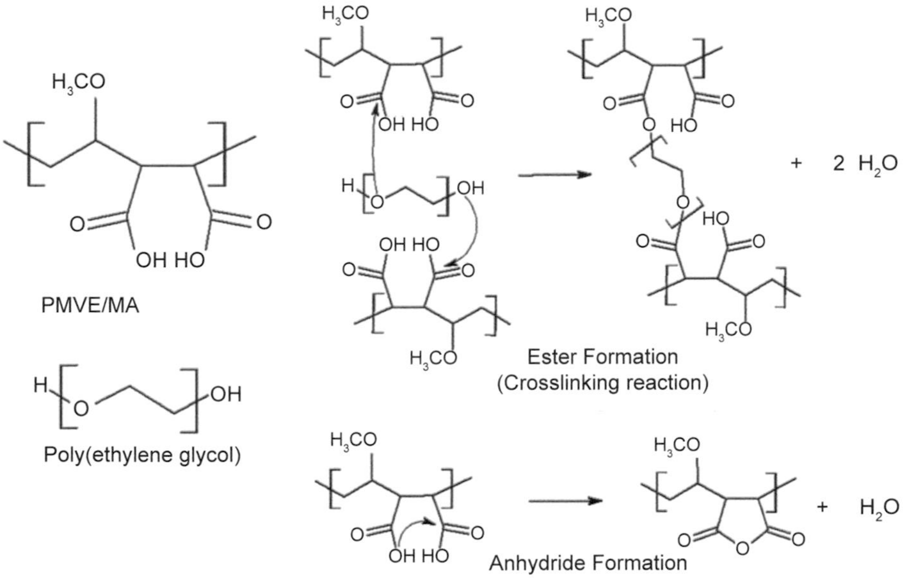

Fig. 3. Chemical structures and proposed chemical reactions that take place during the cross-linking process (Larrañeta et al. 2015).

Daltons) as a cross-linker was found to form a hydrogel with a lower cross-link density and higher average molecular weight between two consecutive cross-links. This was reflected in the higher degree of equilibrium swelling and higher initial swelling rates observed in the hydrogel. This trend was attributed to the greater chain length and relatively fewer reactive hydroxyl groups present in PEG as the molecular weight of the polymer increases. Scanning electron microscopy studies highlighted the porosity of the cross-linked PMVE/MA and PEG 10,000 material, as shown in Fig. 4. Further investigations studied the change in PMVE/MA concentration and the effects on solute permeation across the hydrogel (Thakur et al. 2010). The permeation of model solutes through the hydrogels was demonstrated to be in accordance with the swelling behaviour, the degree of which decreased with increasing PMVE/MA content in the hydrogels. This is explained by the fact that increasing the polymer content also increases the cross-link density of the hydrogels, hence reducing free volume for solute diffusion. Based on the work discussed, subsequent research chose a concentration of 15% w/w PMVE/MA, in combination with 7.5% w/w PEG 10,000, for microneedle preparation (Donnelly et al. 2012). These hydrogel-forming microneedle arrays were prepared by a simple micromoulding technique, using laser-engineered silicone templates. A formulation containing both polymers was cast into female moulds and the microcavities filled under centrifugation, followed by drying at ambient temperature. After 48 h, the filled moulds were placed inside a convection oven at 80°C for a period of 24 h to allow the cross-linking reaction between the polymers to occur. Recently however, cross-linking times for this process have been reduced to around 45 min by using microwave radiation (Larrañeta et al. 2015). The swelling of the resultant formulation can be further modified by the addition of sodium carbonate (Na_2CO_3). The incorporation of Na_2CO_3 into a hydrogel prepared using the

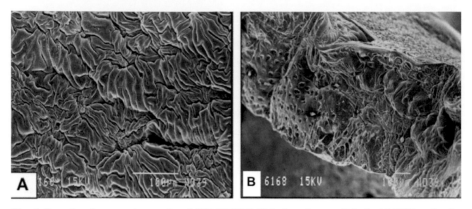

Fig. 4. Scanning electron micrographs of 15% PMVE/MA hydrogels cross-linked with PEG molecular weight 10,000 Daltons in 2:1 ratio (Thakur et al. 2009).

acid form of PMVE/MA and PEG was found to increase the swelling capacity of the resulting material (Donnelly et al. 2014a). For example, after 1 hour, the percentage swelling of what is termed 'super swelling hydrogels' (20% w/w acid form of PMVE/MA, 7.5% w/w PEG 10,000 and 3% w/w Na_2CO_3) was 1119%, compared to only 250% for the original formulation (15% w/w PMVE/MA, 7.5% w/w PEG 10,000). Infrared spectrometry indicated that this action was due to sodium salt formation on free acid groups on the copolymer, thus reducing ester-based cross-linking. The extremely porous structure formed was also evidenced by the average molecular weight between crosslinks, M_c, determined to be 6,793,627 g/mol, highlighting the potential for diffusion of macromolecules through this network.

The glass transition temperature of the PMVE/MA and PEG hydrogel first described for microneedle manufacture ($55.82 \pm 0.97°C$) is well above typical room temperatures, thus, at ambient temperature, the polymer chains within the network are not sufficiently mobile and the material is relatively hard (Donnelly et al. 2012). The mechanical properties of these materials, therefore, allow skin insertion and mechanical resistance to fracture when dry, making this type of hydrogel a good candidate for microneedle manufacture. Insertion forces as low as 0.03 N per needle resulted in 100% needle penetration *in vitro* and regardless of the force applied, none of the needles on the array broke or shattered upon application into the skin. Upon mechanical testing, a force of 23.55 N was required to break the hydrogel microneedle base-plate, with an angle of approximately 79.28° at break point, demonstrating both the strength of the material and, also, its conformability, important for application to the uneven skin surface. The hydrogel-forming microneedle arrays were also demonstrated to retain their mechanical integrity when swollen, being sufficiently robust in this state to ensure the microneedles were removed intact from the skin.

In a different polymeric approach, Hardy et al. (2016) described formation of hydrogel-forming microneedles using 2-hydroxyethyl methacrylate (pHEMA) cross-linked with ethylene glycol dimethacrylate (EGDMA). Prepared using the same micromoulding technique as described by Donnelly et al. (2012), polymerization and cross-linking occurred simultaneously when the monomer gel mixture was placed in the oven at a temperature of 90°C for 2 h. This system displayed a slow swelling rate and low extent of swelling overall, reaching a maximum of approximately a 50% mass increase, beyond the 24 h period, suggesting that this type of material would be more suitable for the production of drug delivery systems for prolonged release.

Besides polyanhydride and acrylate type polymers, only mixtures of polysaccharides (dextran, gelatin) and poly(vinyl alcohol) (PVA) have been reported to be used successfully to produce hydrogel-forming microneedle arrays for drug delivery (Hong et al. 2014). Yang et al. (2012) used PVA, dextran, and carboxymethylcellulose (CMC) to prepare what they have termed 'phase-transition microneedles', using a similar casting method to that described previously, albeit with some key differences. A ceramic material, known as purple clay, was used to form the female microneedle mould and upon addition of the polymer solution, a vacuum was applied to the opposite side of the mould in order to force the formulation into the tips of the microcavities. The filled mould was then frozen at −20°C for 2 hours and thawed at 4°C for 1 hour, with this freeze-thaw cycle repeated twice more, with the aim of forming microcrystalline junctions within the structure, to cross-link and solidify the polymer. Following this process, the arrays possessed sufficient strength to be detached from the mould and dried, before sterilization by steaming in an oxirane vapour. Similarly, Demir et al. (2013) prepared swelling microneedle arrays by crosslinking 20% w/v PVA and 10% w/v gelatin. The formulation was cast into polydimethylsiloxane micromoulds and then frozen at −20°C for 12 h, followed by thawing at 25°C for 12 h, with this cycle repeated three times, creating a physically cross-linked system by cryogelation.

Safety and biocompatibility

In general, hydrogels are highly biocompatible, as reflected in their successful use in the peritoneum (Sutton 2005) and other sites *in vivo*. This is due in part to the high water content and, also, the physiochemical similarity of hydrogels to the native extracellular matrix. With respect to microneedles, the biocompatibility of the materials used for manufacture is considered important, as when applied to the skin, the needles are introduced into the body intradermally. All polymers in the formulations discussed, have been widely used in other pharmaceutical applications, prior to microneedle manufacture. PVA is known to be biocompatible and has been commonly employed as a biomedical excipient, as it is non-toxic and non-carcinogenic, with both swelling properties and bioadhesive characteristics (Baker et al. 2012). Likewise, PMVE/MA and its acid form (Gantrez® type co-polymers) have been extensively used for over 40 years as thickening and suspending agents in topical salves and ointments, as well as in denture adhesives (Mrak et al. 1988).

The biocompatibility of PEG-cross-linked PMVE/MA-based hydrogel microneedle materials was evaluated by Donnelly et al. (2012) using three different cell-lines; fibroblasts (Balb/3T3), keratinocytes (NRERT-1) and a 3D keratinocyte organotypic raft culture. No significant reduction in cell viability was observed in any test, indicating that this type of hydrogel-based microneedle material was likely to be biocompatible. *In vitro* skin irritancy studies showed that the microneedle formulation was likely to also be non-irritant, resulting in significantly less interleukin-1 alpha production in a 3D reconstructed human skin model, when compared to a positive control of 5% w/v sodium dodecyl sulphate. This is in line with other research that has demonstrated the *in vitro* biocompatibility of hydrogels prepared from this type of polymer (Luzardo-Álvarez et al. 2011; Moreno et al. 2014). Hydrogel-forming microneedles prepared from the polymer PMVE/MA have also been shown to exhibit antimicrobial properties, with no microbial growth detected upon storage (Donnelly et al. 2013). This type of hydrogel is, therefore, highly unlikely to cause skin or systemic infection. Indeed, the human studies to date have revealed no skin reactions following use, with swollen arrays removed intact after up to 6 h in place in skin (Donnelly et al. 2014c).

Drug delivery

Hydrogel-forming microneedles been shown to successfully deliver a range of molecules of varying molecular weight *in vivo*, from small, hydrophilic molecules, such as metronidazole, to larger molecular weight peptide and protein molecules, such as insulin and fluorescein isothiocyanate labelled-bovine serum albumin (Donnelly et al. 2012). The combination of the hydrogel-forming microneedles with iontophoresis, with the aim of achieving for pulsatile or bolus delivery, was observed to provoke a marked increase in the rate and extent of in-skin swelling of the arrays. In general, this led to a greater rate and overall extent of transdermal delivery for each of the molecules; however, the difference was only significant for the biomolecules under investigation.

The hydrogel-forming microneedle arrays described as 'super swelling' have also been tested for their drug delivery capabilities (Donnelly et al. 2014a). Paired with a lyophilized drug reservoir, delivery of a clinically relevant dose of a low potency, high dose drug substance (ibuprofen) was achieved, as well as rapid delivery of a model protein (ovalbumin). Hardy et al. (2016) also investigated ibuprofen delivery, using a light-responsive 3,5-dimethoxybenzoin conjugate of the drug incorporated in a pHEMA formulation, in order to test light-triggered transdermal drug delivery. *In vitro*, this hydrogel array was able to deliver up to three doses of 50 mg of ibuprofen upon application of an optical trigger, over a prolonged period of time (up to 160 h). This type of system offers great potential as a stimulus responsive delivery platform, where "on-demand" drug delivery is required, with patient- or physician-controlled analgesia an obvious example.

Application of a 'phase-transition microneedle patch' containing insulin at a dose of 2.0 IU kg^{-1} was able to achieve comparable blood insulin area under curve (AUC) to a 0.4 IU kg^{-1} injection in a diabetic pig model, indicating the relative availability of insulin delivered by the microneedles to be around 20% of the total insulin contained within. In fact, over a 2 month period, the PVA, dextran and CMC microneedle array showed significantly better control of long-term blood glucose over the subcutaneous injection, as measured by HbA1c level, likely due to the post-peak sustained release of insulin from the array. This offers opportunity for non-invasive insulin delivery, with future work hoping to load insulin in selected regions along the microneedle shafts to accommodate the different insulin-dosing regimens. With these alternative polymer systems, however, the drug is included inside the hydrogel-forming microneedle patch rather than in an external reservoir, thus potentially limiting the quantity of drug that can be delivered. The use of a separate drug reservoir, paired with a drug-free hydrogel-forming array, provides flexibility in the formulation of the attached drug reservoir, which inherently confers greater loading capacity than the methods employed in drug loading of an array containing the drug within itself.

Conceptualized and created for transdermal drug delivery, hydrogel-forming microneedles have also found application in other healthcare scenarios. In only a slight aside, in the field of photodynamic therapy, a hydrogel-forming microneedle array composed of 20% w/w PMVE/MA, cross-linked with 6% w/w glycerol, was shown to enhance delivery of the porphyrin precursor 5-aminolevulinic acid and a preformed photosensitizer, meso-tetra (N-methyl-4-pyridyl) porphine tetra tosylate. Moving away from drug delivery completely, however, Yang et al. (2013) have demonstrated that their advanced microneedle system could be used in skin graft adherence, as illustrated in Fig. 5. Biphasic, conical shaped microneedles composed of a non-swelling polystyrene core and a polystyrene-*block*-poly(acrylic acid) swellable tip were inserted into tissue with minimal force and once in place, displayed enhanced tissue adhesion strength in comparison to staples, which are conventionally used in skin graft adherence. Furthermore, there is the opportunity for the swelling tips to be loaded with therapeutic agents, in order to facilitate both local drug delivery and tissue adhesion.

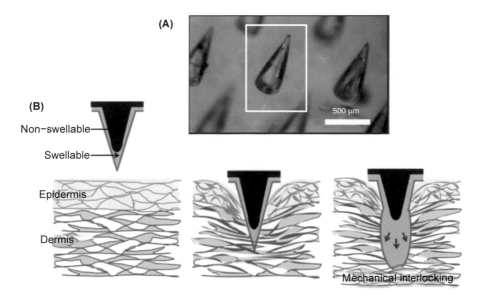

Fig. 5. Concept of the bio-inspired hydrogel microneedle adhesive. Microneedle image showing the poly(styrene)-block-poly(acrylic acid) swellable tip, clearly distinguishable from the non-swellable polystyrene core (A). Illustration showing mechanical interlocking of a water-responsive shape-changeable microneedle, following penetration into tissue (B).

Therapeutic drug monitoring

Therapeutic monitoring is an important tool in patient care, with a role in diagnosing illness, optimising treatment and subsequently tracking progress. This process is typically conducted by the collection of blood samples, followed by the analysis and determination of plasma concentrations of the drug or endogenous substance of interest. However, the use of hypodermic needles for sampling is associated with a number of well-characterized disadvantages, including for example, needle-phobia, the need for trained healthcare staff for administration, sharps disposal, the risk of needle-stick injury and transmission of infection (Simonsen et al. 1999). An alternative method of sampling is, therefore, much needed. Due to the intrinsic capacity of hydrogels to imbibe fluid, there is potential for application of such systems in the collection of specific analytes for screening, diagnostic and monitoring purposes. This concept has been employed in tandem with microneedles, in order to extract interstitial fluid, due to the two-way movement of fluid possible with a microneedle platform (Mukerjee et al. 2004). Interstitial fluid levels can be used as surrogate markers for the blood concentration of an analyte, often enabling accurate comparisons to the free concentrations of drugs and endogenous substances in plasma (Kiang et al. 2012). This can then be converted to relevant clinical information, either in one step by a sensor specific to the particular analyte of interest as part of the array, or in two steps by analysis upon removal of the patch and extraction of the specific substance. Typically the movement of interstitial fluid relies on capillary action, in order to extract the fluid, or indeed, more complex mechanisms such as vacuum or osmotic pressure. The use of a hydrogel for this purpose, however, offers an interesting alternative. This potential process is summarized in Fig. 6. Sakaguchi et al. (2012) described pre-treatment of the skin with a poly(carbonate) plastic microneedle array, followed

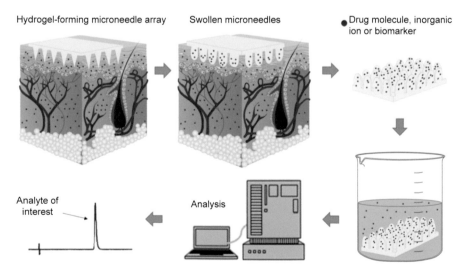

Fig. 6. Schematic representation demonstrating the principle of microneedle-mediated therapeutic drug monitoring. Images display swelling of hydrogel-forming microneedles upon insertion due to interstitial fluid uptake, capture and extraction of analyte of interest and ultimately quantification of analyte (Caffarel-Salvador et al. 2015).

by application of a hydrogel patch, prepared from PVA containing 2% potassium chloride, for accumulation of interstitial fluid. This approach enabled comparison between the interstitial fluid glucose AUC and the plasma glucose AUC in the 2 h following an oral glucose tolerance test, demonstrating a strong correlation between the two values. To further streamline the sampling process, microneedles, to enable interstitial fluid access, and a hydrogel for fluid accumulation, can be combined into one step by the preparation of hydrogel-forming microneedle arrays (Donnelly et al. 2014b). Once inserted, such systems rapidly uptake interstitial fluid, and in so doing, collect a sample of the analyte of interest.

The swelling in skin and the associated fluid uptake are an important consideration in the preparation of a hydrogel microneedle formulation, the volume of fluid particularly of concern for the purposes of sample collection. These parameters were investigated in human volunteers, with microneedle arrays prepared from aqueous blends of hydrolyzed PMVE/MA (15% w/w) and the cross-linking agent, PEG 10,000 (7.5% w/w) (Donnelly et al. 2014c). The microneedle arrays swelled in skin upon insertion and, hence, displayed a percentage mass increase, which increased significantly as in-skin residence time also increased, reaching a maximum of approximately 30% after 6 h. After 1 h, the estimated fluid uptake ranged from 0.9–2.7 mg, comparable to other microneedle-mediated methods of sample extraction, which use more intensive methods to withdraw the sample. Similar results have also been reported by Romanyuk et al. (2014) who found interstitial fluid uptake in rats after 1 h, using a similar hydrogel formulation, to be 0.84 ± 0.24 mg. This demonstrates the ease of sample collection over a short time period, with the likelihood that the patch wear-time may be able to be further reduced in the future.

Eltayib et al. (2016) used hydrogel-forming microneedles to collect interstitial fluid for extraction and analysis of lithium concentration, a treatment for bipolar disorder with a narrow therapeutic window. Following oral administration of lithium to Sprague-Dawley rats and application of microneedle arrays, it was shown that the hydrogel formulation was able to capture a quantifiable amount of lithium from interstitial fluid, following a period of only 1 h. Similarly, Caffarel-Salvador et al. (2015) demonstrated this principal in a similar experiment using theophylline, noting a highly significant difference in the interstitial fluid concentrations measured after oral administration of 5 mg/kg and 10 mg/kg theophylline to Sprague-Dawley rats. This observation, therefore, suggests that microneedles have the potential to differentiate between therapeutic and toxic interstitial fluid concentrations of drug substances. The premise of hydrogel-forming microneedle monitoring has also been demonstrated in human volunteers, using microneedle arrays prepared from the same polymeric materials and both caffeine and glucose as model analytes (Caffarel-Salvador et al. 2015). Whilst not directly correlated with the blood levels achieved, concentrations extracted from hydrogel microneedles were clearly indicative of trends in the human volunteers. Future work in this area will involve reducing microneedle application time in human volunteers while simultaneously investigating the applicability of the method for a wide range of clinically relevant drug compounds and biomarkers. If researchers are successful in these endeavours, there is great potential for hydrogel-forming microneedles in minimally invasive patient monitoring and diagnosis.

Conclusion

Hydrogels have found an important role in formulation of advanced drug delivery systems, with transdermal drug delivery no exception. Transdermal drug delivery is an attractive alternative route to the conventional oral and parenteral preparations, due to the many benefits it offers. Considering transdermal drug delivery and hydrogels together, hydrogel-forming microneedles are one of the most promising innovations, with great potential to yield tangible benefits for both patients and industry in the coming years. Transdermal administration of a wide range of conventional small molecule drugs and biotherapeutics has been demonstrated via a hydrogel-forming microneedle platform, alongside applications in therapeutic drug monitoring, highlighting the versatility of the technology.

References

Ammar, H.O., H.A. Salama, S.A. El-Nahhas and H. Elmotasem. 2008. Design and evaluation of chitosan films for transdermal delivery of glimepiride. Curr. Drug. Deliv. 5(4): 290–298.

Baker, M.I., S.P. Walsh, Z. Schwartz and B.D. Boyan. 2012. A review of polyvinyl alcohol and its uses in cartilage and orthopedic applications. J. Biomed. Mater. Res. Part B Appl. Biomater. 100B(5): 1451–1457.

Caffarel-Salvador, E., A.J. Brady, E. Eltayib, T. Meng, A. Alonso-Vicente, P. Gonzalez-Vazquez et al. 2015. Hydrogel-forming microneedle arrays allow detection of drugs and glucose *in vivo*: potential for use in diagnosis and therapeutic drug monitoring. PLOS ONE. 10(12): e0145644.

Demir, Y., Z. Akan and O. Kerimoglu. 2013. Characterization of polymeric microneedle arrays for transdermal drug delivery. PLOS ONE. 8(10): e77289.

Donnelly, R.F., D.I.J. Morrow, F. Fay, C.J. Scott, S. Abdelghany, R.R.S. Thakur et al. 2010. Microneedle-mediated intradermal nanoparticle delivery: potential for enhanced local administration of hydrophobic pre-formed photosensitisers. Photodiagnosis Photodyn. Ther. 7(4): 222–231.

Donnelly, R.F., R.R.S. Thakur, M.J. Garland, K. Migalska, R. Majithiya, C.M. McCrudden et al. 2012. Hydrogel-forming microneedle arrays for enhanced transdermal drug delivery. Adv. Funct. Mater. 22(23): 4879–4890.

Donnelly, R.F., R.R.S. Thakur, A. Zaid Alkilani, M.T.C. McCrudden, S. O'Neill, C. O'Mahony et al. 2013. Hydrogel-forming microneedle arrays exhibit antimicrobial properties: potential for enhanced patient safety. Int. J. Pharm. 451(1-2): 76–91.

Donnelly, R.F. and A.D. Woolfson. 2014. Patient safety and beyond: what should we expect from microneedle arrays in the transdermal delivery arena? Ther. Deliv. 5(6): 653–662.

Donnelly, R.F., M.T.C. McCrudden, A. Zaid Alkilani, E. Larrañeta, E. McAlister, A.J. Courtenay et al. 2014a. Hydrogel-forming microneedles prepared from "super swelling" polymers combined with lyophilised wafers for transdermal drug delivery. PLOS ONE. 9(10): e111547.

Donnelly, R.F., K. Mooney, E. Caffarel-Salvador, B.M. Torrisi, E. Eltayib and J.C. McElnay. 2014b. Microneedle-mediated minimally invasive patient monitoring. Ther. Drug. Monit. 36(1): 10–17.

Donnelly, R.F., K. Mooney, M.T.C. McCrudden, E.M. Vicente-Pérez, L. Belaid, P. González-Vázquez et al. 2014c. Hydrogel-forming microneedles increase in volume during swelling in skin, but skin barrier function recovery is unaffected. J. Pharm. Sci. 103(5): 1478–1486.

Edens, C., M.L. Collins, J.L. Goodson, P.A. Rota and M.R. Prausnitz. 2015. A microneedle patch containing measles vaccine is immunogenic in non-human primates. Vaccine. 33(37): 4712–4718.

Eltayib, E., A.J. Brady, E. Caffarel-Salvador, P. Gonzalez-Vazquez, A. Zaid Alkilani, H.O. McCarthy et al. 2016. Hydrogel-forming microneedle arrays: potential for use in minimally-invasive lithium monitoring. Eur. J. Pharm. Biopharm. 102: 123–131.

Ghobril, C. and M.W. Grinstaff. 2015. The chemistry and engineering of polymeric hydrogel adhesives for wound closure: a tutorial. Chem. Soc. Rev. 44(7): 1820–1835.

Gill, H.S. and M.R. Prausnitz. 2007. Coating formulations for microneedles. Pharm. Res. 24(7): 1369–80.

Gong, C., Q. Wu, Y. Wang, D. Zhang, F. Luo, X. Zhao et al. 2013. A biodegradable hydrogel system containing curcumin encapsulated in micelles for cutaneous wound healing. Biomaterials. 34(27): 6377–6387.

Guo, L., Y. Qiu, J. Chen, S. Zhang, B. Xu and Y. Gao. 2013. Effective transcutaneous immunization against hepatitis B virus by a combined approach of hydrogel patch formulation and microneedle arrays. Biomed. Microdevices. 15(6): 1077–1085.

Hardy, J.G., E. Larrañeta, R.F. Donnelly, N. McGoldrick, K. Migalska, M.T.C. McCrudden et al. 2016. Hydrogel-forming microneedle arrays made from light-responsive materials for on-demand transdermal drug delivery. Mol. Pharm. 13(3): 907–914.

Hoare, T.R. and D.S. Kohane. 2008. Hydrogels in drug delivery: progress and challenges. Polymer. 49(8): 1993–2007.

Hong, X., Z. Wu, L. Chen, F. Wu, L. Wei and W. Yuan. 2014. Hydrogel microneedle arrays for transdermal drug delivery. Nano-Micro. Lett. 6(3): 191–199.

Jenkins, K. 2014. Needle phobia: a psychological perspective. Br. J. Anaesth. 113(1): 4–6.

Jodar, K.S.P., V.M. Balcão, M.V. Chaud, M. Tubino, V.M.H. Yoshida, J.M. Oliveira et al. 2015. Development and characterization of a hydrogel containing silver sulfadiazine for antimicrobial topical applications. J. Pharm. Sci. 104(7): 2241–2254.

Kiang, T.K.L., V. Schmitt, M.H.H. Ensom, B. Chua and U.O. Häfeli. 2012. Therapeutic drug monitoring in interstitial fluid: a feasibility study using a comprehensive panel of drugs. J. Pharm. Sci. 101(12): 4642–4652.

Kim, M., B. Jung and J.H. Park. 2012. Hydrogel swelling as a trigger to release biodegradable polymer microneedles in skin. Biomaterials. 33(2): 668–678.

Larrañeta, E., R.E.M. Lutton, A.J. Brady, E.M. Vicente-Pérez, A.D. Woolfson, R.R.S. Thakur et al. 2015. Microwave-assisted preparation of hydrogel-forming microneedle arrays for transdermal drug delivery applications. Macromol. Mater. Eng. 300(6): 586–595.

Liu, X., L. Fu, W. Dai, W. Liu, J. Zhao, Y. Wu et al. 2014. Design of transparent film-forming hydrogels of tolterodine and their effects on stratum corneum. Int. J. Pharm. 471(1-2): 322–331.

Luppi, B., T. Cerchiara, F. Bigucci, A.M. Di Pietra, I. Orienti and V. Zecchi. 2003. Crosslinked poly(methyl vinyl ether-co-maleic anhydride) as topical vehicles for hydrophilic and lipophilic drugs. Drug Deliv. 10(4): 239–244.

Luzardo-Álvarez, A., J. Blanco-Méndez, P. Varela-Patiño and B. Martín Biedma. 2011. Amoxicillin-loaded sponges made of collagen and poly[(methyl vinyl ether)-co-(maleic anhydride)] for root canal treatment: preparation, characterization and *in vitro* cell compatibility. J. Biomater. Sci. Polym. Ed. 22(1-3): 329–342.

Martanto, W., J. Moore, O. Kashlan, R. Kamath, P.M. Wang, J.M. O'Neal et al. 2006. Microinfusion using hollow microneedles. Pharm. Res. 23(1): 104–113.

Mazzitelli, S., C. Pagano, D. Giusepponi, C. Nastruzzi and L. Perioli. 2013. Hydrogel blends with adjustable properties as patches for transdermal delivery. Int. J. Pharm. 454(1): 47–57.

Moreno, E., J. Schwartz, E. Larrañeta, P.A. Nguewa, C. Sanmartín, M. Agüeros et al. 2014. Thermosensitive hydrogels of poly(methyl vinyl ether-co-maleic anhydride)—Pluronic® F127 copolymers for controlled protein release. Int. J. Pharm. 459(1-2): 1–9.

Morrow, D.I.J., P.A. McCarron, A.D. Woolfson and R.F. Donnelly. 2007. Innovative strategies for enhancing topical and transdermal drug delivery. TODD J. 1: 36–59.

Mrak, E.M., G.F. Stewart and C.O. Chichester. 1988. Advances in Food Research. Elsevier Science Ltd., London.

Mukerjee, E.V., S.D. Collins, R.R. Isseroff and R.L. Smith. 2004. Microneedle array for transdermal biological fluid extraction and *in situ* analysis. Sensor. Actuat. A-Phys. 114(2-3): 267–275.

Negi, P., B. Singh, G. Sharma, S. Beg, K. Raza and O.P. Katare. 2014. Phospholipid microemulsion-based hydrogel for enhanced topical delivery of lidocaine and prilocaine: QbD-based development and evaluation. Drug Deliv. 23(3): 951–967.

Norman, J.J., J.M. Arya, M.A. McClain, P.M. Frew, M.I. Meltzer and M.R. Prausnitz. 2014. Microneedle patches: Usability and acceptability for self-vaccination against influenza. Vaccine. 32(16): 1856–1862.

O'Mahony, C. 2014. Structural characterization and *in-vivo* reliability evaluation of silicon microneedles. Biomed. Microdevices. 16(3): 333–43.

Peppas, N., P. Bures, W. Leobandung and H. Ichikawa. 2000. Hydrogels in pharmaceutical formulations. Eur. J. Pharm. Biopharm. 50(1): 27–46.

Prausnitz, M.R. and R. Langer. 2008. Transdermal drug delivery. Nature Biotechnol. 26(11): 1261–1268.

Rehman, K. and M.H. Zulfakar. 2014. Recent advances in gel technologies for topical and transdermal drug delivery. Drug Dev. Ind. Pharm. 40(4): 433–440.

Romanyuk, A.V., V.N. Zvezdin, P. Samant, M.I. Grenader, M. Zemlyanova and M.R. Prausnitz. 2014. Collection of analytes from microneedle patches. Anal. Chem. 86(21): 10520–10523.

Sakaguchi, K., Y. Hirota, N. Hashimoto, W. Ogawa, T. Sato, S. Okada et al. 2012. A minimally invasive system for glucose area under the curve measurement using interstitial fluid extraction technology: evaluation of the accuracy and usefulness with oral glucose tolerance tests in subjects with and without diabetes. Diabetes Tech. Ther. 14(6): 485–491.

Scott, L.J. 2016. Fentanyl iontophoretic transdermal system: a review in acute postoperative pain. Clin. Drug Investig. 36(4): 321–330.

Simonsen, L., A. Kane, J. Lloyd, M. Zaffran and M. Kane. 1999. Unsafe injections in the developing world and transmission of bloodborne pathogens: a review. Bull. World Health Organ. 77(10): 789–800.

Suedee, R., C. Bodhibukkana, N. Tangthong, C. Amnuaikit, S. Kaewnopparat and T. Srichana. 2008. Development of a reservoir-type transdermal enantioselective-controlled delivery system for racemic propranolol using a molecularly imprinted polymer composite membrane. J. Control. Release. 129(3): 170–178.

Sutton, C. 2005. Adhesions and their prevention. TOG. 7(3): 168–176.

Thakur, R.R.S., P.A. McCarron, A.D. Woolfson and R.F. Donnelly. 2009. Investigation of swelling and network parameters of poly(ethylene glycol)-crosslinked poly(methyl vinyl ether-co-maleic acid) hydrogels. Eur. Polym. J. 45(4): 1239–1249.

Thakur, R.R.S., A.D. Woolfson and R.F. Donnelly. 2010. Investigation of solute permeation across hydrogels composed of poly(methyl vinyl ether-co-maleic acid) and poly(ethylene glycol). J. Pharm. Pharmacol. 62(7): 829–837.

Tuan-Mahmood, T.-M., M.T.C. McCrudden, B.M. Torrisi, E. McAlister, M.J. Garland, R.R.S. Thakur et al. 2013. Microneedles for intradermal and transdermal drug delivery. Eur. J. Pharm. Sci. 44(5): 623–37.

Wang, Q., G. Yao, P. Dong, Z. Gong, G. Li, K. Zhang et al. 2015. Investigation on fabrication process of dissolving microneedle arrays to improve effective needle drug distribution. Eur. J. Pharm. Sci. 66: 148–156.

Yang, S., Y. Feng, L. Zhang, N. Chen, W. Yuan and T. Jin. 2012. A scalable fabrication process of polymer microneedles. Int. J. Nanomedicine. 7: 1415–1422.

Yang, S.Y., E.D. O'Cearbhaill, G.C. Sisk, K.M. Park, W.K. Cho, M. Villiger et al. 2013. A bio-inspired swellable microneedle adhesive for mechanical interlocking with tissue. Nat. Commun. 4: 1702.

CHAPTER 15

Preparation of Photocurable Hydrogels

Hitomi Shirahama and Bae Hoon Lee*

Introduction

Hydrogels are three-dimensional (3D) polymeric networks confining a substantial fraction of water within the structure (Ahmed 2015); hydrogels are attractive materials for various biomedical applications because they exhibit their structural, compositional similarity to natural tissues (Caló and Khutoryanskiy 2015; Peppas et al. 2006; Van Vlierberghe et al. 2011). They can be divided into reversible physical hydrogels and irreversible chemical hydrogels. Physical hydrogels are formed by non-covalent interactions between molecules such as hydrophobic associations, hydrogen bonding interactions, and ionic interactions, being relatively weak in mechanical strength. In contrast, chemical hydrogels have intermolecular covalent bonds, displaying stable and robust mechanical properties (Ghobril and Grinstaff 2015). In general, chemical hydrogels are prepared by radical photopolymerization or addition/condensation polymerization as presented in Fig. 1.

Photocurable polymers can be polymerized upon light (ultraviolet [UV] or visible) exposure for a few minutes in the presence of a small amount of initiators. This photopolymerization has many advantages over chemical addition/condensation crosslinking method, including a fast and high polymerization, good spatio-temporal control over hydrogel formation, and mild reaction conditions at room temperature in physiological aqueous solutions (Fedorovich et al. 2009; Ki et al. 2013; Mironi-Harpaz et al. 2012). The mechanical properties of photopolymerized hydrogels can be tailored through manipulating their crosslinking density. The degree of crosslinking

School of Biomedical Engineering, Wenzhou Medical University, Wenzhou 325027, China Wenzhou Institute of Biomaterials and Engineering, CNITECH, CAS, Wenzhou 325001, China
E-mail: bhlee@wibe.ac.cn
* Corresponding author

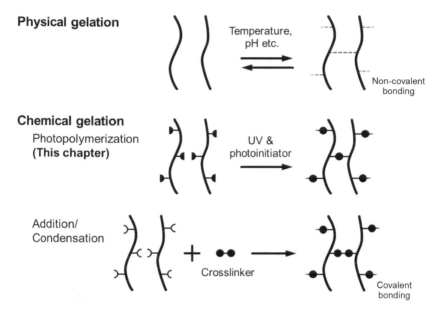

Fig. 1. Classification of hydrogels by polymerization method.

of hydrogels can be influenced by some parameters such as light exposure time, light intensity, photoinitiator concentration, monomer concentration, monomer chain length, and conjugation of various biological molecules (Fedorovich et al. 2009; Mironi-Harpaz et al. 2012).

Photocurable polymers have been extensively utilized for biomedical applications such as 3D hydrogel scaffolds, drug delivery, coatings for biosensors, and bioinks for 3D bio-printing, allowing scientists to fabricate complex, customized configurations in a facile manner (Desai et al. 2010). In addition, they have been explored for *in situ* gelling scaffolds, which can be injected into a body in a minimal invasive way because photopolymerization can convert a liquid monomer to a hydrogel that conforms to the shape of an injection site.

In this chapter, we begin with introducing photoinitiators, which play important roles in the preparation of photocurable hydrogels. Subsequently, we deal with two types of photocurable hydrogels; the first section focuses on those made from synthetic materials (Poly(ethylene glycol)diacrylate, Polyvinyl alcohol, etc.), followed by the second section on photocurable hydrogels from natural materials (collagen/gelatin, alginate, etc.).

Photoinitiators

Photoinitiators are molecules that generate reactive species upon exposure to light, initiating photopolymerization. They exhibit high absorption at a specific wavelength of light and change absorbed light energy into chemical energy, resulting in producing reactive species. Photoinitiators are generally classified into two types (Type 1 and Type 2) by their mechanisms as presented in Fig. 2.

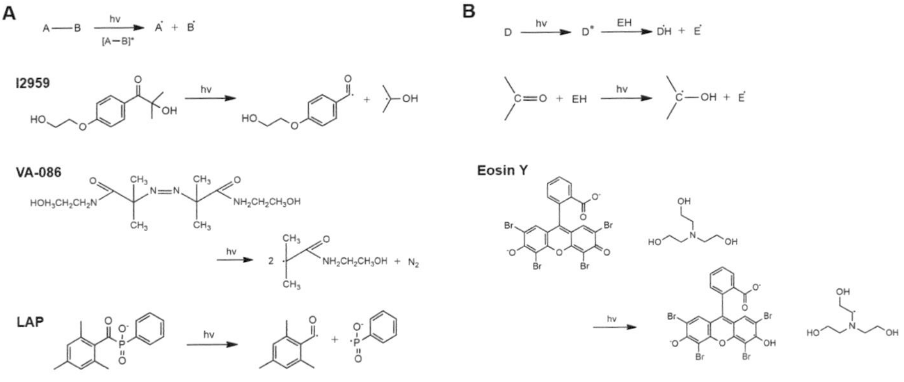

Fig. 2. Photoinitiators start radical polymerization. (A) Type 1 photoinitiators (B) Type 2 photoinitiators.

Type 1 photoinitiators produce two free radicals through a unimolecular bond cleavage upon light exposure. Subsequently, the generated two free radicals initiate polymerization. The photolysis arises at the most fragile bonds in their structures. In most cases, photolabile site is CO-C bond of aromatic carbonyl compounds, such as benzoin compounds, acetophenone compounds, and hydroxylalkylphenones (Green 2010; Nguyen and West 2002).

Type 2 photoinitiators experience a bimolecular reaction in which the excited photoinitiators abstract hydrogen from donor molecules for producing free radicals. These types of photoinitiators are usually aromatic ketone compounds such as benzophenone and thioxanthone, which can be in a triplet excited state by irradiation. The donor molecules include amines, thiols and alcohols that possess active hydrogen (e.g., triethanolamine). The donor radicals initiate polymerization process, whereas the ketyl radicals couple each other (Esen et al. 2014; Kork et al. 2015). In general, Type 2 photoinitiators are less efficient than Type 1 photoinitiators because of the biomolecular reaction, solvent cage influence in aqueous media, and back electron transfer (Qina et al. 2014; Ullrich et al. 2006).

For cell encapsulation and injectable tissue engineering purpose, initiators are required to be water-soluble, less cytotoxic, and highly efficient (He et al. 2011). The most widely used photoinitiators are 2-hydroxy-1-[4-(2-hydroxyethoxy) phenyl]-2-methyl-1-propanone (alias: Irgacure 2959 or I2959) and 2,2'-Azobis[2-methyl-N-(2-hydroxyethyl)propionamide] (alias: VA-086) as presented in Table 1. They led to a high level of crosslinking and significantly high cell viabilities (Mironi-Harpaz et al. 2012; Occhetta et al. 2015). However, in UV exposure, photoinitiators, and free radicals can cause toxicity to cells (Williams et al. 2005). Fairbanks et al. reported that the initiator, lithium phenyl-2,4,6-trimethylbenzoylphosphinate (LAP: lithium acylphosphinate), had advantages over I2959 in terms of better water solubility and visible light polymerization (Benedikt et al. 2016; Fairbanks et al. 2009). Eosin Y also offers visible light polymerisation at 519 nm, as a safer alternative to UV photoinitiators (Fenn and Oldinski 2016). In preparation of hydrogels, researchers should optimise curing conditions such as, types of photoinitiators, concentrations of photoinitiators, and light exposure time/intensity in their experiment setups.

Table 1. Photoinitiators commonly used for photocrosslinking.

Initiators	Name	Type	Wavelength for curing	Curing time	Intensity	Solubility	Concentration for cell encapsulation
Irgacure 2959 (I2959)	2-Hydroxy-4'-(2-hydroxyethoxy)-2-methylpropiophenone	1	365 nm	5~15 min	1~20 mW/cm^2	Water ($\leq 0.5\%$), ethanol (10%)	~0.1%
VA-086	2,2'-Azobis[2-methyl-N-(2-hydroxyethyl) propionamide]	1	365 nm			Water ($\leq 5\%$)	~1.5%
LAP	Lithium phenyl-2,4,6-trimethylbenzoyl phosphinate	1	365 or 405 nm			Water ($\leq 8.5\%$)	~0.1%
Eosin Y	2-(2,4,5,7-Tetrabromo-6-oxido-3-oxo-3H-xanthen-9-yl)benzoate	2	519 nm			Water ($\leq 5\%$)	~0.01%

Synthetic Polymer-based Photocurable Hydrogels

Photocurable synthetic polymer-based hydrogels have been utilized for various bio-applications owing to following advantages: They can be mass-produced at a low cost, their mechanical properties can be easily tailored by some parameters such as their molecular weights and degrees of modification (methacryloylation or acryloylation), and in addition, their biological features can be provided via incorporation of biological molecules. Typical synthetic photocurable hydrogel precursors are poly(ethylene glycol) and poly(vinyl alcohol).

Poly(ethylene glycol)-based photocurable hydrogels

Poly(ethylene glycol) (PEG) is a highly water soluble synthetic polymer which is composed of repeating ethylene glycol (-OCH$_2$CH$_2$-) units. It has been utilized for bio-applications such as drug delivery systems, bio-printing, and tissue engineering because PEG has prominent features such as hydrophilicity, biocompatibility, non-immunogenicity, and anti-fouling properties (Amer et al. 2015; Lee et al. 2016b; Peyton et al. 2006; Turturro and Papavasiliou 2012). PEG has hydroxyl groups at both ends, which can be modified with functional molecules for specific applications (Sawhney et al. 1993b). For photocurable PEG, it is normally modified in the form of PEG diacrylate (PEGDA) or PEG dimethacrylate (PEGDMA) as seen in Fig. 3. PEGDA or PEGDMA can be prepared through the reaction with a small molar excess of acryloyl chloride or methacryloyl chloride in tetrahydrofuran or methylene chloride containing the equimolar triethylamine in an ice bath for overnight (Lee et al. 2004; Li et al. 2010). PEGDA or PEGDMA can be photocrosslinked in the presence of photoinitiators upon light exposure at their corresponding wave lengths (e.g., upon 365 nm UV light exposure in the presence of I2959). PEGDA is faster reactive to light exposure than PEGDMA probably because acrylate radicals are sterically less hindered than methacrylate radicals (reactivity: acrylate > vinyl ester >

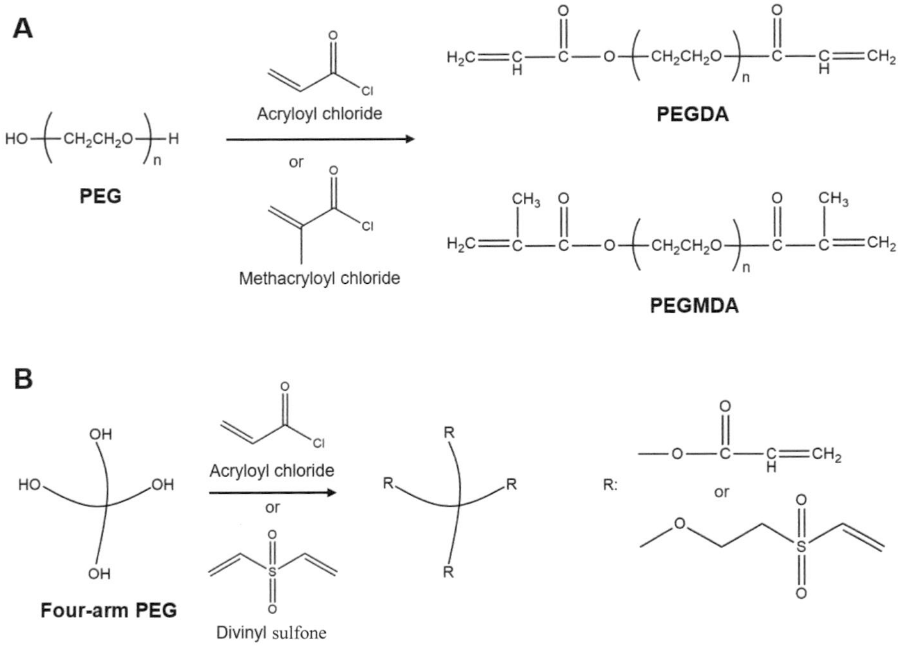

A

B

Fig. 3. Photocurable PEG-based materials (A) PEG diacrylate (PEGDA) and PEG dimethacrylate (PEGDMA) (B) 4-arm PEG acrylate and 4-arm PEG vinyl sulfone.

methacrylate > fumarate) (Husar and Liska 2012; Nguyen et al. 2015). Mechanical properties of photocurable PEG-based hydrogels can be turned by their molecular weights and concentrations. The use of multi-arm PEG derivatives (cf. Fig. 3B) is another option to enhance mechanical properties and can also offer a wide range of functionalization capability (Fairbanks et al. 2009b; Lee et al. 2016b; Wang et al. 2017). In addition, photocrosslinkable multi-arm PEG derivatives can form hydrogels through reaction with multifunctional thiols in a step growth mode upon light exposure without the presence of cytotoxic photoinitiators. This thiol-ene photopolymerization could overcome the light attenuation through the thickness of photocurable hydrogel samples and managed to cure even 10 cm thick samples (Fairbanks et al. 2009b; Rydholm et al. 2005).

PEG hydrogels undergo slow hydrolysis by the cleavage of the ester bonds over time in aqueous solutions. In an attempt to control degradation of PEG-based hydrogels, poly(α-hydroxy acid) as a biodegradable moiety was incorporated into PEG chains (Moeinzadeh et al. 2013). The degradation of PEG-co-poly(α-hydroxy acid) diacrylate hydrogels can be modulated by the length and composition of α-hydroxy acid block (Sawhney et al. 1993a; Sawhney et al. 1994). Their swelling and mechanical properties are influenced by the length of PEG block and the concentration of copolymers. Multi-arm PEG-based hydrogels containing MMP (matrix metalloproteinase) moieties can be degraded by enzymes secreted from cells as presented in Fig. 4 (Mhanna et al. 2014). Cell adhesion onto PEG hydrogels can be enhanced by the incorporation of cell attachment peptides, such as RGD (Arg-Gly-Asp) (Beamish et al. 2009; Yang et al.

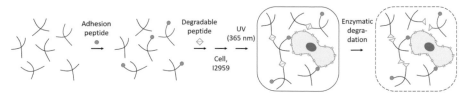

Fig. 4. Photocured PEG-based hydrogels with cell adhesion molecules and enzyme degradable molecules.

Table 2. Photocurable PEG polymers for various applications.

PEG hydrogels with additional features	Functionality
PEG-co-poly(α-hydroxyl acid) hydrogel containing poly(glycolic acid) (PGA) or poly(lactic acid) (PLA) or PLGA	Hydrolytic degradation
MMP (matrix metalloproteinase)-immobilized PEG hydrogels	Enzymatic degradation
Adhesion peptides (RGD, YIGSR, KQAGDV, etc.)-immobilized PEG hydrogels	Cell adhesion/proliferation/differentiation
RGD- and MMP-immobilized PEG hydrogels	Control over adhesion and degradation
TGF-β-immobilized PEG hydrogels	Cartilage regeneration/ECM production
VEGF-immobilized PEG hydrogels	Vascular growth
Phosphate-tethered PEG hydrogels	Osteogenic differentiation
t-Butyl-tethered PEG hydrogels	Adipogenic differentiation
Natural polymer (fibrinogen, gelatin)-conjugated PEG hydrogels	Control over cell adhesion and degradation

2005), a laminin-derived peptide YIGSR (Tyr-Ile-Gly-Ser-Arg) (Coburn et al. 2011), and a fibrinogen-derived KQAGDV (Lys-Gln-Ala-Gly-Asp-Val) (Peyton et al. 2006). Furthermore, PEG hydrogels with specific bioactive peptides have been explored for regenerative medicine applications; the bioactive peptides include VEGF (Vascular endothelial growth factor) and TGF-(transforming growth factor-beta), as seen in Table 2 (Leslie-Barbick et al. 2011; Sridhar et al. 2014; Villanueva et al. 2009; Wacker et al. 2008). In addition, photocurable hydrogels with small chemical groups can guide stem cell fate decisions. Phosphate-tethered PEG hydrogels differentiated human mesenchymal stem cells (hMSCs) into an osteogenic lineage whereas hydrophobic t-butyl group-tethered PEG hydrogels induced adipogenic differentiation of hMSCs (Benoit et al. 2008).

Poly(propylene fumarate)-based photocurable hydrogels

Poly(propylene fumarate) (PPF) is another photocurable material, which has biodegradable properties. PPF has a chemical structure of repeating units with multiple ester groups and carbon-carbon double bonds. It is used mainly in the form of poly(propylene fumarate-co-ethylene glycol) (Poly(PF-co-EG)) or oligo(propylene fumarate-co-ethylene glycol) (oligo(PF-co-EG)) owing to the hydrophilic feature

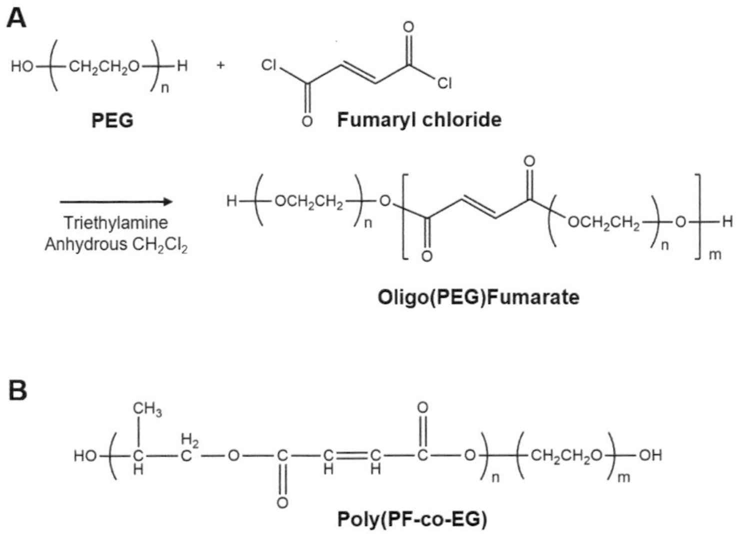

A

PEG + **Fumaryl chloride**

Triethylamine
Anhydrous CH$_2$Cl$_2$

Oligo(PEG)Fumarate

B

Poly(PF-co-EG)

Fig. 5. Photocurable poly(propylene fumarate)-based polymers (A) Oligo(propylene fumarate-co-ethylene glycol) (B) Poly(propylene fumarate-co-ethylene glycol).

of the poly(ethylene glycol) (PEG) chains (Suggs et al. 1998a; Suggs et al. 1998b; Tanahashi et al. 2002). Poly(PF-co-EG) can be obtained through the reaction of fumaryl chloride and triethylamine as seen in Fig. 5. Purified PEG was first dissolved in dichloromethane, and fumaryl chloride and triethylamine (TEA) were added drop-wise over several hours while the reaction flask was maintained near 0°C. The reaction further proceeded for 1–2 days at room temperature. As propylene fumarate has linear unsaturated double bonds, poly(PF-co-EG) undergoes photocrosslinking (Timmer et al. 2003). Photocrosslinking poly(PF-co-EG) containing cell adhesion peptides (RGD) and growth factors (TGF-β) were explored for use of injectable drug delivery systems and tissue engineering (Kallukalam et al. 2009; Shung et al. 2003).

Poly(vinyl alcohol)-based photocurable hydrogels

Poly(vinyl alcohol) (PVA) is a water soluble synthetic polymer with pendant hydroxyl groups, which is a hydrolysed product from poly(vinyl acetate). It is biocompatible and possesses antifouling property against proteins and cells (Murosaki et al. 2011). PVA can be modified for photopolymerization through the reaction of pendant hydroxyl groups with acrylic acid, methacrylic acid, glycidyl acrylate, and 2-isocyanotoethyl methacrylate (ICEMA) (Andrews et al. 2012; Bourke et al. 2003; Bryant et al. 2004; Ichimura and Komatsu 1987; Ichimura and Watanabe 1982; Muhlebach et al. 1997; Nuttelman et al. 2002; Schmedlen et al. 2002). The mechanical properties of photocurable poly(vinyl alcohol) hydrogels can be controlled by their concentration and the number of crosslinking groups per chain. Some representative PVA derivatives are shown in Fig. 6. 'Figure 6 photocurable poly(vinyl alcohol)-based polymers'. Anseth group developed photocurable biodegradable poly(vinyl alcohol) for tissue engineering

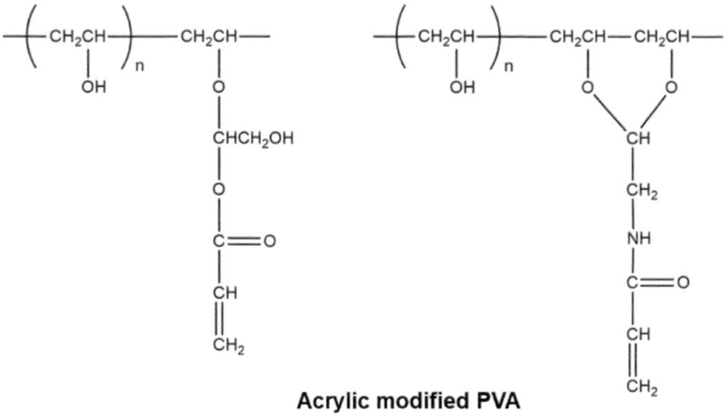

Acrylic modified PVA

Fig. 6. Photocurable poly(vinyl alcohol)-based polymers.

scaffolds (Bryant et al. 2004; Nuttelman et al. 2002). They prepared photocurable poly(lactic acid)-graft-PVA by reaction of HEMA-Lac-Suc (hydroxyethyl methacrylate-lactide-succinic) with the hydroxyl groups of PVA. First, PVA was dissolved in DMSO (dimethyl sulfoxide) and then transferred to HEMA-Lac-Suc in the presence of pyridine and DMAP (4-Dimethylaminopyridine) for reaction of 24 h at room temperature (Nuttelman et al. 2002). Another photocurable PVA derivative, PVA-ICEMA was prepared for drug delivery and cell encapsulation. PVA was dissolved in DMSO and then ICEMA was added dropwise to the PVA solution in a stoichiometric ratio for 5 h in nitrogen atmosphere at 60°C (Bryant et al. 2004; Kundu et al. 2012). PLA-, PEG-, or chondroitin sulfate-incorporated photocurable PVA hydrogels have been tested for diverse tissue engineering applications and drug delivery purpose (Bourke et al. 2003; Bryant et al. 2004; Crispim et al. 2012).

Natural Polymer-based Photocurable Hydrogels

Natural polymers such as collagen, gelatin, hyaluronic acid (HA), and chitosan are attractive materials for a variety of biomedical applications because natural polymers exhibit key features of their bioactivity, biocompatibility and biodegradability. However, their poor mechanical properties often limit their applications. The addition of photocurable moieties to natural polymers can enhance the mechanical properties and structural stability of natural polymers, whereas modified natural polymers can still retain their original bioactivities.

Collagen- and gelatin-based photocurable hydrogels

Collagen is the most abundant protein in the human body (Lullo et al. 2002), providing structural support and regulating cell signalling. Gelatin is denatured collagen, obtained from partial hydrolysis of collagen through acid/base treatment. Collagen and gelatin have been used for a wide area of regenerative studies (skin, bone, cornea, etc.) and drug delivery applications.

Their structure has a repetition of tripeptide, (Gly-X-Y)n, where X and Y are often proline and 4-hydroxyproline, respectively. The major chemical modification method for collagen/gelatin utilizes mainly free amino groups from lysine and hydroxylysine, which can react with methacrylic anhydride (MAA) as shown in Fig. 7A. The pioneered method was to dissolve gelatin in phosphate buffered saline (PBS) at 50°C, followed by drop-wise addition of MAA to yield gelatin methacryloyl (GelMA) (Bulcke et al. 2000). This method was applied to collagen methacryloylation with the use of 10 mM HCl at 4°C as a buffer solution (Brinkman et al. 2003). Recent studies on GelMA showed that the use of carbonate-bicarbonate buffer and pH maintenance at pH 9 produced GelMA with a higher degree of methacryloylation at relatively a low feed ratio of MAA to gelatin since this method minimized protonation of amino groups and allowed gelatin to effectively react with MAA, as seen in Fig. 8 (Lee et al. 2016a; Shirahama et al. 2016). Collagen and gelatin methacryloyl hydrogels have been studied extensively and applied to many bioapplications including 3D printing technologies (Billiet et al. 2014; Chen et al. 2012; Egger et al. 2016; Klotz et al. 2016; Loessner et al. 2016; Nguyen et al. 2016; Prakash Parthiban et al. 2017; Wu et al. 2016; Yue et al. 2015).

There are other chemical functionalization methods for the preparation of photocurable collagen; Dong et al. utilized 6-aminohexyl cinnamate (AHC) to react with glutamic acid and aspartic acid of collagen via EDC (1-ethyl-3-(3-dimethylamino)

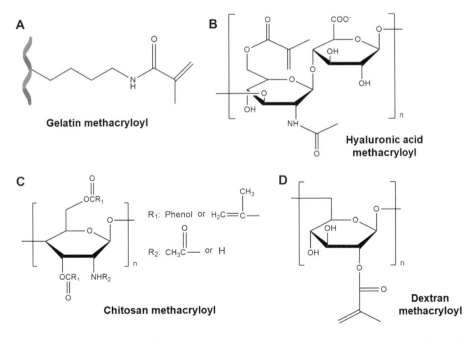

Fig. 7. Examples of chemically modified photocurable natural polymers. (A) Gelatin methacryloyl (GelMA) via reaction of gelatin with methacrylic anhydride (MAA). (B) hyaluronic acid methacryloyl (HAMA) via reaction of HA with MAA. (C) Chitosan benzyol (or methacryloyl) via reaction of Chitosan with benzoyl chloride and methacryloyl chloride. (D) Dextran methacryloyl (DexMA) via reaction of Dextran with MAA.

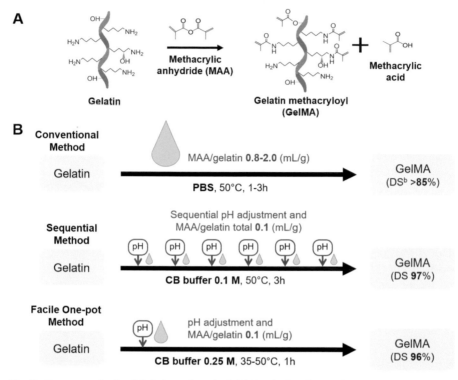

Fig. 8. One-pot synthesis of Gelatin methacryloyl (A) Synthesis scheme of gelatin methacryloyl. (B) Comparison of different methods of gelatin methacryloyl synthesis. Adopted from (Shirahama et al. 2016).

propyl carbodiimide, hydrochloride)/NHS(N-hydroxysuccinimide) conjugation method (Dong et al. 2005). In this reaction, the carboxylic groups of collagen were activated by EDC/NHS in 10 mM HCl at 4°C and then were conjugated with AHC. Also the reaction of gelatin with thymine could produce UV crosslinkable gelatin (Chung and Matsuda 1998).

In addition to UV light curing, photocurable gelatin hydrogels have been also explored in visible light curing methods for developing surgical tissue adhesives. As for visible light curing, xanthene dyes (fluorescein, eosin Y, and rose bengal)-derivatized gelatins or styrene-derivatized gelatin with carboxylated camphorquinone were used (Li et al. 2003; Nakayama and Matsuda 1998). The preparation of photocurable gelatin with vinyl groups was as follows: gelatin was dissolved in PBS at 60°C, and 4-vinylbenzoic acid was dissolved in 1 M sodium hydroxide, separately. Two solutions were then mixed in the presence of EDC for half an hour at 0°C, followed by continuous overnight stirring at room temperature. Photocurable styrene-derivatized gelatin and dye-derivatized gelatins were cured by visible light wave lengths between 400 and 600 nm. Additional PEGDA was utilized to reinforce the mechanical stiffness of the gelatin-based hydrogels, which could serve as a tissue adhesive glue for vascular surgery and endoscopic surgery.

Hyaluronic acid (HA)-based photocurable hydrogels

HA is a non-adhesive glycosaminoglycan, prevalent in connective, epithelial, and neural tissues. Since HA is involved in wound healing and angiogenesis and can interact with cell surface receptors like CD44, CD54 and CD168, it has been used for studies on tissue regeneration as well as drug delivery (Bae et al. 2014; Bae et al. 2011; Bian et al. 2013; Erickson et al. 2009; Khademhosseini et al. 2006).

HA consists of repeating disaccharide units, D-glucuronic acid and D-N-acetylglucosamine, possessing many functional groups such as glucuronic acid carboxylic acid, primary and secondary hydroxyl groups. The major modification method for its photopolymerization (e.g., HA-MA: hyaluronic acid methacrylate) is the methacryloylation of hydroxyl groups of HA by employing MAA, which can be prepared by the reaction of HA with MAA in water of pH 8 at 5°C for 24 h as depicted in Fig. 7B (Chung and Burdick 2009; Levett et al. 2014; Smeds and Grinstaff 2001). Levett et al. reported that the addition of HA-MA to GelMA constructs enhanced chondrogenesis and produced a significant amount of cartilage-specific matrix proteins, which showed a great promise for effective cartilage tissue engineering (Levett et al. 2014). Another method is to use glycidyl methacrylate (GM); GMHA was synthesized by adding GM into HA aqueous solution with triethylamine and tetrabutylammonium bromide at room temperature for overnight (Baier Leach et al. 2003). Photocurable HA can be also obtained via EDC chemistry by the reaction of HA with N-(3-aminopropyl)-methacrylamide hydrochloride or 4-vinylaniline. In this method, first sodium HA was dissolved in PBS and stirred at 4°C for half an hour in the presence of EDC. Aqueous solution of 4-vinylaniline was prepared separately and its pH was adjusted at 3. Finally, styrenated HA was obtained by mixing the two solutions at 4°C for 24 h (Matsuda and Magoshi 2002). Vinylated HA and vinylated gelatin were used for the preparation of tubular photoconstructs. The addition of PEGDA to vinylated HA enhanced the burst strength of the hydrogels.

Chitosan-based photocurable hydrogels

Chitosan is one of the linear polysaccharides, derived from partial deacetylation of chitin (β-1,4-linked N-acetyl-D-glucosamine). It has been applied for tendon, bone and skin regeneration (Abarrategi et al. 2010; Baxter et al. 2013; Freitas et al. 2011; Gingras et al. 2003; Kim et al. 2014; Matsunaga et al. 2006; Olmez et al. 2007; Saraiva et al. 2015; Shim et al. 2008; Wang et al. 2015).

One of the pioneering modification methods for photocurable chitosan is to introduce azide and lactose moieties into chitosan using a two-step condensation method (Ono et al. 2000). Specifically, chitosan was dissolved in N,N,N',N'-tetramethylethylenediamine (TEMED) solution and subsequently EDC and 4-O-b-D-galactopyranosyl-(1,4)-D-gluconic acid (lactobionic acid) were added under stirring at room temperature for 24 h to obtain lactose-linked chitosan (CH-LA). Next, the product (CH-LA), EDC, and 4-azidobenzoic acid were added to the TEMED solution. The mixture was stirred at room temperature for 72 h to obtain the photocrosslinkable chitosan (Az-CH-LA). Photocured Az-CH-LA hydrogels showed better sealing properties as a biological glue when compared with the fibrin glue, having great potential for tissue adhesive applications. Similar to a photocurable gelatin modification method, vinylbenzoic acid-conjugated chitosan can be prepared via reaction between amino groups of chitosan and 4-vinylbenzoic acid in the presence of EDC (Matsuda and Magoshi 2002). Another example of preparing photocurable chitosan is to utilize glucosidic unit of chitosan to be modified with benzoyl chloride and methacryloyl chloride (Gao et al. 2014). In this synthesis method, chitosan was dissolved in methane sulfonic acid at room temperature, and two acyl chlorides was added drop-wise to the chitosan solution, being kept stirred for 3–4 h (Fig. 7C). By varying the ratio of benzoyl chloride and methacryloyl chloride, the photocurable chitosan's curability and solubility in organic solvents could be controlled. Bioscaffolds made from photocurable gelatin/chitosan held great potential for cell-based therapy for many devastating human diseases including spinal cord injury.

Dextran-based photocurable hydrogels

Dextran is a bacterial polysaccharide, which consists of main chains from α-(1,6) D-glucopyranosyl units. The linkages and branches of dextran depend on the original bacterial strain. In general, dextran is rich in hydroxyl group. It has been studied as a carrier for drugs, peptides and proteins (Coessens et al. 1996; He et al. 2015a; He et al. 2015b; Lin et al. 2012; Rowland 1977; Schacht et al. 1985; Schacht et al. 1990; Van Tomme and Hennink 2007; Zhong and Gong 1994).

A photocurable dextran was prepared through the reaction of dextran with bromoacetyl bromide and sodium acrylate via hydroxyl group. In this method, dextran went through bromoacetylation in lithium chloride/dimethylformaide (LiCl/ DMF) with pyridine. Subsequently, sodium acrylate was added into the solution at 40°C. Another type of photocurable dextran, dextran methacrylate, was synthesized through the reaction of dextran with MAA, whose structure is illustrated in Fig. 7D (Kim and Chu 2000, 2009). LiCl/DMF was used as a reaction solvent and MAA was diffused to react with the hydroxyl groups of dextran. A wide range (9~75%) of the DS of dextran methacrylate was obtained through control over some parameters (temperature (40~80°C), reaction time (5~30 h), a molar ratio of MAA (0.0093~0.0370) to hydroxyl groups (0.0185), and a catalyst (triethylamine) concentration (1.85×10^{-4}~1.85×10^{-3}) (Kim and Chu 2000). In addition, dextran methacrylate was explored to be photocrosslinked by visible light using (−)- riboflavin (0.01~0.5 wt%) as a photoinitiator and L-arginine (5~10 wt%) as a co-initiator with a fluorescence light exposure for 15~40 min (Kim and Chu 2009). Photocrosslinkable dextran glycidyl methacrylate was synthesized as follows: dextran was dissolved in anhydrous dimethylsulfoxide (DMSO) containing dimethylaminopyridine (DMAP), and glycidyl methacrylate was added to the dextran solution. The reaction proceeded for 24 h at room temperature. The hydrogel mixture of photocurable dextran glycidyl methacrylate and scleroglucan was explored for injectable drug delivery applications (Corrente et al. 2013).

Alginate-based photocurable hydrogels

Alginate is a polysaccharide from brown seaweeds, composed of a-L-guluronic acid and b-D-mannuronic acid units. It has been studied on bone, cartilage, and skin tissue engineering as well as drug delivery (Chou et al. 2009; Higham et al. 2014; Lewandowska-Lancucka et al. 2017; Rouillard et al. 2011; Samorezov et al. 2015). Alginate can be conjugated with MAA via hydroxyl groups to be photocurable (Chou et al. 2009). The preparation method was first to dissolve alginate in deionized water with pH adjustment at 8. Subsequently, MAA was added into the solution while pH of the reaction solution was maintained at 8 at 4°C. The obtained photocrosslinked alginate hydrogel showed greater maintenance of its mechanical integrity and provided better support for nucleus pulposus repair, compared with the ionically crosslinked alginate hydrogel. To further reinforce the stiffness of photocrosslinked alginate hydrogels, additional ionic crosslinking can be employed (D'Arrigo et al. 2012; Matricardi et al. 2008). The hybrid materials of photocurable alginate methacrylate/gelatin methacryloyl and silica particles induced mineralization under simulated body fluid conditions, showing potential for bone tissue regeneration (Lewandowska-Lancucka et al. 2017).

Conclusions and Outlook

Photocurable hydrogels from synthetic and natural materials have been extensively explored for drug delivery system, cell encapsulation, and 3D printing owing to their biocompatibility, facile and fast fabrication of complex scaffolds, and excellent spatiotemporal control over gelation process. In addition, they are amenable to versatile bio-functional modifications, which further have widened their bioapplications. From a design perspective, researchers need to choose types of photocurable materials, additional features (degradation, biofunctionality, etc.), and a light source based on a photoinitiator for their specific hydrogel applications. Recently, hydrogels for mimicking 3D microenvironments with *in vivo*-like gradients of bio-functionality and mechanical properties have been highly coveted. To this end, the hybrid materials of combining photocurable natural polymers with photocurable synthetic polymers are preferred for engineering 3D constructs with tailorable biofunctionality and mechanical properties.

As to the photocurable hydrogel design for cell encapsulation and implant applications, researchers need to notice that photoinitiators, their reactive species (free radicals) and UV light sources are harmful to cells and tissues, potentially inducing DNA damage. Even the most commonly used I2959 suffers from low water solubility and cellular toxicity of its reactive species as well as UV light, which depends on the concentration of I2959, and the intensity and exposure time of UV light. On the other hand, visible light photoinitiators such as Eosin Y are highly water soluble but show relatively low photoreactive efficiency in polymerization. Thus, researchers should optimize the concentration of photocurable polymers, the concentration of initiators, and the intensity/exposure time of light sources in their experiment setups to obtain the desirable properties of hydrogels and to not compromise cell viability.

Looking forward, highly efficient, water-soluble, visible light photoinitiators are aspired to be developed for cell encapsulation applications and injectable hydrogels for tissue repair.

References

Abarrategi, A., Y. Lopiz-Morales, V. Ramos, A. Civantos, L. Lopez-Duran, F. Marco et al. 2010. Chitosan scaffolds for osteochondral tissue regeneration. J. Biomed. Mater. Res. A. 95A: 1132–1141.

Ahmed, E.M. 2015. Hydrogel: Preparation, characterization, and applications: J. Adv. Res. 6: 105–121.

Almany, L. and D. Seliktar. 2005. Biosynthetic hydrogel scaffolds made from fibrinogen and polyethylene glycol for 3D cell cultures. Biomaterials. 26: 2467–2477.

Amer, L.D., A. Holtzinger, G. Keller, M.J. Mahoney and S.J. Bryant. 2015. Enzymatically degradable poly(ethylene glycol) hydrogels for the 3D culture and release of human embryonic stem cell derived pancreatic precursor cell aggregates. Acta Biomater. 22: 103–110.

Andrews, D.U., B.R. Heazlewood, A.T. Maccarone, T. Conroy, R.J. Payne, M.J. Jordan et al. 2012. Photo-tautomerization of acetaldehyde to vinyl alcohol: a potential route to tropospheric acids. Science. 337: 1203–1206.

Bae, M.S., D.H. Yang, J.B. Lee, D.N. Heo, Y.D. Kwon, I.C. Youn et al. 2011. Photo-cured hyaluronic acid-based hydrogels containing simvastatin as a bone tissue regeneration scaffold. Biomaterials. 32: 8161–8171.

Bae, M.S., J.Y. Ohe, J.B. Lee, D.N. Heo, W. Byun, H. Bae et al. 2014. Photo-cured hyaluronic acid-based hydrogels containing growth and differentiation factor 5 (GDF-5) for bone tissue regeneration. Bone. 59: 189–198.

Baxter, R.M., T.H. Dai, J. Kimball, E. Wang, M.R. Hamblin, W.P. Wiesmann et al. 2013. Chitosan dressing promotes healing in third degree burns in mice: Gene expression analysis shows biphasic effects for rapid tissue regeneration and decreased fibrotic signaling. J. Biomed. Mater. Res. A. 101: 340–348.

Beamish, J.A., A.Y. Fu, A.J. Choi, N.A. Haq, K. Kottke-Marchant and R.E. Marchant. 2009. The influence of RGD-bearing hydrogels on the re-expression of contractile vascular smooth muscle cell phenotype. Biomaterials. 30: 4127–4135.

Benedikt, S., J. Wang, M. Markovic, N. Moszner, K. Dietliker, A. Ovsianikov et al. 2016. Highly efficient water-soluble visible light photoinitiators. J. Polym. Sci. Pol. Chem. 54: 473–479.

Benoit, D.S., M.P. Schwartz, A.R. Durney and K.S. Anseth. 2008. Small functional groups for controlled differentiation of hydrogel-encapsulated human mesenchymal stem cells. Nat. Mater. 7: 816–823.

Bian, L., C. Hou, E. Tous, R. Rai, R.L. Mauck and J.A. Burdick. 2013. The influence of hyaluronic acid hydrogel crosslinking density and macromolecular diffusivity on human MSC chondrogenesis and hypertrophy. Biomaterials. 34: 413–421.

Billiet, T., E. Gevaert, T. De Schryver, M. Cornelissen and P. Dubruel. 2014. The 3D printing of gelatin methacrylamide cell-laden tissue-engineered constructs with high cell viability. Biomaterials. 35: 49–62.

Bourke, S.L., M. Al-Khalili, T. Briggs, B.B. Michniak, J. Kohn and L.A. Poole-Warren. 2003. A photo-crosslinked poly(vinyl alcohol) hydrogel growth factor release vehicle for wound healing applications. AAPS PharmSci. 5: E33.

Brinkman, W.T., K. Nagapudi, B.S. Thomas and E.L. Chaikof. 2003. Photo-cross-linking of type I collagen gels in the presence of smooth muscle cells. Biomacromolecules. 4: 890–895.

Bryant, S.J., K.A. Davis-Arehart, N. Luo, R.K. Shoemaker, J.A. Arthur and K.S. Anseth. 2004. Synthesis and characterization of photopolymerized multifunctional hydrogels: Water-soluble poly(vinyl alcohol) and chondroitin sulfate macromers for chondrocyte encapsulation. Macromolecules. 37: 6726–6733.

Bulcke, A.I.V.D., B. Bogdanov, N.D. Rooze, E.H. Schacht, M. Cornelissen and H. Berghmans. 2000. Structural and rheological properties of methacrylamide modified gelatin hydrogels. Biomacromolecules. 1: 31–38.

Caló, E. and V.V. Khutoryanskiy. 2015. Biomedical applications of hydrogels: A review of patents and commercial products. Eur. Polym. J. 65: 252–267.

Cao, Y., B.H. Lee, H.B. Peled and S.S. Venkatraman. 2016. Synthesis of stiffness-tunable and cell-responsive gelatin-Poly (ethylene glycol) hydrogel for 3-dimensional cell encapsulation. J. Biomed. Mater. Res. A.

Chen, Y.C., R.Z. Lin, H. Qi, Y. Yang, H. Bae, J.M. Melero-Martin et al. 2012. Functional human vascular network generated in photocrosslinkable gelatin methacrylate hydrogels. Adv. Funct. Mater. 22: 2027–2039.

Chou, A.I., S.O. Akintoye and S.B. Nicoll. 2009. Photo-crosslinked alginate hydrogels support enhanced matrix accumulation by nucleus pulposus cells *in vivo*. Osteoarthr. Cartilage. 17: 1377–1384.

Chung, C. and J.A. Burdick. 2009. Influence of three-dimensional hyaluronic acid microenvironments on mesenchymal stem cell chondrogenesis. Tissue Eng. Pt. A. 15: 243–254.

Chung, D.J. and T. Matsuda. 1998. Gelatin modification with photocuring thymine derivative and its application for hemostatic aid. J. Ind. Eng. Chem. 4: 340–344.

Coburn, J., M. Gibson, P.A. Bandalini, C. Laird, H.Q. Mao, L. Moroni et al. 2011. Biomimetics of the extracellular matrix: An integrated three-dimensional fiber-hydrogel composite for cartilage tissue engineering. Smart Struct. Syst. 7: 213–222.

Coessens, V., E. Schacht and D. Domurado. 1996. Synthesis of polyglutamine and dextran conjugates of streptomycin with an acid-sensitive drug-carrier linkage. J. Control Release. 38: 141–150.

Corrente, F., H.M. Abu Amara, S. Pacelli, P. Paolicelli and M.A. Casadei. 2013. Novel injectable and *in situ* cross-linkable hydrogels of dextran methacrylate and scleroglucan derivatives: preparation and characterization. Carbohyd. Polym. 92: 1033–1039.

Crispim, E.G., J.F. Piai, A.R. Fajardo, E.R.F. Ramos, T.U. Nakamura, C.V. Nakamura et al. 2012. Hydrogels based on chemically modified poly(vinyl alcohol) (PVA-GMA) and PVA-GMA/chondroitin sulfate: Preparation and characterization. Express Polym. Lett. 6: 383–395.

D'Arrigo, G., C. Di Meo, L. Pescosolido, T. Coviello, F. Alhaique and P. Matricardi. 2012. Calcium alginate/dextran methacrylate IPN beads as protecting carriers for protein delivery. J. Mater. Sci.-Mater. M. 23: 1715–1722.

Desai, P.N., Q. Yuan and H. Yang. 2010. Synthesis and characterization of photocurable polyamidoamine dendrimer hydrogels as a versatile platform for tissue engineering and drug delivery. Biomacromolecules. 11: 666–673.

Dikovsky, D., H. Bianco-Peled and D. Seliktar. 2006. The effect of structural alterations of PEG-fibrinogen hydrogel scaffolds on 3-D cellular morphology and cellular migration. Biomaterials. 27: 1496–1506.

Dong, C.M., X. Wu, J. Caves, S.S. Rele, B.S. Thomas and E.L. Chaikof. 2005. Photomediated crosslinking of C6-cinnamate derivatized type I collagen. Biomaterials. 26: 4041–4049.

Egger, M., G.E. Tovar, E. Hoch and A. Southan. 2016. Gelatin methacrylamide as coating material in cell culture. Biointerphases. 11: 021007.

Erickson, I.E., A.H. Huang, S. Sengupta, S. Kestle, J.A. Burdick and R.L. Mauck. 2009. Macromer density influences mesenchymal stem cell chondrogenesis and maturation in photocrosslinked hyaluronic acid hydrogels. Osteoarthr. Cartilage. 17: 1639–1648.

Esen, D.S., G. Temel, D.K. Balta, X. Allonas and N. Arsu. 2014. One-component thioxanthone acetic acid derivative photoinitiator for free radical polymerization. Photochem. Photobiol. 90: 463–469.

Fairbanks, B.D., M.P. Schwartz, C.N. Bowman and K.S. Anseth. 2009a. Photoinitiated polymerization of PEG-diacrylate with lithium phenyl-2,4,6-trimethylbenzoylphosphinate: polymerization rate and cytocompatibility. Biomaterials. 30: 6702–6707.

Fairbanks, B.D., M.P. Schwartz, A.E. Halevi, C.R. Nuttelman, C.N. Bowman and K.S. Anseth. 2009b. A versatile synthetic extracellular matrix mimic via thiol-norbornene photopolymerization. Adv. Mater. 21: 5005–5010.

Fedorovich, N.E., M.H. Oudshoorn, D. van Geemen, W.E. Hennink, J. Alblas and W.J. Dhert. 2009. The effect of photopolymerization on stem cells embedded in hydrogels. Biomaterials. 30: 344–353.

Fenn, S.L. and R.A. Oldinski. 2016. Visible light crosslinking of methacrylated hyaluronan hydrogels for injectable tissue repair. Biomed. Mater. Res. B. 104: 1229–1236.

Freitas, R.M., R. Spin-Neto, L.C. Spolidorio, S.P. Campana, R.A.C. Marcantonio and E. Marcantonio. 2011. Different molecular weight chitosan-based membranes for tissue regeneration. Materials. 4: 380–389.

Gao, S., P. Zhao, C. Lin, Y.X. Sun, Y.L. Wang, Z.C. Zhou et al. 2014. Differentiation of human adipose-derived stem cells into neuron-like cells which are compatible with photocurable three-dimensional scaffolds. Tissue Eng. Pt. A. 20: 1271–1284.

Ghobril, C. and M.W. Grinstaff. 2015. The chemistry and engineering of polymeric hydrogel adhesives for wound closure: a tutorial. Chem. Soc. Rev. 44: 1820–1835.

Gingras, M., I. Paradis and F. Berthod. 2003. Nerve regeneration in a collagen-chitosan tissue-engineered skin transplanted on nude mice. Biomaterials. 24: 1653–1661.

Green, W.A. 2010. A little chemistry. pp. 17–46. In Industrial Photoinitiators. CRC Press.

He, C., F. Li, J.I. Ahn, M. Latorre and M. Griffith. 2011. Photo-induced *in situ* forming hydrogels based on collagen and a biocompatible macromolecular photoinitiator. J. Control Release. 152 Suppl 1: e207–208.

He, S.S., Y.W. Cong, D.F. Zhou, J.Z. Li, Z.G. Xie, X.S. Chen et al. 2015a. A dextran-platinum(IV) conjugate as a reduction-responsive carrier for triggered drug release. J. Mater. Chem. B. 3: 8203–8211.

He, S.S., D.F. Zhou, H.H. Kuang, Y.J. Wu, X.B. Jing and Y.B. Huang. 2015b. Dextran-platinum(IV) conjugate as drug carrier for triggered drug release. J. Control Release. 213: E96–E96.

Higham, A.K., C.A. Bonino, S.R. Raghavan and S.A. Khan. 2014. Photo-activated ionic gelation of alginate hydrogel: real-time rheological monitoring of the two-step crosslinking mechanism. Soft Matter. 10: 4990–5002.

Husar, B. and R. Liska. 2012. Vinyl carbonates, vinyl carbamates, and related monomers: synthesis, polymerization, and application. Chem. Soc. Rev. 41: 2395–2405.

Ichimura, K. and S. Watanabe. 1982. Preparation and characteristics of photocrosslinkable polyvinyl-alcohol. J. Polym. Sci. Pol. Chem. 20: 1419–1432.

Ichimura, K. and T. Komatsu. 1987. Novel method for preparation of photocrosslinkable polyvinyl-alcohol. J. Polym. Sci. Pol. Chem. 25: 1475–1480.

Kallukalam, B.C., M. Jayabalan and V. Sankar. 2009. Studies on chemically crosslinkable carboxy terminated-poly(propylene fumarate-co-ethylene glycol)-acrylamide hydrogel as an injectable biomaterial. Biomed. Mater. 4: 015002.

Khademhosseini, A., G. Eng, J. Yeh, J. Fukuda, J. Blumling, 3rd, R. Langer et al. 2006. Micromolding of photocrosslinkable hyaluronic acid for cell encapsulation and entrapment. J. Biomed. Mater. Res. A. 79: 522–532.

Ki, C.S., H. Shih and C.C. Lin. 2013. Facile preparation of photodegradable hydrogels by photopolymerization. Polymer. 54: 2115–2122.

Kim, S., H. Lee, Y. Kim and G. Kim. 2014. Multi-layered alginate/chitosan-based biocomposites for hard tissue regeneration. J. Tissue Eng. Regen. M. 8: 161–162.

Kim, S.H. and C.C. Chu. 2000. Synthesis and characterization of dextran-methacrylate hydrogels and structural study by SEM. J. Biomed. Mater. Res. 49: 517–527.

Kim, S.H. and C.C. Chu. 2009. Visible light induced dextran-methacrylate hydrogel formation using (–)-riboflavin vitamin B2 as a photoinitiator and L-arginine as a co-initiator. Fiber Polym. 10: 14–20.

Klotz, B.J., D. Gawlitta, A.J. Rosenberg, J. Malda and F.P. Melchels. 2016. Gelatin-methacryloyl hydrogels: Towards biofabrication-based tissue repair. Trends Biotechnol. 34: 394–407.

Kork, S., G. Yilmaz and Y. Yagci. 2015. Poly(vinyl alcohol)-thioxanthone as one-component type II photoinitiator for free radical polymerization in organic and aqueous media. Macromol. Rapid Comm. 36: 923–928.

Kundu, J., L.A. Poole-Warren, P. Martens and S.C. Kundu. 2012. Silk fibroin/poly(vinyl alcohol) photocrosslinked hydrogels for delivery of macromolecular drugs. Acta Biomater. 8: 1720–1729.

Leach, B.J., K.A. Bivens, C.W. Patrick, Jr. and C.E. Schmidt. 2003. Photocrosslinked hyaluronic acid hydrogels: natural, biodegradable tissue engineering scaffolds. Biotechnol. Bioeng. 82: 578–589.

Lee, B., N. Lum, L. Seow, P. Lim and L. Tan. 2016a. Synthesis and characterization of types A and B gelatin methacryloyl for bioink applications. Materials. 9: 797.

Lee, B.H., M.H. Kim, J.H. Lee, D. Seliktar, N.J. Cho and L.P. Tan. 2015. Modulation of huh7.5 spheroid formation and functionality using modified peg-based hydrogels of different stiffness. PLOS ONE. 10.

Lee, B.P., K. Huang, F.N. Nunalee, K.R. Shull and P.B. Messersmith. 2004. Synthesis of 3,4-dihydroxyphenylalanine (DOPA) containing monomers and their co-polymerization with PEG-diacrylate to form hydrogels. J. Biomat. Sci.-Polym. E. 15: 449–464.

Lee, S., X. Tong and F. Yang. 2016b. Effects of the poly(ethylene glycol) hydrogel crosslinking mechanism on protein release. Biomater. Sci. 4: 405–411.

Leslie-Barbick, J.E., J.E. Saik, D.J. Gould, M.E. Dickinson and J.L. West. 2011. The promotion of microvasculature formation in poly(ethylene glycol) diacrylate hydrogels by an immobilized VEGF-mimetic peptide. Biomaterials. 32: 5782–5789.

Levett, P.A., F.P. Melchels, K. Schrobback, D.W. Hutmacher, J. Malda and T.J. Klein. 2014. A biomimetic extracellular matrix for cartilage tissue engineering centered on photocurable gelatin, hyaluronic acid and chondroitin sulfate. Acta Biomater. 10: 214–223.

Lewandowska-Lancucka, J., K. Mystek, A. Mignon, S. Van Vlierberghe, A. Latkiewicz and M. Nowakowska. 2017. Alginate- and gelatin-based bioactive photocross-linkable hybrid materials for bone tissue engineering. Carbohyd. Polym. 157: 1714–1722.

Li, C., T. Sajiki, Y. Nakayama, M. Fukui and T. Matsuda. 2003. Novel visible-light-induced photocurable tissue adhesive composed of multiply styrene-derivatized gelatin and poly(ethylene glycol) diacrylate. J. Biomed. Mater. Res. B. 66B: 439–446.

Li, Y., H.D. Tolley and M.L. Lee. 2010. Monoliths from poly(ethylene glycol) diacrylate and dimethacrylate for capillary hydrophobic interaction chromatography of proteins. J Chromatogr A. 1217: 4934–4945.

Lin, Y.S., R. Radzi, M. Morimoto, H. Saimoto, Y. Okamoto and S. Minami. 2012. Characterization of chitosan-carboxymethyl dextran nanoparticles as a drug carrier and as a stimulator of mouse splenocytes. J. Biomat. Sci.-Polym. E.. 23: 1401–1420.

Loessner, D., C. Meinert, E. Kaemmerer, L.C. Martine, K. Yue, P.A. Levett et al. 2016. Functionalization, preparation and use of cell-laden gelatin methacryloyl-based hydrogels as modular tissue culture platforms. Nat. Protoc. 11: 727–746.

Lullo, G.A.D., S.M. Sweeney, J. Korkko, L. Ala-Kokko and J.D. San Antonio. 2002. Mapping the ligand-binding sites and disease-associated mutations on the most abundant protein in the human, type I collagen. J. Biol. Chem. 277: 4223–4231.

Matricardi, P., M. Pontoriero, T. Coviello, M.A. Casadei and F. Alhaique. 2008. *In situ* cross-linkable novel alginate-dextran methacrylate IPN hydrogels for biomedical applications: mechanical characterization and drug delivery properties. Biomacromolecules. 9: 2014–2020.

Matsuda, T. and T. Magoshi. 2002. Preparation of vinylated polysaccharides and photofabrication of tubular scaffolds as potential use in tissue engineering. Biomacromolecules. 3: 942–950.

Matsunaga, T., K. Yanagiguchi, S. Yamada, N. Ohara, T. Ikeda and Y. Hayashi. 2006. Chitosan monomer promotes tissue regeneration on dental pulp wounds. J. Biomed. Mater. Res. A. 76A: 711–720.

Mhanna, R., E. Ozturk, Q. Vallmajo-Martin, C. Millan, M. Muller and M. Zenobi-Wong. 2014. GFOGER-modified MMP-sensitive polyethylene glycol hydrogels induce chondrogenic differentiation of human mesenchymal stem cells. Tissue Eng Pt. A. 20: 1165–1174.

Mironi-Harpaz, I., D.Y. Wang, S. Venkatraman and D. Seliktar. 2012. Photopolymerization of cell-encapsulating hydrogels: crosslinking efficiency versus cytotoxicity. Acta Biomater. 8: 1838–1848.

Mironi-Harpaz, I., A. Berdichevski and D. Seliktar. 2014. Fabrication of PEGylated fibrinogen: a versatile injectable hydrogel biomaterial. pp. 61-68. *In*: Radisic, M. and L.D. Black [eds.]. Cardiac Tissue Engineering: Methods and Protocols. Springer New York, New York, NY, USA.

Moeinzadeh, S., D. Barati, S.K. Sarvestani, O. Karaman and E. Jabbari. 2013. Nanostructure formation and transition from surface to bulk degradation in polyethylene glycol gels chain-extended with short hydroxy acid segments. Biomacromolecules. 14: 2917–2928.

Muhlebach, A., B. Muller, C. Pharisa, M. Hofmann, B. Seiferling and D. Guerry. 1997. New water-soluble photo crosslinkable polymers based on modified poly(vinyl alcohol). J. Biomed. Mater. Res. A. 35: 3603–3611.

Murosaki, T., N. Ahmed and J. Ping Gong. 2011. Antifouling properties of hydrogels. Sci. Technol. Adv. Mater. 12: 064706.

Nakayama, Y. and T. Matsuda. 1998. Photocurable surgical tissue adhesive glues composed of photoreactive gelatin and poly(ethylene glycol) diacrylate. J. Biomed. Mater. Res. 48: 511–521.

Nguyen, A.H., Y. Wang, D.E. White, M.O. Platt and T.C. McDevitt. 2016. MMP-mediated mesenchymal morphogenesis of pluripotent stem cell aggregates stimulated by gelatin methacrylate microparticle incorporation. Biomaterials. 76: 66–75.

Nguyen, K.T. and J.L. West. 2002. Photopolymerizable hydrogels for tissue engineering applications. Biomaterials. 23: 4307–4314.

Nguyen, Q.V., D.P. Huynh, J.H. Park and D.S. Lee. 2015. Injectable polymeric hydrogels for the delivery of therapeutic agents: A review. Eur Polym. 72: 602–619.

Nuttelman, C.R., S.M. Henry and K.S. Anseth. 2002. Synthesis and characterization of photocrosslinkable, degradable poly(vinyl alcohol)-based tissue engineering scaffolds. Biomaterials. 23: 3617–3626.

Occhetta, P., R. Visone, L. Russo, L. Cipolla, M. Moretti and M. Rasponi. 2015. VA-086 methacrylate gelatine photopolymerizable hydrogels: A parametric study for highly biocompatible 3D cell embedding. J. Biomed. Mater. Res. A. 103: 2109–2117.

Oliveira, M.B., O. Kossover, J.F. Mano and D. Seliktar. 2015a. A continuous solvent- and oil-free method to prepare injectable pegylated fibrinogen cell-laden microparticles. Tissue Eng. Pt. A. 21: S287–S287.

Oliveira, M.B., O. Kossover, J.F. Mano and D. Seliktar. 2015b. Injectable PEGylated fibrinogen cell-laden microparticles made with a continuous solvent- and oil-free preparation method. Acta Biomater. 13: 78–87.

Olmez, S.S., P. Korkusuz, H. Bilgili and S. Senel. 2007. Chitosan and alginate scaffolds for bone tissue regeneration. Pharmazie. 62: 423–431.

Ono, K., Y. Saito, H. Yura, K. Ishikawa, A. Kurita, T. Akaike et al. 2000. Photocrosslinkable chitosan as a biological adhesive. J. Biomed. Mater. Res. 49: 289–295.

Peppas, N.A., J.Z. Hilt, A. Khademhosseini and R. Langer. 2006. Hydrogels in biology and medicine: from molecular principles to bionanotechnology. Adv. Materi. 18: 1345–1360.

Peyton, S.R., C.B. Raub, V.P. Keschrumrus and A.J. Putnam. 2006. The use of poly(ethylene glycol) hydrogels to investigate the impact of ECM chemistry and mechanics on smooth muscle cells. Biomaterials. 27: 4881–4893.

Prakash Parthiban, S., D. Rana, E. Jabbari, N. Benkirane-Jessel and M. Ramalingam. 2017. Covalently immobilized VEGF-mimicking peptide with gelatin methacrylate enhances microvascularization of endothelial cells. Acta Biomater. 51: 330–340.

Qina, X.-H., A. Ovsianikov, J. Stampfl and R. Liska. 2014. Additive manufacturing of photosensitive hydrogels for tissue engineering applications. BioNanoMaterials. 15: 49–70.

Rouillard, A.D., C.M. Berglund, J.Y. Lee, W.J. Polacheck, Y. Tsui, L.J. Bonassar et al. 2011. Methods for photocrosslinking alginate hydrogel scaffolds with high cell viability. Tissue Eng. Pt C. 17: 173–179.

Rowland, G.F. 1977. Effective antitumour conjugates of alkylating drug andantibody using dextran as intermediate carrier. Eur. J. Cancer. 13: 593–596.

Rydholm, A.E., C.N. Bowman and K.S. Anseth. 2005. Degradable thiol-acrylate photopolymers: polymerization and degradation behavior of an *in situ* forming biomaterial. Biomaterials. 26: 4495–4506.

Samorezov, J.E., C.M. Morlock and E. Alsberg. 2015. Dual ionic and photo-crosslinked alginate hydrogels for micropatterned spatial control of material properties and cell behavior. Bioconjug. Chem. 26: 1339–1347.

Saraiva, S.M., S.P. Miguel, M.P. Ribeiro, P. Coutinho and I.J. Correia. 2015. Synthesis and characterization of a photocrosslinkable chitosan-gelatin hydrogel aimed for tissue regeneration. RSC Adv. 5: 63478–63488.

Sawhney, A.S., C.P. Pathak and J.A. Hubbell. 1993a. Bioerodible hydrogels based on photopolymerized poly(ethylene glycol)-co-poly(alpha-hydroxy acid) diacrylate macromers. Macromolecules. 26: 581–587.

Sawhney, A.S., C.P. Pathak and J.A. Hubbell. 1993b. Interfacial photopolymerization of poly(ethylene glycol)-based hydrogels upon alginate-poly(l-lysine) microcapsules for enhanced biocompatibility. Biomaterials. 14: 1008–1016.

Sawhney, A.S., C.P. Pathak, J.J. van Rensburg, R.C. Dunn and J.A. Hubbell. 1994. Optimization of photopolymerized bioerodible hydrogel properties for adhesion prevention. J. Biomed. Mater. Res. 28: 831–838.

Schacht, E., J. Vermeersch and R. Duncan. 1985. Biodegradation studies of dextran, a frequently used drug carrier. Pharm. Weekblad. 7: 225–225.

Schacht, E.H., S. Vansteenkiste, J. Loccufier and D. Permentier. 1990. Use of dextran as drug carrier. Abstr. Pap. Am. Chem. S. 199: 300-POLY.

Schmedlen, K.H., K.S. Masters and J.L. West. 2002. Photocrosslinkable polyvinyl alcohol hydrogels that can be modified with cell adhesion peptides for use in tissue engineering. Biomaterials. 23: 4325–4332.

Shim, I.K., S.Y. Lee, Y.J. Park, M.C. Lee, S.H. Lee, J.Y. Lee et al. 2008. Homogeneous chitosan-PLGA composite fibrous scaffolds for tissue regeneration. J. Biomed. Mater. Res. A. 84A: 247–255.

Shirahama, H., B.H. Lee, L.P. Tan and N.J. Cho. 2016. Precise tuning of facile one-pot gelatin methacryloyl (GelMA) synthesis. Sci Rep. 6: 31036.

Shung, A.K., E. Behravesh, S. Jo and A.G. Mikos. 2003. Crosslinking characteristics of and cell adhesion to an injectable poly(propylene fumarate-co-ethylene glycol) hydrogel using a water-soluble crosslinking system. Tissue Eng. 9: 243–254.

Smeds, K.A. and M.W. Grinstaff. 2001. Photocrosslinkable polysaccharides for in situ hydrogel formation. J. Biomed. Mater. Res. 54: 115–121.

Sridhar, B.V., N.R. Doyle, M.A. Randolph and K.S. Anseth. 2014. Covalently tethered TGF-beta1 with encapsulated chondrocytes in a PEG hydrogel system enhances extracellular matrix production. J. Biomed. Mater. Res. A. 102: 4464–4472.

Suggs, L.J., E.Y. Kao, L.L. Palombo, R.S. Krishnan, M.S. Widmer and A.G. Mikos. 1998a. Preparation and characterization of poly(propylene fumarate-co-ethylene glycol) hydrogels. J. Biomat. Sci.-Polym. E. 9: 653–666.

Suggs, L.J., R.S. Krishnan, C.A. Garcia, S.J. Peter, J.M. Anderson and A.G. Mikos. 1998b. *In vitro* and *in vivo* degradation of poly(propylene fumarate-co-ethylene glycol) hydrogels. J. Biomed. Mater. Res. 42: 312–320.

Tanahashi, K., S. Jo and A.G. Mikos. 2002. Synthesis and characterization of biodegradable cationic poly(propylene fumarate-co-ethylene glycol) copolymer hydrogels modified with agmatine for enhanced cell adhesion. Biomacromolecules. 3: 1030–1037.

Timmer, M.D., C.G. Ambrose and A.G. Mikos. 2003. Evaluation of thermal- and photo-crosslinked biodegradable poly(propylene fumarate)-based networks. J. Biomed. Mater. Res. A. 66: 811–818.

Turturro, M.V. and G. Papavasiliou. 2012. Generation of mechanical and biofunctional gradients in PEG diacrylate hydrogels by perfusion-based frontal photopolymerization. J. Biomat. Sci.-Polym. E. 23: 917–939.

Ullrich, G., P. Burtscher, U. Salz, N. Moszner and R. Liska. 2006. Phenylglycine derivatives as coinitiators for the radical photopolymerization of acidic aqueous formulations. J. Biomed. Mater. Res. A. 44: 115–125.

Van Tomme, S.R. and W.E. Hennink. 2007. Biodegradable dextran hydrogels for protein delivery applications. Expert Rev. Med. Devic. 4: 147–164.

Van Vlierberghe, S., P. Dubruel and E. Schacht. 2011. Biopolymer-based hydrogels as scaffolds for tissue engineering applications: a review. Biomacromolecules. 12: 1387–1408.

Villanueva, I., C.A. Weigel and S.J. Bryant. 2009. Cell-matrix interactions and dynamic mechanical loading influence chondrocyte gene expression and bioactivity in PEG-RGD hydrogels. Acta Biomater. 5: 2832–2846.

Wacker, B.K., S.K. Alford, E.A. Scott, M. Das Thakur, G.D. Longmore and D.L. Elbert. 2008. Endothelial cell migration on RGD-peptide-containing PEG hydrogels in the presence of sphingosine 1-phosphate. Biophys. J. 94: 273–285.

Wang, C., X. Tong, X. Jiang and F. Yang. 2017. Effect of matrix metalloproteinase-mediated matrix degradation on glioblastoma cell behavior in 3D PEG-based hydrogels. J. Biomed. Mater. Res. A. 105: 770–778.

Wang, D.M., F. Romer, L. Connell, C. Walter, E. Saiz, S. Yue et al. 2015. Highly flexible silica/chitosan hybrid scaffolds with oriented pores for tissue regeneration. J. Mater. Chem. B. 3: 7560–7576.

Williams, C.G., A.N. Malik, T.K. Kim, P.N. Manson and J.H. Elisseeff. 2005. Variable cytocompatibility of six cell lines with photoinitiators used for polymerizing hydrogels and cell encapsulation. Biomaterials. 26: 1211–1218.

Wu, Y., Y.X. Chen, J. Yan, D. Quinn, P. Dong, S.W. Sawyer et al. 2016. Fabrication of conductive gelatin methacrylate-polyaniline hydrogels. Acta Biomater. 33: 122–130.

Yang, F., C.G. Williams, D.-a. Wang, H. Lee, P.N. Manson and J. Elisseeff. 2005. The effect of incorporating RGD adhesive peptide in polyethylene glycol diacrylate hydrogel on osteogenesis of bone marrow stromal cells. Biomaterials. 26: 5991–5998.

Yue, K., G. Trujillo-de Santiago, M.M. Alvarez, A. Tamayol, N. Annabi and A. Khademhosseini. 2015. Synthesis, properties, and biomedical applications of gelatin methacryloyl (GelMA) hydrogels. Biomaterials. 73: 254–271.

Zhong, B.H. and X.Q. Gong. 1994. Synthesis of antibody-drug conjugates via dextran as an intermediate carrier. Abstr. Pap. Am. Chem. S. 208: 66-Medi.

CHAPTER 16

Stimuli-Responsive Biomolecular Hydrogels for Medical Applications

Garry Laverty

Introduction

The success of hydrogels as a biomedical platform is demonstrated by their current wealth of applications. They stand at the forefront of biomaterial, medical device, drug delivery and regenerative health applications due to their versatility and biocompatibility. Their hydrophilic nature enables the uptake of copious amounts of water, mimicking the extracellular matrix and providing tissue-like characteristics in three-dimensions (3D). The properties of the overall hydrogel polymer are highly influenced by their corresponding monomer units allowing unique tailoring of hydrogel motifs to selective functional requirements. Common synthetic hydrogel motifs include: poly(acrylic acid), poly(acrylamide), poly(ethylene glycol) (PEG), poly(vinyl alcohol) (PVA), poly(2-hydroxyethyl methacrylate) (PHEMA), poly(2-hydroxypropyl methacrylate) (PHPMA) and poly(N-isopropylacrylamide) (PNIPAm). Polymers are manipulated further by: combining monomer units to form co-polymer blends of varying ratios; altering the method of manufacture; varying cross-linking density and controlling amorphous/crystalline morphology. Whilst research into synthetic hydrogels are ongoing and has led to the clinical translation of a number of successful platforms, there has been a re-emergence in the study of natural-based hydrogels with inherent biodegradability and improved biofunctional properties. Hydrogels abundant throughout nature include agarose, alginate, elastin, collagen, gelatin, chitosan, fibrin,

Lecturer in Pharmaceutical Science, Biofunctional Nanomaterials Group, School of Pharmacy, Medical Biology Centre, Queen's University Belfast, 97 Lisburn Rd, Belfast, BT9 7BL.
E-mail: garry.laverty@qub.ac.uk

silk and hyaluronan. In the 21st century scientists have endeavoured to define and replicate nature's biological structures via a bottom-up approach whereby biomolecule monomers of the natural building blocks of life (lipids, peptides, nucleic acids and carbohydrates) are uniquely tailored to meet clinical and mechanical needs. These so-called biomolecular hydrogels possess numerous advantages over synthetic polymers including: increased chemical versatility, tunable biodegradability, reduced immunogenicity, tailored gelation in response to stimuli and enhanced biocompatibility. Biomolecules demonstrate inherent inter and intramolecular interactions which are commonly found in monomers capable of hydrogel formation. For example, long chain hydrocarbon chains of lipids generate van der Waals forces and hydrophobic interactions. Carbohydrates consist of multiple hydroxyl moieties ($-OH$) capable of hydrogen bonding. Nucleobases (cytosine, guanine, adenine, thymine and uracil) demonstrate specific hydrogen bonds and pi-pi (π-π) electrostatic interactions. Protein and peptide molecules have the advantage of being easily functionalized due to an available array of chemical groups granted by the presence of a variety of R-groups. High specific intermolecular interactions (hydrogen bonds, ionic, electrostatic, hydrophobic, dipole-dipole, van der Waals) can be developed by modifying the primary sequence, alleviating the need for toxic chemical cross-linkers such as glutaraldehyde, phenol and formaldehyde. Non-native chemistries and functional groups are easily incorporated into the primary structure at the sequence level, as are synthetic monomers (forming polymeric hybrid), enabling biomolecular hydrogels to be tailored to specific functional requirements. This is an important attribute that widens their scope of applications in the medical field (McCloskey et al. 2014).

There has been significant interest in developing hydrogels with tunable properties and the ability to respond to changes in environmental stimuli. Introducing stimuli sensitivity to hydrogelators broadens their range of applications as biomaterials. The human body presents a diverse environment for physical, biological and chemical stimuli allowing hydrogel properties to be controlled in response to external conditions at different sites throughout the body. A variety of stimuli have been harnessed for biomedical applications including: pH, ionic strength, oxidation/reduction, temperature, enzymes, light, shear stress, magnetism, and electricity, with resultant physicochemical changes in the hydrogel network and supramolecular structure enabling tailored delivery of drugs, increased/decreased gel strength and optimal mechanical behaviour. Responsive hydrogels are highly desirable as evidenced by a rapid expansion of research into these technologies. Self-assembling peptides are particularly promising molecules in the creation of hydrogels that form in response to specific environmental conditions. The following chapter will explore each of these stimuli in greater detail, focusing on the unique potential of biomolecular, mainly peptide-based, hydrogel platforms and their development as "smart", environmentally-responsive materials with diverse applications particular within the fields of drug delivery, 3D cell culture, tissue repair and regenerative medicine.

pH-Responsive Hydrogels

The human body displays a vast diversity of pH ranges which serve as a popular method for the hydrogel targeted delivery of drugs. Disease has also been implicated in increasing the acidic or alkalinity of the local cellular environment and scientists have been keen to exploit differences in healthy and diseased pH characteristics to enable localized drug delivery. For example, certain cancers are associated with a decrease in local tumour environment pH serving as a target for the delivery of chemotherapeutic payloads, selectively reducing damage to healthy cells (Kato et al. 2013). Urinary catheter associated infections are commonly accompanied with an increase in alkalinity due to the conversion of urea in the urine to highly basic ammonia by the enzyme urease, produced by pathogenic bacteria such as *Proteus mirabilis* (Stickler et al. 2006). Healthy human body systems and tissues also demonstrate localized diversity in pH (Table 1). In the gastrointestinal tract the pH of the stomach is attributed to be between pH 1.0–3.0, whilst the upper small intestine has an increased pH of 4.8–8.2, with the colon averaging pH 7.0 (Schmaljohann 2006). Oral dosage formulations make use of this variation to control the site of drug release, and optimize absorbance (Philip and Philip 2010). For example enteric-coating utilized in active ingredients such as aspirin and omeprazole are insoluble in acid media (stomach) but soluble in neutral/alkaline media (intestine). The active ingredients are protected from release in the stomach where conditions may cause stability issues (omeprazole) or side effects (aspirin) (Becker et al. 2004).

Hydrogels respond to the pH of their surrounding environments by either swelling or deswelling. This process is dependent on the presence of ionisable functional groups within the polymeric backbone and their respective logarithmic acid dissociation constant (pKa), resulting in an overall charge density (Ninawe and Parulekar 2011). The pH and ionic composition of the solution in direct contact with the hydrogel is also an important consideration in determining the charge density and overall swelling/deswelling effect. Swelling results from absorption of water into the hydrogel whilst expulsion causes deswelling guided by electrostatic interacts with the aqueous environment. Anionic hydrogels possess functional groups that are ionized in solutions with a pH greater than their respective pKa. Anionic hydrogels therefore become ionized and swell, due to electrostatic repulsions, in solutions where pH is greater than pKa (Kim et al. 2003). The opposite is true of cationic moieties which become ionized and swollen at pH lower than pH. Acrylic acid and methacrylic acid are the most commonly utilized synthetic anionic monomers governed primarily by the presence of a carboxylic functional group. Acrylamide, diethylaminoethyl methacrylate

Table 1. pH of various human systems, tissue and cellular compartments. Adapted from Scmaljohann 2006.

Tissue/cellular compartment	pH
Blood	7.34–7.45
Stomach	1.0–3.0
Upper small intestine	4.8–8.2
Colon	7.0–7.5
Tumour, extracellular	7.2–6.5
Early endosome	6.0–6.5
Late endosome	4.5–5.0
Vagina	3.8–4.5
Inflamed tissue/wound	5.4–7.4

and dimethylaminoethyl methacrylate are synthetic cationic monomers with basicity due to amino groups (Koetting et al. 2015). The importance of carboxylic acids and amino functional groups in determining swelling/deswelling and overall charge (pKa) of the molecule lead scientists to hypothesizing a role for amino acid molecules in hydrogel applications.

Amino acids are excellent monomers for controlling pH dependent self-assembly and hydrogelation. Comprising of at least one amino group and one acid functionality as a minimum, a variety of properties and charge/pKa are endowed by variation in respective R-groups. The naturally occurring amino acids aspartic acid and glutamic acid become ionized in solutions with a pH greater than their respective pKa. Basic amino acids, for example histidine, arginine and lysine, provide the potential for cationic behaviour. Charged amino acids are utilized to create highly specific charge-charge interactions to drive (opposing charges) or prevent (equal charge) self-assembly and hydrogel formation (Fig. 1) (McCloskey et al. 2014). The influence of the amino acid R-group is increased further when respective amino and carboxylic acid groups (attached to the α-carbon) covalently attach via a condensation reaction forming an amide bond and the peptide chain.

Biomolecules are also able to self-organize and assemble into nanostructures. The formation of a nanofibrous architecture can allow supramolecular hydrogel formation. The Schneider group demonstrated that pH could be utilized as a trigger for the self-assembly of β-hairpin peptides forming a cytocompatible, mechanically

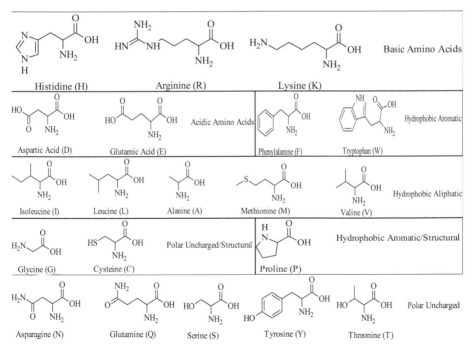

Fig. 1. The structures and codes for the 20 naturally occurring amino acids. Each amino acid shares a carboxylic acid (−COOH) and a primary amine group (−NH₂). The properties of the individual amino acids are governed by the nature and functionality of the R-group attached to the α-carbon. Adapted from (McCloskey et al. 2014).

rigid hydrogel with antibacterial activity. The synthetic peptide MAX1 (H₂N-VKVKVKVKVᴰPPTKVKVKVKV-CONH₂) is composed of 20 amino acid units of alternating valine (V) and lysine (K) molecules with a central D-valine-diproline-threonine sequence (VᴰPPT) driving the formation of a type-II β-turn (Schneider et al. 2002). At acidic pH, below the pKa of lysine, assembly does not occur due to charge repulsion. At basic pH, above the pKa of lysine, a β-hairpin forms due to lack of repulsion driving self-assembly and molecular interactions. The β-hairpin secondary structure motif forms two faces of varying character. An outlying hydrophobic face composed of valines and an internal hydrophilic lysine face. Hydrophobic interactions (van der Waal's, dipole-dipole) and hydrogen bonding (between respective amide/peptide bonds) are responsible for driving intermolecular self-assembly and hydrogel formation.

Modification of MAX1 peptide also allows thermo-responsiveness to be introduced. The potential applications of MAX1 were expanded for use as three dimensional biomineralization scaffolds (Altunbas et al. 2010). Lysine groups provided sufficient cationicity to allow the addition of tetraethoxysilane and silica on the fibril surface forming defined silica shells with increased mechanical properties when compared to MAX1 alone. At increased pH (above pH 7) silicic acid (from tetraethoxysilane) dissociates into its silicate anion, $[SiO(OH)_3]^-$, catalysed by the presence of a polycationic lysine surface. This dissociation increases as the pH is elevated resulting in greater electrostatic interactions between anionic silicate and cationic lysine and an increased density of silicate anions at the peptide fibril surface. The successful production of a silica-peptide hydrogel material holds great promise for future use as tissue engineering scaffolds.

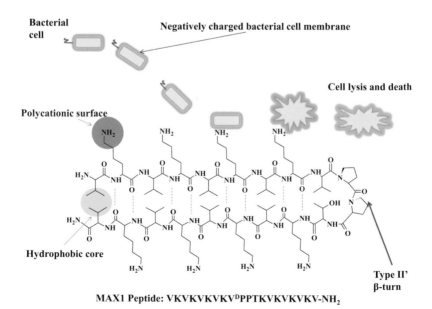

MAX1 Peptide: VKVKVKVKVᴰPPTKVKVKVKV-NH₂

Fig. 2. Primary amino acid sequence and structural organization of MAX1 peptide at basic pH. The presence of cationic lysine molecules endow antimicrobial activity to the peptide. Adapted from (McCloskey et al. 2014).

Our own group pioneered the development of an ultrashort cationic peptide nanomaterials which demonstrates potent activity against resistant biofilm forms of medical device related pathogens including: staphylococci, *Escherichia coli* and *Pseudomonas aeruginosa* (Laverty et al. 2014). This group of peptides utilize a carboxylic acid terminated naphthalene-diphenylalanine (NapFF) backbone to provide pH-responsive hydrogel formation whilst the addition of two units of cationic charge (lysine, ornithine) allows the molecule to selectively target negatively charged bacterial membranes. NapFFKK proved particularly promising as an anti-biofilm hydrogel with potential future use as a biomaterial in wound-healing or as an infection-responsive hydrogel coating in medical implants such as intravascular catheters and hip replacements. A nanofibrous architecture is derived from β-sheet stacking of NapFF motifs. Highly aromatic naphthalene allows intermolecular π-π electrostatic interactions between delocalized π-electrons. Amide groups present as part of the peptide linkage allow formation of hydrogen bonds between peptide molecules but also with water. The overall hydrophobic-hydrophilic balance of the molecule will determines whether the peptide precipitates (too hydrophobic), dissolves (too hydrophilic) or forms a hydrogel (optimum balance) in solution. The presence of a terminal carboxylic acid moiety is also critical to driving the self-assembly process and supramolecular hydrogel formation. Basic pH, above the pKa of the carboxylic acid, results in removal of a proton (H^+) from the hydroxyl group of the carboxylic acid creating a carboxylate anion (COO^-) allowing full dissolution of the peptide in aqueous solution. Gradual acidification of this solution, using for example dilute hydrochloric acid or utilizing the hydrolysis of glucono-δ-lactone to gluconic acid in aqueous solution, to physiological pH (in the case of our NapFFKK peptide) or acidic pH (NapFF), results in the formation of a homogenous hydrogel at concentrations of ~ 0.5% w/v and above. The pH responsiveness of the NapFF motifs may have important applications as hydrogels in cancer therapeutics and infection. Some infections, for example those related to the presence of intravascular catheters, are associated with decreased local pH due to a combination of host inflammation, phagocytosis and microbial anaerobic fermentation owing to low oxygen tension. Local pH can be reduced to as low as pH 5.5 (Radovic-Moreno et al. 2012). This may serve as a stimulus to trigger self-assembly of a protective hydrogel surface when it is most required (infection development) extending the antimicrobial profile beyond the approximate one to two week protection granted by current medical device strategies (McCloskey et al. 2014).

Ionic Strength-Responsive Hydrogels

Ionic strength relates closely to pH in that they dictate formation and properties of hydrogels due to fundamental differences in molecular charge. At physiological pH (7.4) and low ionic strength, the MAX1 peptide does not gelate as it forms a random coil conformation even at concentrations as high as 4% w/v in water (Ozbas et al. 2004). An increase in ionic strength, corresponding to 150 mM buffered saline (NaCl) and cell culture media, promotes self-assembly and hydrogelation at 2% w/v due to β-hairpin formation. Increased ionic strength results in dampening of positive charged lysine residues in the MAX1 backbone allowing hydrogelation to proceed.

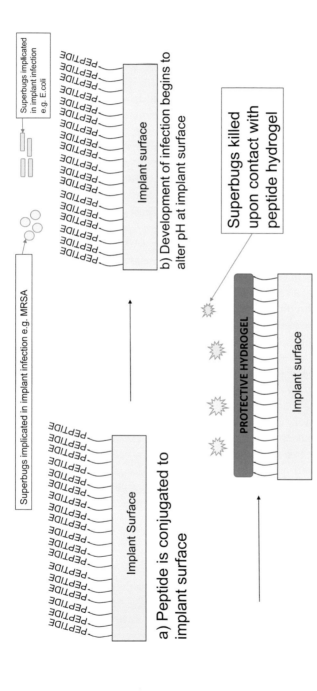

Fig. 3. pH responsive self-assembling hydrogels for the long-term prevention of medical device related infection. (a) Self-assembling peptide is conjugated to surface of a medical device. (b) pH change, initiated by infection (e.g., increase in urinary catheter infection) drives formation of antimicrobial peptide hydrogel formation only when infection begins. (c) Formation of an antimicrobial and biocompatible hydrogel layer in response to infectious stimuli provides prolonged protection from superbug colonization/biofilm formation. This process replicates the evolutionary advantage awarded to organisms such as amphibians/frogs that secrete a thin peptide mucus on their skin to protect against infection with the hypothesis that this will provide protection against implant infection for longer than existing products.

Addition of MAX1 to the common cell culture Dunlbecco's Modified Eagle's Medium (DMEM) of 165 mM salinity and pH 7.4, results in hydrogelation after 30 minutes (Kretsinger et al. 2005). Inclusion of cells in DMEM allows entrapment in MAX1 but forms a cell sediment due to a lengthened gelation time. Replacement of one cationic lysine at position 15 with an anionic glutamic acid residue was sufficient to allow self-assembled hydrogelation within one minute of mixing with DMEM ensuring homogenous entrapment of encapsulated cells. Its cytocompatibility and ability to promote cell proliferation highlights the potential use of the MAX peptides in biomedical engineering particularly within the tissue regeneration and 3D cell culture fields. This is further evidence of the sensitivity and responsiveness of this group of peptides to a variety of physiological conditions.

A group of ionic self-complementary β-sheet oligopeptides (RAD16-I and RAD16-II), derived from the model ionically complementary EAK16 peptide (Jun et al. 2004), are composed of a primary sequence of alternating cationic arginine, alanine and anionic aspartate residues (Holmes et al. 2000). This RAD sequence resembles the RGD cell adhesion motif often utilized to promote cell attachment and growth. This allows complementary electrostatic interactions and formation of β-sheet secondary structures. Optimal hydrogelation occurs at an ionic strength and pH (7.4) similar to that utilized in tissue culture media (RPMI 1640: 24 mM $NaHCO_3$/103 mM NaCl) and phosphate buffered saline (5 mM NaPO4/150 mM NaCl). Therefore RAD16-I and RAD16-II have potential application in both tissue and cell regeneration. Most promisingly, RAD peptides allow neuronal cell attachment, differentiation and significant outgrowth with the same degree of success as extracellular matrix proteins such as laminin, fibronectin, and collagen but without the need for synthetic materials to increase mechanical strength and tissue-like properties. This has successfully translated to the Puramatrix® technology (CH_3CO-[RADA]$_4$-$CONH_2$) widely used as a cell culture media but is also set to undergo clinical testing for use as a haemostasis product (as PuraStat®); an aid in endoscopic mucosal resection and to promote tissue regeneration as a filler for voids in dental bone. Similar research by the Aggeli group developed β-sheet-forming peptide hydrogels (QQRFEWEFEQQ) responsive to pH/ionic strength and capable of hydroxyapatite nucleation, leading to enamel remineralization and repair of dental decay in the oral cavity (Kirkham et al. 2007). Delivery to the area as a peptide-based solution aided administration. Anionic groups on the peptide side chain were capable of binding to calcium resulting in phosphate salt precipitation within dental caries.

The Stupp group developed a separate group of gelators termed peptide amphiphiles. As their name suggests these molecules are composed to two separate hydrophobic and hydrophilic sections. Amphiphilic peptides are composed of a 6–12 amino acid segment coupled via an amide bond to a fatty acid chain that varies from 10 to 22 carbon atoms in length. The hydrophilic section often provides biofunctionality with most containing an aliphatic hydrophobic portion enabling self-assembly (Hartgerink et al. 2001). A hydrophilic peptide, $C_{16}H_{33}$-VVVAAAEEE-COOH, shows promise as a hydrogel tissue scaffold for brain, spinal cord and heart regeneration. Gelation results from screening of charged amino acid residues, in the case of $C_{16}H_{33}$-VVVAAAEEE-COOH, positively charged divalent calcium (from calcium chloride, $CaCl_2$) negated anionic charge of glutamic acids (E). The Stupp group also discovered that negatively charged peptide amphiphiles hydrogels were non-toxic when formed using divalent metal cations and interestingly served as nutrient source for cells such as MC3T3-E1 (murine, bone fibroblast) (Beniash et al. 2005). Peptide amphiphiles can also be modified to contain bioactive residues. For example self-assembling amphiphiles containing the neuroactive amino acid motif IKVAV, derived from laminin, enhanced axon regeneration, reduced glial scar formation and led improved hindlimb movement in mouse models after spinal cord injury (Tysseling-Mattiace et al. 2008). Heparin-binding peptide amphiphiles, containing a Cardin-Weintraub heparin-binding domain, were shown to specifically bind to heparin sulphate-like glycosminoglycans leading to self-assembly and hydrogel formation (Ghanaati et al. 2009). This hydrogel promoted angiogenesis and healing of chronic wounds. As the peptide hydrogel degraded the growth of vascularized connective tissue was observed over 30 days.

The importance of charge within the primary molecular structure was confirmed by the Hartgerink group who formed a peptide-based ABA block system. The A blocks are composed of charged amino acid residues with B composed of alternating hydrophobic and hydrophilic residues. Addition of multivalent ions of opposing charge, such as magnesium cation (Mg^{2+}) and phosphate anion ($PO_4)^{-3}$, to the A block are utilized to trigger hydrogelation (Dong et al. 2007). For example lysine containing multi-domain peptide 1 (MDP1) (KK-SLSLSLSLSLSL-KK) successfully formed a hydrogel in the presence of negatively charged PO_4^{-3} anions (Aulisa et al. 2009). Serine acted as a neutral, hydrophilic amino acid with B and increased hydrogen bonding between nanofibers and therefore improved gel strength. MDPs was demonstrated to have application as a tissue scaffold with inclusion of an enzyme cleavable KGRGDS bioactive motif (as part of terminal A block) improving cell proliferation in dental mesenchymal stem cells (Galler et al. 2010).

Oxidation/Reduction-Responsive Hydrogels

An area of emerging interest is the use of reducing conditions to stimulate self-assembly and hydrogelation, harnessing relative conformational changes in cysteines disulphide bonds. Bowerman and Nilsson demonstrated the cyclized disulphide bonding of the peptide $CH3COC-(FKFE)_2CG-NH_2$ could prevent self-assembly to a β-sheet, nanofibrous architecture in an oxidized state (Bowerman and Nilsson 2010). Reduction of the disulphide bond allows the peptide to switch to a thermodynamically preferred, low energy, β-sheet conformation forming a viscoelastic hydrogel. As the authors suggested such peptides could be of value for localized delivery of chemotherapeutic drugs to tumours which often possess an extracellular reducing environment.

Thermo-Responsive Hydrogels

The MAX group of peptides were also demonstrated to possess temperature responsive hydrogel formation. Alteration of the pH responsive MAX1 motif by substitution of one (position 16) or two (and position 7) valines of the peptide primary sequence with the less hydrophobic amino acid threonine, creates MAX2 (H_2N-VKVKVKVKV^{D}PPTKVKTKVKV-CONH$_2$) and MAX3 (H_2N-VKVKVKTKV^{D}PPTKVKTKVKV-CONH$_2$) peptides (Pochan et al. 2003). These subtle changes increased the temperature of gelation to 40°C for one substitution (MAX2) and 60°C for two substitutions from 25°C (recorded for MAX1, pH 9). Increased hydrophobicity of the peptide motif results in greater hydrophobic interactions, increased intramolecular folding of MAX and self-assembled gelation at lower temperatures. Further work by the Schneider group lead to the development of TSS1, a three stranded β-sheet peptide that undergoes thermo-responsive hydrogelation at physiological temperature (37°C), supports cell adhesion, cell migration and is non-toxic to mesenchymal stem cells (Rughani et al. 2009).

β-sheet peptides and their variants are the most popular form of short self-assembled peptide hydrogels. However the Woolfson group pioneered several self-assembling fibre peptides based on a heptad repeat (seven amino acids) that forms an alternative α-helical coiled-coil secondary structure (Banwell et al. 2009). An amino acid sequence of *abcdefg*, forms the heptad template where position *a* and *d*, are occupied by hydrophobic residues, and *e* and *g* are charged moieties. Assembly and hydrogel formation are driven by a hydrophobic: charge balance where *a* and *d* are buried within the coiled-coil interface and electrostatic interactions between *e* and *g* stabilize the structure. Successful hydrogelation was demonstrated when two separate cationic and anionic (*g* and *e*) heptads were mixed. A thermo-responsive α-helical coiled-coil system was created by introducing hydrophobic alanine at positions *b*, *c* and *f*. As *b*, *c* and *f* are responsible for the interactions of coiled-coils at the interface between heptad dimers, the presence of alanine at these positions increased hydrophobic interactions at the exposed coiled-coil surface. Mixing of alanine containing peptide self-assembling fibres IAALKAK-IAALKAE-IAALEAE-NAALEAK with IAALKAK-NAALKAE-IAALEAE-IAALEAK forms a hydrogel with increased gel strength at higher temperatures due to mainly hydrophobic interactions. Replacing alanine with glutamines at positions *b*, *c* and *f* (to form a mixture of: IQQLKQK-IQQLKQE-IQQLEQE-NQQLEQK with IQQLKQK-NQQLKQE-IQQLEQE-IQQLEQK) increases hydrogen bond formation between coiled-coil dimers and reduces hydrophobic interactions. Upon heating these hydrogels melt due to breaking of hydrogen bonds thus reversing the peptide's response to temperature. Mixing of two different self-assembling fibre peptides also serves to allow greater control over gelation temperature. Stupp's hydrophilic peptide $C_{16}H_{33}$-VVVAAAEEE-COOH forms a hydrogel when subjected to increased temperature/heat treatment at 80°C and cooling to 25°C (Hartgerink et al. 2001). Heating drives alignment of fibrils over macroscopic scales, increasing solubilization and allowing hydrogel formation upon return to 25°C. The contribution of the hydrophobic tail to the overall hydrophobic: hydrophilic balance, and thus its importance to thermo-responsive hydrogelation of peptide amphiphiles cannot be underestimated (Gore et al. 2001).

Silk-elastin-like polymers (SELP) are a class of larger polypeptides of repeating silk fibroin (GAGAGS) and mammalian elastin (GVGVP) amino acid residues often synthesized by genetic engineering techniques. SELP hydrogels have been studied for a variety of drug delivery purposes, including delivery of plasmid DNA, adenoviral vectors, vitamin B_{12} cytochrome C and theophylline (Dinerman et al. 2002; Megeed et al. 2004). Substitution of glutamic acid for valine in the elastin segment has been proven to induce thermo-responsive. Replacement of the ionisable glutamic acid with more hydrophobic valine results in a more hydrophobic polymer that requires a lower temperature to precipitate into a hydrogel (Nagarsekarn et al. 2003). A greater state of ionization, induced by pH and ionic strength considerations, also increases hydrophilicity therefore thermo-responsiveness requires an appreciation of these factors also. Amino acids, such as glutamic acid, with ionisable R-groups are more influenced by changes in pH and ionic strength.

Thermo-responsive hydrogelation takes advantage of the ability of water to solubilize hydrophobic moieties at reduced temperatures. Increasing temperature decreases the solubility of the hydrophobic species resulting in phase separation of these groups creating hydrogels due to formation of physically cross-linked networks (Badiger et al. 1998). Peptide folding is also sensitive to temperature changes. A transition from α-helix to β-sheet secondary structure was utilized by Zhang and colleagues to induce temperature responsive gelation in EAK-12 (AEAEAEAEAKAK) and DAR16-IV (ADADADADARARARAR) peptides. β-sheet formation and gelation predominantly occur at 25°C for EAK-12 with α-helix conformation at 85°C. DAR16-IV was proven to transform to an α-helix nature at 75°C. An increase in temperature to trigger an α-helix to β-sheet conformational change was also used by Kammerer to trigger gelation in short coiled-coil peptides (Kammerer and Steinmetz 2006). There is increased interest in developing biomolecular hydrogels that mimic human tissue. The ability to tailor hydrogelation to a specific temperature may be of benefit for tissue regeneration and wound healing applications. The temperature of external human skin varies depending on a range of factors including health status and location but is estimated to be between 31 and 40°C (Benedict et al. 1919). A formulation that was liquid at room temperature would allow ease of application to the highly varied shape of wound cavities. Rapid gelation at skin temperature would enable a biomolecular hydrogel to fill this cavity, potentially promoting healing and preventing infection. Such a product would be highly valued by emergency services and within conflict zones.

Enzyme-Responsive Hydrogels

Self-assembly in biological systems is tightly controlled by spatially confined molecular mechanisms, often catalysed by enzymes, to form cellular architecture such as microtubules, actin filaments, DNA, vesicles and micelles (Rasale and Das 2015). Enzymes are viable molecules for instructing localized assembly of biomolecules, resulting in hydrogel formation. They are particularly promising as hydrogelation can be triggered within a cell by utilizing an activating enzyme that is not found extracellularly. Enzymatic responsive systems involving hydrolysis of a peptide (amide) bond (Guilbaud et al. 2013), phosphate ester (Yang et al. 2006) or methyl ester (Hirst et al. 2010) are more commonly utilized for research purposes. Enzyme instructed self-assembly can be achieved by either catalysing the addition or removal of a group to/from a molecule to form a self-assembling motif (Yang et al. 2004; Toledano et al. 2006). Enzymatic synthesis of a self-assembling molecule has been proven for peptides whereby an amide linkage forms from the reversible condensation/hydrolysis reaction of an amine and carboxylic acid under conditions that govern thermodynamic control. The laws of thermodynamics ensure that condensation will be favoured over peptide hydrolysis only for molecules that self-assemble to form stable structures (e.g., hydrogels) and have sufficient free energy to overcome hydrolysis (Williams et al. 2009). The Xu group demonstrated reversible enzymatic formation of supramolecular hydrogels, proving enzymatic reactions can modulate the balance of hydrophobicity and hydrophilicity of small peptide molecules (Yang et al. 2006). Cleavage of a hydrophilic phosphate group from NapFFGEY-P(O)(OH)$_2$ in the presence of a phosphatase enzyme results in the formation of the more hydrophobic hydrogelator NapFFGEY. Addition of a kinase to the NapFFGEY hydrogel in the presence of adenosine triphosphate (ATP) converts the terminal tyrosine (Y) to tyrosine phosphate resulting in the restoration of NapFFGEY-P(O)(OH)$_2$ and the soluble phase. The level of control provided by this kinase/phosphatase switch demonstrates how simple it is to regulate the formation of supramolecular hydrogels by enzymatic approaches and is of great promise in the development of biomaterials for localized drug delivery and tissue engineering. Enzyme instructed reversible self-assembly and gelation is advantageous as it allows the hydrogels to respond to the presences of specific enzymes within specific tissues or diseases. Cancer (Saha et al. 2001), Alzheimer's (Yuan and Yankner 2000), diabetes (Hutton and Eisenbarth 2003), and multiple sclerosis (Auch et al. 2004) are associated with the abnormal kinase and/or phosphatase activity and are therefore viable biological targets for future therapies. The Xu group demonstrated the therapeutic potential of this approach by conjugating the antineoplastic drug paclitaxel to NapFFKY-P(O)(OH)$_2$ via a succinic acid linker (Gao et al. 2009). Alkaline phosphate transformed this precursor into the hydrogelating variant whilst providing localized antitumour activity and cytocompatibility. Intracellular hydrogel formation may also be exploited to direct cell death in cancerous cells. Xu also synthesized an ester-containing NapFF peptide precursor that only self-assembles intracellularly in response to endogenous esterase enzymes (Yang et al. 2007). HeLa cells, an immortalized cell line of cervical cancer, were demonstrated to possess increased intracellular esterase levels relative to NIH3T3 standard fibroblast cells. The intracellular formation of a nanofibrous hydrogel induces stresses on the HeLa cell preventing biochemical transport and triggering cell death.

Enzymes may also be utilized to mediate degradation of hydrogel networks for drug delivery and tissue remodelling. The Hartgerink group proved the matrix metalloproteinase protease (MMP) family, specifically MMP-2, was able to recognize and cleave the GTAGLIGQ amino acid sequence between glycine (G) and leucine (L) in a mixture of peptide amphiphiles (Jun et al. 2005). This resulted in cell-mediated proteolytic degradation of the hydrogel network, allowing cell migration through the hydrogel matrix and remodelling of the matrix with natural extracellular matrix. They hypothesized this would be of benefit for dental use with encapsulation of dental pulp cells feasible within the hydrogel matrix and inclusion of aspartic acid in the peptide primary sequence promoting calcium binding.

Shear-Responsive Hydrogels

Hydrogels can vary in their response to an applied shear force. Shear-thinning hydrogels demonstrate a reduced viscosity in response to the application of shear stress. Shear thickening express an opposing increased viscosity in response to shear and are exemplified by ceramic systems such as hydroxyapatite, utilized commonly as bone constructs (Cyster et al. 2005). In biomolecular peptide hydrogels shear-thinning hydrogels are more common due to their self-assembled nature with hydrophobic and electrostatic interactions, and hydrogen bonding important for developing cross-links (Aulisa et al. 2009). As these molecular forces are weaker than covalent bonds they can be disrupted allowing the hydrogel network to flow. Shear-thinning is an optimal property for the precise delivery of a hydrogel to wound site, for example using a simple syringe. The shear force require to move the hydrogel out of the syringe is sufficient to enable the formulation to display liquid-like, flowing properties. These subsequently recover their elastic gel-like properties upon removal of shear force after application. MAX8 was proven to be an excellent shear thinning gel for the potential encapsulation and delivery of mesenchymal stem cells (Haines-Butterick et al. 2007). When an appropriate shear stress is applied, the MAX8 hydrogel shear-thins resulting in a low-viscosity gel. However, when shear has stopped, the gel quickly recovers its initial mechanical rigidity and gel-like properties. Shear-thickening natural-based hydrogels do exist, for example the Craig group developed a cysteine containing elastin-like polypeptide which formed covalent disulphide cross-linked networks in hydrogen peroxide and increased shear thickening up to an applied threshold force at concentration of 2.5% w/v (Xu et al. 2012). An applied force above a maximal defined threshold leads to shear-thinning properties and limits the wider use of these gels in medical context.

Light-Triggered Hydrogels

Light can also be used as an external stimulus to trigger the process of self-assembly and photopolymerization is commonly employed throughout the polymer industry to create a vast library of synthetic industrial and medical materials. Its use within peptide self-assembly has also been studied. Cui and colleagues incorporated a photoacid generator into liposomes which acted to lower the pH upon exposure to light. This was a successful approach in triggering the self-assembly of peptides by light activation within a spatially confined acidic environment (Lee et al. 2008). Schneider and Pochan have also developed a light triggered β-hairpin system based on the MAX peptide motif, termed MAX7CNB. A cysteine residue was introduced into the hydrophobic face of the peptide primary structure and a photocage (α-carboxy-2-nitrobenzyl) was then attached to the thiol group of this cysteine. Self-assembly could be controlled via specific wavelengths of UV light ($260 < \lambda < 360$ nm). The photocage prevented the folding of the peptide to a β-hairpin until exposure to light in the UV spectrum caused decaging and self-assembly (Haines et al. 2005). Using light to drive the self-assembly process has the advantage that it should not perturb the solution but interacts only with the material, meaning that it should not cause localized changes in the environment (e.g., pH) which may affect parameters such as drug release. However, the widespread use of light as a trigger throughout biomedicine is limited by its inability to effectively cross dense tissues (Carling et al. 2015).

Electrical-Responsive Hydrogels

Electronic signals are fundamental to the optimum functioning of human systems however there is a major challenge in combining biofunctional hydrogel materials with electronic engineering due to the reliance and abundance of water in the hydrogel structures and its negative effect on electronics. The opportunity to significantly advance biosensing platforms to monitor health and electronic signalling components for the nervous system makes research efforts in this area valuable. Peptide-based conducting hydrogel materials have been produced by incorporation of aromatic ligands such as 1,4,5,8-naphthalenetetracarboxylic acid diimide (NDI) at optimal locations. Shao and Parquette developed a transparent NDI hydrogel FmocKK (NDI) which formed β-sheets in aqueous solution driven by hydrophobic π-π interactions of NDI and Fmoc chromophores (Shao and Parquette 2010). Electrostatic repulsions governed by the neighbouring cationic charge of dilysines prevented aggregation and promoted an optimal hydrophobic: hydrophilic balance. The presence of NDI, which can control long-range charge migration, means this hydrogel may have potential applications within bioelectronic devices that source, detect and control light. Electrically-responsive hydrogels are also thought to be of benefit as future artificial muscle fibres replicating the response to electrical signals applied by neurons (Osada et al. 1992), or for tailored drug-delivery in the form of implanted pulsatile subcutaneous implants (Murdan 2003).

Future Perspectives

The development of bioinspired hydrogel materials have accelerated in the past decade however there remain a number of barriers that have to be overcome to ensure their widespread clinical translation. Despite some progress, cost-effective pharmaceutical scale-up of biomolecules, in line with current Good Manufacturing Practice (cGMP) (Fosgerau and Hoffmann 2015). Up-scaling from the laboratory to the industrial setting is a major challenge especially for large protein molecules of hundreds of amino acids and more complicated chemically modified biomolecules (e.g., peptide-sugar-nucleic acid conjugates) (Du et al. 2014). Sequences over 35 amino acids are not currently acknowledge to be economically feasible to mass produce by chemical methods alone (Sato et al. 2006). Recombinant production by transgenic means (bacteria, fungi, animals) is a viable alternative but face challenges related to long lead times, ethical considerations (animals) and efficient production purification of self-assembling molecules which may precipitate during manufacture (Kyle et al. 2009). Despite these challenges there is still a therapeutic appetite for hydrogel biomaterials composed of biomolecular building blocks. Great confidence can be taken from the research advances outlined in this chapter and the clinical translation of self-assembling peptide therapies such as lanreotide (Valery et al. 2003). The potential applications of hydrogel formats are expanding rapidly in the medical field with some of the most exciting recent developments using hydrogels as scaffolds for 3D printing of replacement organs (Bhattacharjee et al. 2015), and to form magnetic-responsive, noodle-like fibres for artificial muscle formation (Li et al. 2015). Such exciting approaches will only reaffirm the importance of hydrogels platforms in advancing future healthcare and biomaterial strategies.

Acknowledgements

The author acknowledges funding provided by the Queen's University Research Support Package for New Academic Staff and a Royal Society Research Grant (RG150171).

References

Altunbas, A., N. Sharma, M.S. Lamm, C. Yan, R.P. Nagarkar, J.P. Schneider et al. 2010. Peptide—silica hybrid networks: biomimetic control of network mechanical behavior. ACS Nano. 4: 181–188.

Auch, C.J., R.N. Saha, F.G. Sheikh, X. Liu, B.L. Jacobs and K. Pahan. 2004. Role of protein kinase R in double-stranded RNA-induced expression of nitric oxide synthase in human astroglia. FEBS Lett. 563: 223–228.

Aulisa, L., H. Dong and J.D. Hartgerink. 2009. Self-assembly of multidomain peptides: sequence variation allows control over cross-linking and viscoelasticity. Biomacromolecules. 10: 2694–2698.

Badiger, M.V., A.K. Lele, V.S. Bhalerao, S. Varghese and R.A. Mashelkar. 1998. Molecular tailoring of thermoreversible copolymer gels: some new mechanistic insights. J. Chem. Phys. 109: 1175–1184.

Banwell, E.F., E.S. Abelardo, D.J. Adams, M.A. Birchall, A.M. Corrigan, A. Donald et al. 2009. Rational design and application of responsive alpha-helical peptide hydrogels. Nat. Mater. 8: 596–600.

Becker, J.C., W. Domschke and T. Pohle. 2004. Current approaches to prevent NSAID-induced gastropathy-COX selectivity and beyond. Br. J. Clin. Pharmacol. 58: 587–600.

Benedict, F.G., W.R. Miles and A. Johnson. 1919. The temperature of the human skin. Proc. Natl. Acad. Sci. USA. 5: 218–222.

Beniash, E., J.D. Hartgerink, H. Storrie, J.C. Stendahl and S.I. Stupp. 2005. Self-assembling peptide amphiphile nanofiber matrices for cell entrapment. Acta Biomater. 1: 387–397.

Bhattacharjee, T., S.M. Zehnder, K.G. Rowe, S. Jain, R.M. Nixon, W.G. Sawyer et al. 2015. Writing in the granular gel medium. Science Advances. 1: 1–6.

Bowerman, C.J. and B.L. Nilsson. 2010. A reductive trigger for peptide self-assembly and hydrogelation. J. Am. Chem. Soc. 132: 9526–9527.

Carling, C.J., M.L. Viger, V.A. Huu, A.V. Garcia and A. Almutairi. 2015. Visible light-triggered drug release from an implanted depot. Chem. Sci. 6: 335–341.

Cyster, L.A., D.M. Grant, S.M. Howdle, F.R. Rose, D.J. Irvine, D. Freeman et al. 2005. The influence of dispersant concentration on the pore morphology of hydroxyapatite ceramics for bone tissue engineering. Biomaterials. 26: 697–702.

Dinerman, A.A., J. Cappello, H. Ghandehari and S.W. Hoag. 2002. Solute diffusion in genetically engineered silk-elastin like protein polymer hydrogels. J. Control. Release. 82: 277–287.

Dong, H., S.E. Paramonov, L. Aulisa, E.L. Bakota and J.D. Hartgerink. 2007. Self-assembly of multidomain peptides: balancing molecular frustration controls conformation and nanostructure. J. Am. Chem. Soc. 129: 12468–12472.

Du, X., J. Zhou and B. Xu. 2014. Supramolecular hydrogels made of basic biological building blocks. Chem. Asian J. 9: 1446–1472.

Fosgerau, K. and T. Hoffmann. 2015. Peptide therapeutics: current status and future directions. Drug Discov. Today. 20: 122–128.

Galler, K.M., L. Aulisa, K.R. Regan, R.N. D'Souza and J.D. Hartgerink. 2010. Self-assembling multidomain peptide hydrogels: designed susceptibility to enzymatic cleavage allows enhanced cell migration and spreading. J. Am. Chem. Soc. 132: 3217–3223.

Gao, Y., Y. Kuang, Z.F. Guo, Z. Guo, I.J. Krauss and B. Xu. 2009. Enzyme-instructed molecular self-assembly confers nanofibers and a supramolecular hydrogel of taxol derivative. J. Am. Chem. Soc. 131: 13576–13577.

Ghanaati, S., M.J. Webber, R.E. Unger, C. Orth, J.F. Hulvat, S.E Kiehna et al. 2009. Dynamic *in vivo* biocompatibility of angiogenic peptide amphiphile nanofibers. Biomaterials. 30: 6202–6212.

Gore, T., Y. Dori, Y. Talmon, M. Tirrell and H. Bianco-Peled. 2001. Self-assembly of model collagen peptide amphiphiles. Langmuir. 17: 5352–5360.

Guilbaud, J.B., C. Rochas, A.F. Miller and A. Saiani. 2013. Effect of enzyme concentration of the morphology and properties of enzymatically triggered peptide hydrogels. Biomacromolecules. 14: 1403–1411.

Haines, L.A., K. Rajagopal, B. Ozbas, D.A. Salick, D.J. Pochan and J.P. Schneider. 2005. Light-activated hydrogel formation via the triggered folding and self-assembly of a designed peptide. J. Am. Chem. Soc. 127: 17025–17029.

Haines-Butterick, L., K. Rajagopal, M. Branco, D. Salick, R. Rughani, M. Pilarz et al. 2007. Controlling hydrogelation kinetics by peptide design for three-dimensional encapsulation and injectable delivery of cells. Proc. Natl. Acad. Sci. USA. 104: 7791–7796.

Hartgerink, J.D., E. Beniash and S.I. Stupp. 2001. Self-assembly and mineralization of peptide-amphiphile nanofibers. Science. 294: 1684–1688.

Hirst, A.R., S. Roy, M. Arora, A.K. Das, N. Hodson, P. Murray et al. 2010. Biocatalytic induction of supramolecular order. Nat. Chem. 2: 1089–1094.

Holmes, T.C., S. de Lacalle, X. Su, G. Liu, A. Rich and S. Zhang. 2000. Extensive neurite outgrowth and active synapse formation on self-assembling peptide scaffolds. Proc. Natl. Acad. Sci. USA. 97: 6728–6733.

Hutton, J.C. and G.S. Eisenbarth. 2003. A pancreatic beta-cell-specific homolog of glucose-6-phosphatase emerges as a major target of cell-mediated autoimmunity in diabetes. Proc. Natl. Acad. Sci. USA. 100: 8626–8628.

Jun, H.W., V. Yuwono, S.E. Paramonov and J.D. Hartgerink. 2005. Enzyme-mediated degradation of peptide-amphiphile nanofiber networks. Adv. Mater. 17: 2612–2617.

Jun, S., Y. Hong, H. Imamura, B.Y. Ha, J. Bechhoefer and P. Chen. 2004. Self-assembly of the ionic peptide EAK16: the effect of charge distributions on self-assembly. Biophys. J. 87: 1249–1259.

Kammerer, R.A. and M.O. Steinmetz. 2006. *De novo* design of a two-stranded coiled-coil switch peptide. J. Struct. Biol. 155: 146–153.

Kato, Y., S. Ozawa, C. Miyamoto, Y. Maehata, A. Suzuki, T. Maeda et al. 2013. Acidic extracellular microenvironment and cancer. Cancer. Cell. Int. 13: 89-2867-13-89.

Kim, B., K. La Flamme and N.A. Peppas. 2003. Dynamic swelling behavior of pH-sensitive anionic hydrogels used for protein delivery. J. Appl. Polym. Sci. 89: 1606–1613.

Kirkham, J., A. Firth, D. Vernals, N. Boden, C. Robinson, R.C. Shore et al. 2007. Self-assembling peptide scaffolds promote enamel remineralization. J. Dent. Res. 86, 5: 426–430.

Koetting, M.C., J.T. Peters, S.D. Steichen and N.A. Peppas. 2015. Stimulus-responsive hydrogels: theory, modern advances and applications. Mater. Sci. Eng. 93: 1–49.

Kretsinger, J.K., L.A. Haines, B. Ozbas, D.J. Pochan and J.P. Schneider. 2005. Cytocompatibility of self-assembled beta-hairpin peptide hydrogel surfaces. Biomaterials. 26: 5177–5186.

Kyle, S., A. Aggeli, E. Ingham and M.J. McPherson. 2009. Production of self-assembling biomaterials for tissue engineering. Trends Biotechnol. 27: 423–433.

Laverty, G., A.P. McCloskey, B.F. Gilmore, D.S. Jones, J. Zhou and B. Xu. 2014. Ultrashort cationic naphthalene-derived self-assembled peptides as antimicrobial nanomaterials. Biomacromolecules. 15: 3429–3439.

Lee, H.K., S. Soukasene, H. Jiang, S. Zhang, W. Feng and S.I. Stupp. 2008. Light-induced self-assembly of nanofibers inside liposomes. Soft Matter. 4: 962–964.

Li, Y., C.T. Poon, M. Li, T.J. Lu, B.P. Murphy and F. Xu. 2015. Chinese-noodle-inspired muscle myofiber fabrication. Adv. Funct. Mater. 25: 5999–60008.

McCloskey, A.P., B.F. Gilmore and G. Laverty. 2014. Evolution of antimicrobial peptides to self-assembled peptides for biomaterial applications. Pathogens. 3: 791–821.

Megeed, Z., M. Haider, D. Li, B.W. O'Malley Jr, J. Cappello and H. Ghandehari. 2004. *In vitro* and *in vivo* evaluation of recombinant silk-elastin like hydrogels for cancer gene therapy. J. Controlled Release. 94: 433–445.

Murdan, S. 2003. Electro-responsive drug delivery from hydrogels. J. Control. Release. 92: 1–17.

Nagarsekar, A., J. Crissman, M. Crissman, F. Ferrari, J. Cappello and H. Ghandehari. 2003. Genetic engineering of stimuli-sensitive silk elastin-like protein block copolymers. Biomacromolecules. 4: 602–607.

Ninawe, P.R. and S.J. Parulekar. 2011. Drug loading into and drug release from pH- and temperature-responsive cylindrical hydrogels. Biotechnol. Prog. 27: 1442–1454.

Osada, Y., H. Okuzaki and H. Hori. 1992. A polymer gel with electrically driven motility. Nature. 355: 242–244.

Ozbas, B., J. Kretsinger, K. Rajagopal, J.P. Schneider and D.J. Pochan. 2004. Salt-triggered peptide folding and consequent self-assembly into hydrogels with tunable modulus. Macromolecules. 37: 7331–7337.

Philip, A.K. and B. Philip. 2010. Colon targeted drug delivery systems: a review on primary and novel approaches. Oman Med. J. 25: 79–87.

Pochan, D.J., J.P. Schneider, J. Kretsinger, B. Ozbas, K. Rajagopal and L. Haines. 2003. Thermally reversible hydrogels via intramolecular folding and consequent self-assembly of a *de novo* designed peptide. J. Am. Chem. Soc. 125: 11802–11803.

Radovic-Moreno, A.F., T.K. Lu, V.A. Puscasu, C.J. Yoon, R. Langer and O.C. Farokhzad. 2012. Surface charge-switching polymeric nanoparticles for bacterial cell wall-targeted delivery of antibiotics. ACS Nano. 6: 4279–4287.

Rasale, D.B. and A.K. Das. 2015. Chemical reactions directed peptide self-assembly. Int. J. Mol. Sci. 16: 10797–10820.

Rughani, R.V., D.A. Salick, M.S. Lamm, T. Yucel, D.J. Pochan and J.P. Schneider. 2009. Folding, self-assembly, and bulk material properties of a *de novo* designed three-stranded beta-sheet hydrogel. Biomacromolecules. 10: 1295–1304.

Saha, S., A. Bardelli, P. Buckhaults, V.E. Velculescu, C. Rago, B. St Croix et al. 2001. A phosphatase associated with metastasis of colorectal cancer. Science. 294: 1343–1346.

Sato, A.K., M. Viswanathan, R.B. Kent and C.R. Wood. 2006. Therapeutic peptides: technological advances driving peptides into development. Curr. Opin. Biotechnol. 17: 638–642.

Schmaljohann, D. 2006. Thermo- and pH-responsive polymers in drug delivery. Adv. Drug Deliv. Rev. 58: 1655–1670.

Schneider, J.P., D.J. Pochan, B. Ozbas, K. Rajagopal, L. Pakstis and J. Kretsinger. 2002. Responsive hydrogels from the intramolecular folding and self-assembly of a designed peptide. J. Am. Chem. Soc. 124: 15030–15037.

Shao, H. and J.R. Parquette. 2010. A pi-conjugated hydrogel based on an Fmoc-dipeptide naphthalene diimide semiconductor. Chem. Commun. 46: 4285–4287.

Stickler, D.J., S.M. Jones, G.O. Adusei and M.G. Waters. 2006. A sensor to detect the early stages in the development of crystalline *Proteus mirabilis* biofilm on indwelling bladder catheters. J. Clin. Microbiol. 44: 1540–1542.

Toledano, S., R.J. Williams, V. Jayawarna and R.V. Ulijn. 2006. Enzyme-triggered self-assembly of peptide hydrogels via reversed hydrolysis. J. Am. Chem. Soc. 128: 1070–1071.

Tysseling-Mattiace, V.M., V. Sahni, K.L. Niece, D. Birch, C. Czeisler, M.G. Fehlings et al. 2008. Self-assembling nanofibers inhibit glial scar formation and promote axon elongation after spinal cord injury. J. Neurosci. 28: 3814–3823.

Valery, C., M. Paternostre, B. Robert, T. Gulik-Krzywicki, T. Narayanan, J.C. Dedieu et al. 2003. Biomimetic organization: octapeptide self-assembly into nanotubes of viral capsid-like dimension. Proc. Natl. Acad. Sci. USA. 100: 10258–10262.

Williams, R.J., A.M. Smith, R. Collins, N. Hodson, A.K. Das and R.V. Ulijn. 2009. Enzyme-assisted self-assembly under thermodynamic control. Nat. Nanotechnol. 4: 19–24.

Xu, D., D. Asai, A. Chilkoti and S.L. Craig. 2012. Rheological properties of cysteine-containing elastin-like polypeptide solutions and hydrogels. Biomacromolecules. 13: 2315–2321.

Yang, Z., G. Liang, L. Wang and B. Xu. 2006. Using a kinase/phosphatase switch to regulate a supramolecular hydrogel and forming the supramolecular hydrogel *in vivo*. J. Am. Chem. Soc. 128: 3038–3043.

Yang, Z., K. Xu, Z. Guo, Z. Guo and B. Xu. 2007. Intracellular enzymatic formation of nanofibers results in hydrogelation and regulated cell death. Adv. Mater. 19: 3152–3156.

Yang, Z.M., H.W. Gu, D.G. Fu, P. Gao, J.K. Lam and B. Xu. 2004. Enzymatic formation of supramolecular hydrogels. Adv. Mater. 16: 1440–1444.

Yuan, J. and B.A. Yankner. 2000. Apoptosis in the nervous system. Nature. 407: 802–809.

CHAPTER 17

Bioengineering Complexity and Tuneability in Hydrogels

Alvaro Mata,[1,*] *Helena S. Azevedo,*[1,a] *John Connelly*[2] and *Julien Gautrot*[1,b]

Introduction

Hydrogels are water swollen polymeric chains that are cross-linked through different chemical or physical mechanisms (Utech and Boccaccini 2016). Given the hydrated nature and potential for physical and chemical tuneability, these materials have been explored and applied for applications in medicine since the 1960s (Buwalda et al. 2014). While initial work was mainly focused on developing bioinert structures and improving stability for drug delivery applications (Lee et al. 2013), our growing capacity to engineer at the molecular level has resulted in an increasingly diverse and powerful tool-kit to synthesize hydrogels with unprecedented chemical and physical properties (Peppas et al. 2006).

Hydrogels are being developed with a diverse set of properties including the capacity to be easily synthesized and modulated (Alakpa et al. 2016), elicit specific biological responses (Mata et al. 2010); display chemical and physical anisotropy (Mendes et al. 2013b); and adapt, change, and respond to different stimuli (Mortisen et al. 2010). These materials are opening opportunities to recreate *in vivo* environments *in vitro* to study for example biological processes or more effectively test drugs and to more

[1] School of Engineering and Materials Science, Institute of Bioengineering, Queen Mary University of London, Mile End Road, London, E1 4NS.
[a] E-mail: h.azevedo@qmul.ac.uk
[b] E-mail: j.gautrot@qmul.ac.uk
[2] Centre for Cell Biology and Cutaneous Research, Institute of Bioengineering, Queen Mary University of London, 4 Newark Street, London, E1 2AT.
   E-mail: j.connelly@qmul.ac.uk
* Corresponding author: a.mata@qmul.ac.uk

efficiently deliver drugs, cells, or therapeutic agents as well as guide tissue repair or regeneration *in vivo*.

This chapter presents strategies used to molecularly engineer hydrogel materials and enhance their complexity and functionality. We first present opportunities to create hydrogels through either thiol-ene radical coupling or peptide self-assembly and then describe ways to tune them to exhibit bioactivity with both spatial and temporal control.

Thiol-ene Hydrogels

In addition to the requirements for good cytocompatibility, defined and reproducible composition, controlled cell adhesion and mechanical properties and degradability, 3D hydrogels should be easy to engineer and design (e.g., allowing the independant control of mechanical properties and cell adhesion) (Tibbitt et al. 2013; Anseth et al. 2002), be compatible with a range of patterning, printing and cell encapsulation technologies to allow their micro-structuring (Lowe et al. 2014) and should rely on very specific coupling chemistry for the precise control of molecular structure (Porel and Alabi 2014). Several "click" chemistry approaches have been proposed to achieve such goals (Beria et al. 2014; Jiang et al. 2014; Campos et al. 2008), but thiol-ene radical coupling displays important features that are particularly well suited for the design of biomaterials for tissue engineering and regenerative medicine: it does not require metal catalysts, it is fast and relatively insensitive to oxygen, it can be controlled by light (to avoid overheating the cell microenvironment during curing and for patterning and microfabrication) and it is based on relatively simple abundant functionalities (alkene and thiol moieties) yet is very chemoselective.

Thiol-ene radical coupling and structural design

Thiol-ene radical reactions occur between a thiol moiety and an alkene (or alkyne (Fairbanks et al. 2010)) in two stages (Fig. 1a) (Hoyle and Bowman 2010; Hoyle et al. 2004). Unlike Michael additions of thiols requiring the activation of alkenes, thiol-ene radical reactions occur at unactivated alkenes (Cramer and Bowman 2001). This confers to the reaction an improved chemoselectivity as other nucleophiles (i.e., primary amines) cannot react. This is attractive for the coupling of peptides or proteins to hydrogels and other biomaterials as the low abundance of cysteines in most proteins ensures the control of the reaction site without protection of other amino acids. The typical absence of alkene residues in proteins and many biomacromolecules also ensures very little cross-reactivity with other components of the system studied (during the formation of hydrogels in the presence of cells for example).

The parameters affecting the coupling efficiency and its kinetics have been studied, in particular for hydrophobic monomers. The chemical structure of the alkene was found to determine the rates of propagation (thiyl radical reacting with an alkene) and chain transfer (hydrogen abstraction to another thiol molecule) (Cramer et al. 2003b). Infrared spectroscopy allowed the quantification of the rates of reaction of different alkenes (Cramer et al. 2003a; Cramer and Bowman 2001). It was found that terminal

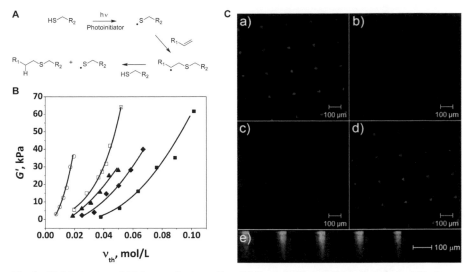

Fig. 1. (A) Mechanism of thiol-ene radical coupling. (B) Control of the mechanical properties (G', storage modulus) of poly(acrylamide) gels (open symbols) and thiol-ene gels (filled symbols) as a function of network density (vth) and molecular weight (Grube and Oppermann 2013). (C) Thiol-ene patterned hydrogels using three subsequent patterning steps and distinct tagged peptides (Gramlich et al. 2013).

monosubstituted alkenes react faster than those bisubstituted or than internal alkenes, suggesting that steric hindrance plays an important role in determining reaction kinetics (Roper et al. 2004). In the case of cyclic alkene molecules (e.g., norbornene), strain energy significantly increase reaction rates. Finally, increased electron density close to the alkene moiety speeds the rate of propagation (Cramer et al. 2003b). Hence the following coupling rates were proposed for different alkenes: norbornene > vinyl ether > vinyl silazane > acrylate > ally ether. These results are in agreement with computational models highlighting the importance of the stability of the carbon radicals formed (Northrop and Coffey 2012).

The initiation and termination stages are other important steps in thiol-ene coupling and play important roles for the design of thiol-ene based hydrogels. Several types of initiators have been proposed: scission-based initiators, activated by light or thermally, and hydrogen abstraction initiators. Photo-activated scission initiators such as 2,2-dimethoxy-2-phenyl acetophenone perform better in thiol-ene systems (Uygun et al. 2010; Campos et al. 2008). However, the hydrophobicity of this molecule does not allow its use for hydrogel formation and the hydrophilic and relatively cytocompatible 2-Hydroxy-4′-(2-hydroxyethoxy)-2-methylpropiophenone is usually preferred (Costa et al. 2014). Similarly, the photoactivated co-initiating system formed of Eosin Y and triethanolamine allowed the fast formation of hydrogels (Fu et al. 2015; Boyer and Xu 2015). Termination steps via bimolecular radical recombinations have important implications for the use of thiol-ene reactions for macromolecular design (Reddy et al. 2006; Koo et al. 2010). However, it should be noted that these effects were only important for large end-functionalised macromolecules and are not reported for smaller molecules. Oxygen is also expected to contribute to terminations, depending on the respective rates of propagation and chain transfer, although this has not been systematically quantified.

Hydrogel formation and control of mechanical properties

Considering the mild conditions required for thiol-ene coupling and the chemoselectivity of this reaction, it is not surprising to find that it has been used for bioconjugation to polymers and surfaces (Dondoni 2008; Bacinello et al. 2014; Jonkheijm et al. 2008). In addition, thiol-ene coupling displays important features for the design of biofunctional hydrogels as it allows the generation and control of polymer networks and their decoration with bioactive moieties. Initial work in this field has focused on the development of mixed acrylate/thiol systems. The incorporation of cysteine-terminated peptides at different ratios in a poly(ethylene glycol) (PEG) diacrylate matrix afforded biofunctionalised gels with high conversions and peptide incorporation (>94%) (Salinas and Anseth 2008). The presence of mono-thiols decreased conversion rates, as expected from the presence of mono-functional building blocks, and a retardation effect was observed with tryptophan residues. To confer degradability, a PEG-poly(lactide) diacrylate was used instead of simple PEG-diacrylates and comparison was made between pure chain-growth gelation and mixed chain growth/thiol-ene polymerizations (Rydholm et al. 2005). The addition of multi-functional thiols increased the rate of conversion and that of hydrolytic degradation. Similar systems were developed based on oligo(poly(ethylene glycol)fumarate) and PEG-dithiol (Brink et al. 2009) or on thiolated gelatin and PEG diacrylate (Fu et al. 2012), with similar conclusions on the evolution of hydrolytic degradability.

In the case of pure thiol-ene systems (e.g., with terminal alkenes or norbornene derivatives), several parameters were found to impact on the mechanical properties of the networks. Varying the concentration of polymer in the solution prior to crosslinking allowed the control of bulk rheological properties. The shear storage modulus (500–10,000 Pa) of dextran polymers modified with pentenoate side chains crosslinked with PEG dithiol was readily tuned by the concentration of starting polymers (Mergy et al. 2012). Similar observations were made for a PEG trithiol and PEG dialkene system (Fig. 1b) (Grube and Oppermann 2013). The molecular weight of the polymers used, their degree of substitution with crosslinkable moieties and hydrophilicity were also important parameters controlling mechanical properties. Poly(2-oxazolines) with longer chains but identical functionality ratios or with higher hydrophilicity displayed higher swelling (Dargaville et al. 2012). In addition, the ratio of thiol to alkene functions, and therefore the degree of crosslinking, were used to tailor mechanical properties. Hence, norbornene-terminated 8-arm PEG molecules were crosslinked with varying ratios of dithiol peptide crosslinker to afford gels with shear moduli in the range of 5–30 kPa for 20 kDa PEG monomer and 1–6 kPa for its 40 kDa counterpart (Gould et al. 2012).

The majority of thiol-ene gels has been generated using UV light curing and the use of the water soluble initiator 1-[4-(2-Hydroxyethoxy)-phenyl]-2-hydroxy-2-methyl-1-propane-1-one (known as Irgacure 2959). Although this initiator is well tolerated by cells, the exposure to UV light can result in cytotoxicity and is a source of genetic mutation. Hence, systems allowing the curing of hydrogels with visible light have been designed. Camphorquinone-10-sulfonic acid was used for the curing of PEG trithiol and PEG dialkene (Grube and Oppermann 2013) using blue light. Others have used green light to activate thiol-ene chemistry with Eosin Y and triethanolamine (Xu and Boyer 2015). Thiolated heparin was crosslinked with PEG diacrylate using Eosin Y and the modulus of the resulting gel was varied in the range of 0.3–11 kPa by changing the polymer concentration, the ratio of crosslinker and the functionality number of the PEG acrylate (Fu et al. 2015).

Biofunctionalization and micropatterning of thiol-ene hydrogels

The availability of cysteine residues in peptides and proteins allows their chemoselective oriented coupling to biomaterials via thiol-ene chemistry (Costa et al. 2014; Dondoni 2008). This concept has been applied for the biofunctionalization of hydrogels, making use of residual alkene moieties to couple peptides such as the cell adhesive RGD sequence. PEG-norbornene derived gels were functionalised with the CGRGDS, CGVGVAPG and CGGTPGPQGIAGQRGVV peptides mimicking the properties of fibronectin, elastin and collagen 1, respectively (Gould et al. 2012). This allowed the modulation of the expression of α-smooth muscle actin by valvular interstitial cells. Spotted microarrays of peptides and dyes were generated using thiol-ene coupling at the surface of hydrogels and could allow the development of high throughput microarrays for *in vitro* cell-based assays (Gupta et al. 2010). Similar strategies have been applied to dextran (Mergy et al. 2012) and hyaluronic acid (Khetan et al. 2009) hydrogels. Poly(2-oxazoline) hydrogels are also attractive platforms for *in vitro* cell culture and tissue engineering as they display similar cytocompatibility and bioinertness to PEG hydrogels and can be designed to display controllable alkene levels (Dargaville et al. 2014; Schenk et al. 2014). In particular, the antifouling properties of poly(2-methyl oxazoline) allowed the control of cell adhesion after functionalization with an RGD peptide. Cell adhesion was correlated with peptide density, confirming the specificity (integrin mediated) of this platform (Farrugia et al. 2015).

The ability to control thiol-ene chemistry by light also offers interesting opportunities for the patterning of hydrogels chemistry and mechanical properties. Burdick and co-workers micropatterned norbornene-functionalised hyaluronic acid with fluorescently tagged peptides (Gramlich et al. 2013). Peptide patterns were generated with high resolution (20 µm, Fig. 1c) and a good penetration depth (100–200 µm). A similar strategy was used to chemically pattern alkyne-azide hydrogels in 3D with tagged thiols and peptides (DeForest et al. 2009). Therefore thiol-ene chemistry, potentially in combination with other click chemistry approaches, offers attractive features for the control of hydrogel chemistry in 3D and the direction of cell behaviour and tissue formation. The ability to control the crosslinking density and mechanics of hydrogels with light was exploited to pattern the mechanical properties of hyaluronic acid-based hydrogels (Marklein and Burdick 2010; Khetan et al. 2013; Khetan et al. 2009) and control cell spreading in 2D and regulate stem cell phenotype in 3D.

Thiol-ene based hydrogels are attractive systems to control the chemical and mechanical properties of the cell microenvironment in 3D. These platforms are compatible with micropatterning and microfluidics technologies, which should contribute to their wider use in the biomedical field. Some important issues remain to be tackled however, as the precise understanding of the impact of the chemical structure on this coupling (especially in buffered conditions) have not been systematically explored. In addition, the use of visible light curing should be further studied to reduce cell toxicity and allow the use of these biomaterials for clinical applications. Such developments will enable the study of cell biology and tissue formation in 3D, with better control of important parameters such as the density of cell adhesion motifs, matrix mechanics, degradability and matrix remodelling.

Self-assembling Peptide Hydrogels

Hydrogels can be formed by the self-assembly of certain peptide molecules which are rationally designed to assemble into nanofibers under specific conditions. To trigger self-assembly, different stimuli and methods have been used, including pH (controlled pH adjustments), ionic strength (addition of counterions), temperature (heating or cooling), enzyme-catalyzed reactions (hydrolysis of self-assembling peptide precursors), and light (selective irradiation). At sufficiently high concentration, the entanglement of these nanofibers leads to gel formation (Fig. 2).

A number of building blocks have been explored for developing hydrogels by self-assembly, but peptides offer many important advantages. They can be designed to incorporate structural and bioactive domains and form discrete nanostructures that emulate not only the physical architecture but also the chemistry of the extracellular matrix (ECM). Researchers have been using self-assembling motifs—β-sheets (Freeman et al. 2015), α-helices and coiled-coils (Woolfson 2010)—found in structural proteins (amyloidogenic proteins, silk fibroin, collagen) to drive peptide self-assembly and short peptide sequences (RGDS, IKVAV, YIGSR, DGEA, GFOGER) derived from cell-adhesive proteins (fibronectin, laminin, collagen) to signal cells and guide regenerative processes. Due their small size, they can be easily obtained through

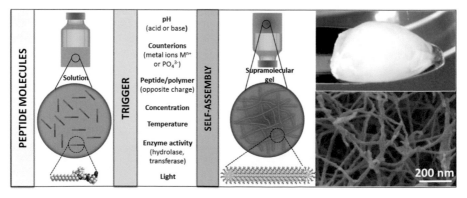

Fig. 2. Peptide self-assembly and the formation of a supramolecular gel. Peptide molecules are initially in solution and when a trigger is applied they are able to associate with each other and assemble into ordered nanofibers that entangle to form a 3D nanofiber network.

automated solid-phase synthesis methods and purified by standard reverse phase high performance liquid chromatography.

Preparing hydrogels by peptide self-assembly requires reliable design rules and excellent reviews have been published describing the chemistry and designs of various self-assembling peptides (Mendes et al. 2013a; Maude et al. 2013; Rubert Perez et al. 2015; Boekhoven and Stupp 2014; Fichman and Gazit 2014). Some self-assembling peptide gels have made the transition to *in vivo* studies, notably the ionic self-complementary peptides (KLD12, RADA16—PuraMatrix™) proposed by Zhang and co-workers at MIT (Gelain et al. 2007) and peptide amphiphiles (PAs) designed by the Stupp group at Northwestern University (Cui et al. 2010). Here, we focus on their application in regenerative medicine.

Neural regeneration

Self-assembling peptide gels are promising for central nervous system (CNS) regeneration as they can be easily injected into the injury site and functionalized to support regrowth of the nervous tissue (Liu et al. 2015b). A PA gel containing the IKVAV epitope (derived from laminin responsible for neurite growth) was used to encapsulate neural progenitor cells (Silva et al. 2004) and shown to induce their differentiation into neurons, while discouraging the development of astrocytes comparatively to laminin. A similar PA molecule containing the IKVAV epitope was tested *in vivo* in a mouse model of spinal cord injury (SCI) (Tysseling-Mattiace et al. 2008). The peptide solution was injected directly at the injury site and the PA treatment reduced astrogliosis and cell death, while increasing the number of oligodendroglia. Regeneration of injured motor and sensory axons was also promoted, while axons were unable to traverse the lesion in injured spinal cords treated with peptide gel without the IKVAV sequence. The injection of IKVAV PA on the animal functional recovery was also investigated using two SCI models (compression and contusion) and two different species (mice and rats) (Tysseling et al. 2010). This PA improved behavioural outcome by stimulating axon regeneration through the lesion. The same PA gel was applied, in combination with embryonic stem cells and neurotrophic factors, as replacement therapy for lesions of the auditory nerve (Palmgren et al. 2012). By promoting the localization and controlled release of neurotrophic factors, the PA gel increased cell survival and neuronal differentiation. Aligned monodomain PA gels containing IKVAV and RGDS epitopes enhanced the growth of neurites from neurons encapsulated in the gel with neurite aligned along the direction of the nanofibers (Berns et al. 2014). After two weeks of culture in the monodomain PA gels, neurons displayed spontaneous electrical activity and established synaptic connections. PA gels, encapsulating neural progenitor cells, were formed *in situ* within the spinal cord and resulted in the growth of oriented processes *in vivo* and extensive migration of dorsal root ganglion cells inside the gel with the direction of their movement guided by the nanofiber orientation.

RADA16 peptide gels have also performed successfully in neurorepair strategies (Holmes et al. 2000). They were able to support neuronal cell attachment, differentiation and extensive neurite outgrowth, being permissive substrates for functional synapse formation between the attached neurons. Neural stem cells (NSCs), encapsulated into RADA16-I gels functionalized with different functional motifs (SKPPGTSS, PFSSTKT and RGDS), and cultured in serum-free medium were able to differentiate into progenitor neural cells, neurons, astrocytes and oligodendrocytes (Koutsopoulos and Zhang 2013). The brain repair ability of these gels was also demonstrated using a severed optic tract in a hamster model. Injection of peptide solution at the lesion site created a permissive environment for regenerated axons to reconnect to target tissues with sufficient density to promote functional recovery, as demonstrated by the return of lost vision (Ellis-Behnke et al. 2006). Reconstruction of acutely injured brain with these peptide gels was also observed (Guo et al. 2009). RADA16-I peptide gel was also used for transplantation of neural progenitor cells and Schwann cells into the transected dorsal column of spinal cord of rats (Guo et al. 2007). The gel was shown to promote survival, migration and differentiation of both cells, as well as migration of host cells, and growth of blood vessels and axons into the gels.

Other functional motifs, such as the bone marrow homing peptide 1 (BMHP1) motif (PFSSTKT) obtained by phage display, were also used to functionalize RADA16 and KLD12 peptides (Caprini et al. 2013; Gelain et al. 2006; Gelain et al. 2012), or to derive new self-assembling peptides (Cigognini et al. 2014; Gelain et al. 2011), for culturing and controlling NSC behavior for nervous tissue regeneration. Promising results were obtained in terms of *in vitro* NSC differentiation and *in vivo* nervous tissue regrowth.

Bone regeneration

The application of PAs for bone regeneration has been reviewed elsewhere (Matson et al. 2011) and some of the functional motifs incorporated in the PA design include peptide sequences containing the phosphoserine (S(P)) residue to induce hydroxyapatite mineralization and the RGD for cell adhesion (Hartgerink et al. 2001). A nanofiber gel combining these signalling epitopes was tested in a rat femoral critical size defect and significant bone formation was observed (Mata et al. 2010). To induce osteoblast differentiation and stimulate bone formation, PAs were functionalized at the N-terminal with a phage-derived peptide (TSPHVPY) that binds to bone morphogenetic protein 2 (BMP-2) (Lee et al. 2015a). *In vivo* studies, using the BMP-2-binding nanofibres in a translational model of bone regeneration (rat posterolateral lumbar intertransverse spinal fusion model), showed that this system allowed a 10-fold reduction in the BMP-2 dose to achieve 100% fusion rate. The observed efficacy was explained by the ability of the BMP-2-binding peptide nanofibres to both capture exogenously delivered or endogenously expressed BMP-2.

RADA16 peptide-based gels have also been demonstrated to be valuable in enhancing bone regeneration (Semino 2008; Misawa et al. 2006; Horii et al. 2007). When functionalized with RGDS and DGEA sequences, human mesenchymal stem cells (MSCs) cultured on these gels showed osteogenic differentiation with and without the addition of osteogenic media (Anderson et al. 2011). RADA peptides containing BMP receptor-binding peptides (Hosseinkhani et al. 2007; Lee et al. 2009) were also explored due to its osteoinductive potential to be applied in bone repair therapies.

Cartilage regeneration

Adult articular cartilage has limited capacity of regeneration. Transforming growth factor β1 (TGF-β1) is known to regulate the formation of connective tissues and the Stupp group has designed self-assembled peptide nanofibers containing a phage-derived peptide sequence (HSNGLPL) with binding affinity to TGF-β1 (Shah et al. 2010). When implanted in a full thickness chondral defect in a rabbit model, these gels were shown to promote the regeneration of articular cartilage with or even without the addition of exogenous TGF-β1, as detected by formation of hyaline-like tissue within the defect space. The KLD-12 peptide hydrogel was used for encapsulating chondrocytes (Kisiday et al. 2002) and showed to support cell survival and to retain the chondrocytic phenotype with increased production of cartilage ECM components (glycosaminoglycans, type II collagen). Bone marrow stromal cells (BMSCs) were encapsulated within KLD-12 and RAD16-I peptide hydrogels (Kopesky et al. 2010). Chondrogenesis was shown to be superior when compared with agarose hydrogels, as shown by cartilage-specific ECM production. The effect of KLD-12 peptide hydrogel, with or without chondrogenic factors and allogenic BMSCs, on osteochondral repair was tested *in vivo* in a critically-sized rabbit cartilage defect model (Miller et al. 2010) and KLD-12 hydrogel alone could fill full-thickness osteochondral defects and improve cartilage repair.

Collagen-mimetic peptides ((GPO)$_5$) were conjugated to the C-terminal of KLD-12 peptide and the chondrogenic differentiation of BMSCs investigated *in vitro* (Kim et al. 2015). These gels promoted the expression of chondrogenic marker genes (collagen type II, aggrecan). In a different study, KLD-12 was coupled to a neuropeptide (RPKPQQFFGLM) and the gel injected in osteoarthritis (OA) rat knee model. After 6 weeks, the gel accelerated cartilage regeneration through recruitment of MSCs (Kim et al. 2016), demonstrating the potential of this conjugated hydrogel to delay the progression of OA and restore articular joint function without cell transplantation.

The chondrogenic differentiation of human adipose-derived stem cells (ADSCs) was investigated *in vitro* by 3D culture in RAD16-I gels combined with heparin (Fernández-Muiños et al. 2015). This bicomponent gel enhanced the chondrogenic commitment of ADSCs, as detected by the expression of cartilage specific markers.

Vascular regeneration

There is a need of cell-based therapies for ischemic tissue repair in cardiovascular diseases, as result of limited regeneration of cardiomyocytes. To overcome this limitation, a biocompatible matrix is normally required to support cell functions during the transplantation, once the direct cell transplantation (embryonic stem or endothelial progenitor cells) results in low cellular viability and minimal retention (Webber et al. 2010b). A gel made of PA nanofibers containing the RGDS sequence was used to encapsulate bone marrow-derived stem and progenitor cells *in vivo* (Webber et al. 2010b). Enhanced viability, proliferation and adhesion of encapsulated cells suggested the potential of these gels to be applied in cell therapies for ischemic diseases. In a subsequent study, incubation of bone marrow-derived pro-angiogenic cells (BMPACs) with these PA nanofibers *in vitro* enhanced cell adhesion and proliferation, while attenuating apoptosis (Tongers et al. 2014). In a murine model of hind limb ischemia, an intramuscular injection of BMPACs within the RGDS containing PA gel, resulted in greater retention of cells, enhanced capillary density, increased limb perfusion and reduced necrosis/amputation, when compared to treatment with cells alone. PA gels with binding ability to heparin were observed to have binding ability for paracrine factors from hypoxic conditioned stem cell media (Webber et al. 2010a). When injected in coronary artery ligation, the preservation of hemodynamic function in a mouse ischemia (reperfusion model of acute myocardial infarction) was observed and revascularization in chronic rat ischemic hind limb models was stimulated.

RADA16 gels have also shown to support the survival of encapsulated endothelial and myocardial cells (Narmoneva et al. 2004) and the potential to create a 3D micro-environment when injected in myocardium by recruiting both endogenous endothelial and smooth muscle cells with stimulation of vascularization (Davis et al. 2005). When injected into the heart tissue after myocardial infarction, RADA16-I nanofiber gel containing vascular endothelial growth factor was shown to create a microenvironment for arteriogenesis and cardiac repair (Lin et al. 2012).

Hydrogel Functionalization

Many types of natural and synthetic hydrogels possess inherently low bioactivity, which is advantageous for avoiding immunogenic responses and improving biocompatibility. However, this lack of bioactivity limits the ability to control or direct cell behaviour for tissue engineering and regenerative medicine applications. Biofunctionalization is therefore an important top-down strategy for creating instructive hydrogels capable of eliciting specific cellular responses.

To date, a range of different materials have been modified with small molecules, peptides, and polysaccharides, as well as larger recombinant proteins. Examples of hydrogel materials amenable to bio-functionalization include synthetic polymers such as poly(ethylene glycol) (PEG) (Hern and Hubbell 1998; Shin et al. 2002; DeForest et al. 2009; Phelps et al. 2012), poly(hydroxyethylene methacrylate) (Bi et al. 2004; Jacob et al. 2005), and polyvinyl alcohol (Schmedlen et al. 2002). PEG-based hydrogels have been extensively studied due to their excellent anti-fouling properties and ease of modification (Hern and Hubbell 1998; Mann et al. 2001; Lee et al. 2008). A number of natural hydrogels, such as alginate (Rowley et al. 1999), chitosan (Ho et al. 2005), and hyaluronic acid (Shu et al. 2004; Gramlich et al. 2013) can also functionalised using similar strategies. Short synthetic peptides are one of the most common molecules used to improve bioactivity of hydrogels as they are stable and easily synthesized with sequence specificity. Peptides containing the fibronectin-mimetic arginine-glycine-aspartic (RGD) motif have been frequently used to create cell adhesive hydrogels and improve cell viability (Hern and Hubbell 1998; Shin et al. 2002; Mann et al. 2001; Rowley et al. 1999). Other peptides used to modify cell function within hydrogel materials include collagen mimetic sequences (Lee et al. 2008; Reyes and García 2003; Connelly et al. 2011), laminin-mimetic sequences (Bellamkonda et al. 1995; Yu and Shoichet 2005; Chung et al. 2008), and matrix metalo-proteinase (MMP) degradable sequences (Phelps et al. 2012; Mann et al. 2001; Gilbert et al. 2010). Finally, modification of hydrogels with small molecules can be used to modulate gel chemistry and cell fate (Benoit et al. 2008; Frith et al. 2014; Zhu et al. 2015), while other studies have even functionalised hydrogels with larger proteins such as growth factors (Fan et al. 2007; Mehta et al. 2010) and recombinant extracellular matrix (ECM) proteins (Connelly et al. 2011; Martino et al. 2011; Martino et al. 2013).

The specific cross-linking strategies employed for bio-functionalization depends both on the chemistry of the material and the biomolecule itself. These reactions require good specificity, efficiency and stability in order to link a sufficient number of molecules to the right location on the hydrogel polymer and for the linkage to remain intact under physiologic conditions. Common reactive groups on the polymer include hydroxyl (Trmcic-Cvitas et al. 2009; Petrie et al. 2006; Costa et al. 2014), carboxyl (Rowley et al. 1999), and acrylate groups (Shin et al. 2002; Mann et al. 2001; Lee et al. 2008), while peptides are often accessed through primary amines or thiols (DeForest et al. 2009; Mann et al. 2001; Rowley et al. 1999; Lutolf et al. 2003). The carboiimide EDC (1-ethyl-3-(3-dimethylaminopropyl) carbodiimide hydrochloride) reacts with carboxyl groups under aqueous conditions, and when combined with amine-reactive sulfo-N-hydroxysuccinimide (sulfo-NHS) (Hermanson 2008), it can be used to couple peptides to carboxyl-containing hydrogels (e.g., sodium alginate (Rowley et al. 1999)). Similarly, the compounds 4-nitrophenyl chloroformate (NPC) and N,N-disuccinimidyl carbonate (DSC) react with hydroxyl groups and can be used to couple primary amines of peptides to polymers (Hermanson 2008). Another key bio-functionalization reaction is the Michael-type addition of thiol groups in cysteinc-containing peptides to methyacrylate groups in PEG-based polymers (Heggli et al. 2003). Likewise, derivatization of hydrogel materials with maleimide groups supports highly efficient coupling with thiols (Phelps et al. 2012; Hermanson 2008). These reactions, although not an extensive list, are some of the most common strategies for bio-functionalization and highlight the diversity of chemistries available for tuning hydrogel bioactivity.

Efficiency and specificity are key considerations when selecting a functionalization strategy, and recent developments in 'click-chemistry' reactions have made significant advances in this area. 'Click chemistry' refers to a class of reactions characterised by high selectivity, minimal by-products, and high efficiency under mild reaction conditions (e.g., physiological temperature and pressure). They include the azide-alkyne cycloaddition (Rostovtsev et al. 2002), as well as the copper-free variation (Baskin et al. 2007; Agard et al. 2004), which uses strained alkynes to avoid the need for toxic copper catalysts. In addition, radical-mediated thiol-ene reactions between free thiol groups and unstatured carbon-carbon bonds are also considered click chemistry type reactions and have been to functionalise a range of different biomaterials (DeForest et al. 2009; Costa et al. 2014; Hensarling et al. 2009). Recent work using norbornene reactive groups to covalently bind thiols and tetrazines have also shown great promise for dual hydrogel cross-linking and functionalization (Gramlich et al. 2013). Thus, there is currently a wide range of strategies for functionalization of hydrogels with biomolecules, and this toolbox provides great flexibility for engineering bio-active hydrogels.

The ultimate goal for bio-functionalization is to specifically control cellular responses to the hydrogel. For example, the presentation of cell adhesive ligands, such as the RGD motif, is particularly important for cell viability within hydrogels designed for tissue engineering (Hern and Hubbell 1998; Burdick and Anseth 2002; Nuttelman et al. 2005; Salinas and Anseth 2008). Adhesion to the RGD motif also facilitates cell migration and vasculogenesis (DeForest et al. 2009; Phelps et al. 2012; Mann et al. 2001; Zisch et al. 2003; Lee et al. 2015b) and enhances osteogenic differentiation of mesenchymal stem cells (MSC) in 3D hydrogels (Shin et al. 2002; Burdick and Anseth 2002; Yang et al. 2005; Alsberg et al. 2001). The addition of collagen-mimetic peptides and recombinant fragments of fibronectin have similarly been used to stimulate osteogenesis (Lee et al. 2008; Reyes and García 2003; Connelly et al. 2011; Petrie et al. 2008). In addition to adhesive peptides and proteins, bio-functionalization can be used to regulate ECM deposition and new tissue formation. For example, functionalization of PEG hydrogels with chondroitin sulphate promotes MSC chondrogenesis and deposition of a cartilaginous ECM (Varghese et al. 2008), while cross-linking of synthetic polymers with MMP-degradable peptides facilitates matrix remodelling (Lutolf et al. 2003; Mann et al. 2001). Finally, covalent binding of growth factors or growth factor binding proteins is a powerful approach to regulating cell fate and function within engineered constructs (Martino et al. 2011; Martino et al. 2013; Watarai et al. 2015). Tethering of epidermal growth factor (EGF) to synthetic scaffolds improves cell survival and is actually more effective than saturating concentrations of EGF in solution (Fan et al. 2007; Mehta et al. 2010; Platt et al. 2009). Moreover, the incorporation of growth-factor binding domains derived from fibrinogen allows multiple growth factors to be simultaneously activated and significantly improves wound repair (Martino et al. 2011; Martino et al. 2013). Together, these studies demonstrate how bio-functionalization of hydrogels can be used to direct cell fate and function and improve their use in regenerative medicine applications.

Bioengineering Functionality with Spatial Control

As described above, hydrogels can be synthesized through different molecular mechanisms and tuned to exhibit specific bioactive properties. However, the successful application of these materials in medical applications requires significant control of both physical and chemical properties in both space and time (Tibbitt et al. 2015; Webber et al. 2016). For example, the ECM plays a crucial role in our body regulating cell adhesion, migration, and differentiation; cell-cell communication, mechanostransduction; tissue development, regeneration, and degeneration; and in general our body's functionality and homoeostasis. This ECM can be thought of as a hydrated matrix material capable of optimizing molecular presentation and providing structural hierarchy, chemical anisotropy, selectivity, and adaptability. Therefore, hydrogels for biomedical applications that are designed to replace, recreate, interact with, or stimulate elements of the ECM, would require a high level of tuneability of their properties, including the ability to exhibit specific signalling capabilities hierarchically and with spatial control.

Anisotropic hydrogels

Most human tissues, like skeletal muscle or liver lobules, as well as evolving biological environments present an anisotropic organization with distinctive chemical (i.e., chemotactic gradients of soluble and insoluble proteins) and/or physical (i.e., aligned fibres or stiffness gradients) environments during processes such as embryogenesis and wound healing (Perez-Castillejos 2010). Hydrogels are being designed to recreate such environments.

Strategies to create topographical anisotropy

Given the importance of surfaces in most biomaterials, a relatively simple way to provide physical anisotropy to hydrogels is through surface topographies (Verhulsel et al. 2014). Topographical patterns can be easily fabricated with a high level of precision thanks to techniques derived from microlithography (Whitesides 2005) including nanoimprint lithography, electron beam lithography, focused ion beam lithography (Smith et al. 2011). Of all, however, the most important and influential technique that has been exploited to create surface patterns is soft lithography due to its simplicity, accessibility, and versatility (Xia and Whitesides 1998). This method has been extensively exploited to create surface topographies on a large variety of hydrogel materials and subsequently provide an additional level of functionalization.

Chitosan substrates (Fukuda et al. 2006b), hyaluronic acid materials (Fukuda et al. 2006a), or elastin-like polymer membranes (Tejeda-Montes et al. 2012; Tejeda-Montes et al. 2014) have been topographically patterned using soft lithographic techniques to guide cell behaviour in different ways through physical hydrogel surface anisotropy. Other methods have been developed for example taking advantage of the surface folds that form during shrinkage of PHEMA-based hydrogels, which were shown to promote osteoblastic differentiation (Guvendiren and Burdick 2010) or photopatterning dynamic PEG-based hydrogels capable of modifying surface topographies in real time and studying how cells respond to these changes (Kirschner and Anseth 2013). The combination of lithographic techniques, such as e-beam lithography and soft lithography, have been used to create surface topographies down to nanometer scales (Mata et al. 2009). However, hydrogels made from self-assembling molecules offer the possibility to provide surface topographies at different scales by taking advantage of the bottom-up assembly of nanostructures. In this way, a higher level of bioactivity and functionalization may be achieved. For example, combining soft lithography with self-assembling peptides enables the fabrication of various surface microtopographies, which are made from well-defined and organized nanofibres. By modulating the assembly process, it is possible to create surface microtopographies made from aligned nanofibres. This process may be exploited to fabricate hydrogels with surface topographies while co-assembling different molecules such as self-assembling peptides and hyaluronic acid (Mendes et al. 2013b) (Fig. 3a).

Strategies to create structural anisotropy

In spite of the capabilities to surface pattern hydrogel materials, these materials are particularly attractive to provide synthetic ECM-like environments for cell encapsulation. Therefore, there is great potential in creating physical and chemical anisotropy within the 3D hydrogel material. Different hydrogels can exhibit a spectrum of porosity and nano/micro-architecture. Those made from entangled fibres

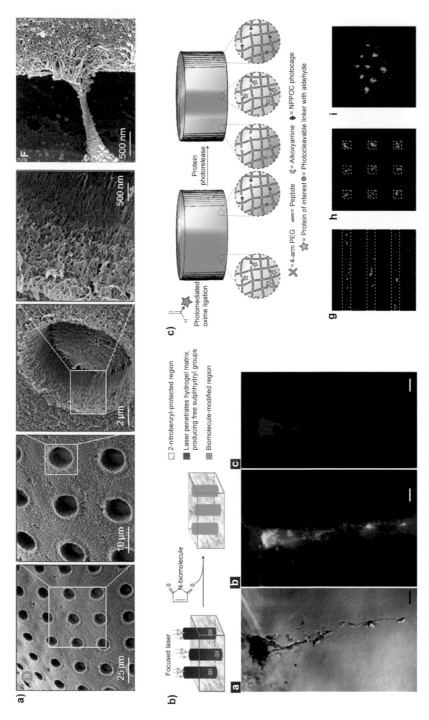

Fig. 3. a) Bioactive hierarchical surface topographies including well-defined nanofibres assembled into precise micro-topographies by integrating soft-lithography and molecular co-assembly between peptides and hyaluronic acid). b) Cell adhesive patterns guiding the growth of neurons within a hydrogel. c) Vitronectin patterns within PEG hydrogels by multiphoton laser scanning lithography.

are particularly well positioned to provide structural anisotropy. Electrospinning techniques have been used to create hydrogel materials with aligned fibres of various sizes and composition. For example, taking advantage of the process of electrospinning, hydrogels formed by aligned fibres have been used to align cells such as myoblasts (Wang et al. 2015) and endothelial cells (Eslami et al. 2014).

Another approach to create fibrous-hydrogels takes advantage of molecular self-assembly. Peptide-based hydrogels are particularly attractive given the possibility to control epitope presentation while creating well-defined nanostructures such as nanoscale fibres, tapes, and ribbons (Zhang 2003). However, controlling self-assembly hierarchically beyond the low nanoscale formation of one-dimensional structures and into the required 3D organization of hydrogels has been a difficult challenge (Smith et al. 2011). Stupp and colleagues have developed strategies based on the application of shear stresses (Mata et al. 2009) or evolving bilayer-to-nanofibre assemblies (Zhang et al. 2010), resulting in 3D hydrogels with domains of aligned nanofibres capable of guiding cell migration and growth. Molecular self-assembly has also been used to assemble nanostructures at higher scales including membranes made from nanofibres organized in precise microscale structures including layers (Inostroza-Brito et al. 2015; Ladet et al. 2008) or orthogonally assembled fibres (Capito et al. 2008; Zha et al. 2016). Other approaches to provide physical anisotropy have included the use of additional materials, for example in the form of particles, to the hydrogel to reinforce their mechanical properties (Liu et al. 2015a) and better control the final hydrogel structure (Studart 2015) and more sophisticated methods involving for example acoustic waves to create 3D patterns (Bouyer et al. 2016). Hydrogels exhibiting environments with distinct mechanical properties can also be created employing top-down techniques such as microfluidics (Orsi et al. 2014) or by creating composites including for example blends of chitosan, gelatine, hyaluronic acid, and ß-tricalcium phosphate capable of recreating articular cartilage (Walker and Madihally 2015) or silk and cardiac-derived ECM composites to be used for cardiac tissue engineering (Stoppel et al. 2015).

Strategies to create chemical anisotropy

In addition to creating structural anisotropy, the development of hydrogels with precise chemical anisotropy is a major goal. The groups of Molly Shoichet, Jennifer West, and Kristy Anseth have pioneered leading photo-patterning strategies capable of immobilizing signalling molecules within 3D hydrogels. For example, using a laser beam, cylindrical patterns of the peptide GRGDS have been generated within modified agarose hydrogels, creating one-dimensional cell-adhesive patterns capable of guiding neuronal growth (Fig. 3b) (Luo and Shoichet 2004). Similar patterns have been created using either a two-photon laser scanning to create RGDS patterns within polyethylene-glycol (PEG) hydrogels (Hoffmann and West 2013) or a multiphoton laser scanning lithography technique to immobilise vitronectin within PEG hydrogels (Fig. 3c) (DeForest and Tirrell 2015).

These approaches take advantage of the opportunities of using light as a patterning tool in order to maximize precision and develop 3D hydrogel environments with distinct and precise chemical patterns. However, in order to provide a more robust approach capable of enabling chemical anisotropy within a broader spectrum of hydrogel materials, electrical fields have been used as a patterning vehicle. This approach exploits the inherent charge and permanent dipole moment characteristics exhibited by many molecules in order to enable direct (DC) or alternating (AC) current to manipulate and localize them within the 3D hydrogel space. For example, Ahadian et al. used dielectrophoresis to create 50 μm-deep cylindrical patterns of aligned carbon nanotubes within a methacrylated gelatin hydrogel in order to create muscle myofibre structures (Ahadian et al. 2014) while Dai et al. used a modified electrophoresis-based device including a porous membrane to define and create 20 μm-deep patterns of nanoparticles within agarose hydrogels (Dai et al. 2012). These electric field-based techniques have been limited to using non-biological molecules and creating relatively shallow patterns.

Mata's group has recently developed a 3D-electrophoresis-assisted-lithography (3DEAL) platform that integrates fundamental principles from native polyacrylamide gel electrophoresis by using electric fields to manipulate proteins in their native state; affinity chromatography by immobilizing molecules within a hydrogel; and microfabrication by using a porous mask to define the printing regions. The 3DEAL technique is simple and affordable, and enables printing within multiple types of hydrogels and using multiple kinds of molecules, including native proteins. The main design element is the capacity to control the electric fields to allow the migration of water molecules, buffer ions, and printing molecules, while selectively preventing the movement of printing molecules. Functional patterns of parallel and perpendicular columns, curved lines, gradients of molecular composition, and patterns of various proteins ranging from tens of microns to centimeters in size and depth can be generated within a large number of hydrogels (Aleman et al. 2014).

References

Agard, N.J., J.A. Prescher and C.R. Bertozzi. 2004. A strain-promoted [3 + 2] azide-alkyne cycloaddition for covalent modification of biomolecules in living systems. J. Am. Chem. Soc. 126(46): 15046–7.

Ahadian, S., J. Ramon-Azcon, M. Estili, X.B. Liang, S. Ostrovidov, H. Shiku et al. 2014. Hybrid hydrogels containing vertically aligned carbon nanotubes with anisotropic electrical conductivity for muscle myofiber fabrication. Scientific Reports. 4.

Alakpa, E.V, V. Jayawarna, A. Lampel, K.V. Burgess, C.C. West, S.C.J. Bakker et al. 2016. Tunable supramolecular hydrogels for selection of lineage-guiding metabolites in stem cell cultures. Chem. 1(2): 298–319.

Aleman, J.P.A., E.E.L. Bernal, J.M.F. Pradas, A. Yaroshchuk, F. Albericio and A. Mata. 2014. 3D electrophoresis-assisted lithography (3DEAL) for patterning hydrogel environments. J. Tissue Eng. Regen. M. 8: 375–375.

Alsberg, E., K.W. Anderson, A. Albeiruti, R.T. Franceschi and D.J. Mooney. 2001. Cell-interactive alginate hydrogels for bone tissue engineering. J. Dent. Res. 80(11): 2025.

Anderson, J.M., J.B. Vines, J.L. Patterson, H. Chen, A. Javed and H.W. Jun. 2011. Osteogenic differentiation of human mesenchymal stem cells synergistically enhanced by biomimetic peptide amphiphiles combined with conditioned medium. Acta Biomater. 7(2): 675–682.

Anseth, K., A.T. Metters, S.J. Bryant, P.J. Martens, J.H. Elisseef and C.N. Bowman. 2002. *In situ* forming degradable networks and their application in tissue engineering and drug delivery. J. Control. Release. 78: 199–209.

Bacinello, D., E. Garanger, D. Taton, K.C. Tam and S. Lecommandoux. 2014. Enzyme-degradable self-assembled nanostructures from polymer-peptide hybrids. Biomacromolecules. 15: 1882–1888.

Baskin, J.M., J.A. Prescher, S.T. Laughlin, N.J. Agard, P.V. Chang, I.A. Miller et al. 2007. Copper-free click chemistry for dynamic *in vivo* imaging. Proc. Natl. Acad. Sci. USA. 104(43): 16793.

Bellamkonda, R., J.P. Ranieri and P. Aebischer. 1995. Laminin oligopeptide derivatized agarose gels allow three-dimensional neurite extension *in vitro*. J. Neurosci. Res. 41(4): 501.

Benoit, D.S.W., M.P. Schwartz, A.R. Durney and K.S. Anseth. 2008. Small functional groups for controlled differentiation of hydrogel-encapsulated human mesenchymal stem cells. Nat. Mater. 7(10): 816.

Beria, L., T.N. Gevrek, A. Erdog, R. Sanyal, D. Pasini and A. Sanyal. 2014. "Clickable" hydrogels for all: facile fabrication and functionalization. Biomater. Sci. 2: 67–75.

Berns, E.J., S. Sur, L. Pan, J.E. Goldberger, S. Suresh, S. Zhang et al. 2014. Aligned neurite outgrowth and directed cell migration in self-assembled monodomain gels. Biomaterials. 35(1): 185–195.

Bi, J., J.C. Downs and J.T. Jacob. 2004. Tethered protein/peptide-surface-modified hydrogels. J. Biomat. Sci.-Polym. E. 15(7): 905.

Boekhoven, J. and S.I. Stupp. 2014. 25th anniversary article: supramolecular materials for regenerative medicine. Adv. Mater. 26(11): 1642–59.

Bouyer, C., P. Chen, S. Guven, T.T. Demirtas, T.J.F. Nieland, F. Padilla et al. 2016. A bio-acoustic levitational (BAL) assembly method for engineering of multilayered, 3d brain-like constructs, using human embryonic stem cell derived neuro-progenitors. Adv. Mater. 28(1): 161–+.

Boyer, C. and J. Xu. 2015. Visible light photocatalytic thiol-ene reaction: an elegant approach for fast polymer postfunctionalization and step-growth polymerization. Macromolecules. 48: 520–529.

Brink, K.S., P.J. Yang and J.S. Temenoff. 2009. Degradative properties and cytocompatibility of a mixed-mode hydrogel containing oligo(poly(ethylene glycol) fumarate) and poly(ethylene glycol) dithiol. Acta Biomater. 5: 570–579.

Burdick, J.A. and K.S. Anseth. 2002. Photoencapsulation of osteoblasts in injectable RGD-modified PEG hydrogels for bone tissue engineering. Biomaterials. 23(22): 4315.

Buwalda, S.J., K.W.M. Boere, P.J. Dijkstra, J. Feijen, T. Vermonden and W.E. Hennink. 2014. Hydrogels in a historical perspective: from simple networks to smart materials. J. Control. Release. 190: 254–273.

Campos, L.M., K.L. Killops, R. Sakai, J.M.J. Paulusse, D. Damiron, E. Drockenmuller et al. 2008. Development of thermal and photochemical strategies for thiol-ene click polymer functionalization. Macromolecules. 41: 7063–7070.

Capito, R.M., H.S. Azevedo, Y.S. Velichko, A. Mata and S.I. Stupp. 2008. Self-assembly of large and small molecules into hierarchically ordered sacs and membranes. Science. 319(5871): 1812–1816.

Caprini, A., D. Silva, I. Zanoni, C. Cunha, C. Volonte, A. Vescovi et al. 2013. A novel bioactive peptide: assessing its activity over murine neural stem cells and its potential for neural tissue engineering. N. Biotechnol. 30(5): 552–62.

Chung, I.M., N.O. Enemchukwu, S.D. Khaja, N. Murthy, A. Mantalaris and A.J. García. 2008. Bioadhesive hydrogel microenvironments to modulate epithelial morphogenesis. Biomaterials. 29(17): 2637.

Cigognini, D., D. Silva, S. Paloppi and F. Gelain. 2014. Evaluation of mechanical properties and therapeutic effect of injectable self-assembling hydrogels for spinal cord injury. J. Biomed. Nanotechnol. 10(2): 309–323.

Connelly, J.T., T.A. Petrie, A.J. García and M.E. Levenston. 2011. Fibronectin- and collagen-mimetic ligands regulate bone marrow stromal cell chondrogenesis in three-dimensional hydrogels. Eur. Cells Mater. 22: 168.

Costa, P., J.E. Gautrot and J. Connelly. 2014. Directing cell migration using micropatterned and dynamically adhesive polymer brushes. Acta Biomater.:10.1016/j.actbio.2014.01.029.

Costa, P., J.E. Gautrot and J.T. Connelly. 2014. Directing cell migration using micropatterned and dynamically adhesive polymer brushes. Acta biomaterialia.

Cramer, N.B. and C.N. Bowman. 2001. Kinetics of thiol-ene and thiol-acrylate photopolymerizations with real-time fourier transform infrared. J. Polym. Sci., A: Polym. Chem. 39: 3311–3319.

Cramer, N.B., T. Davies, A.K. O'Brien and C.N. Bowman. 2003a. Mechanism and modelling of a thiol-ene photopolymerization. Macromolecules. 36: 4631–4636.

Cramer, N.B., S.K. Reddy, A.K. O'Brien and C.N. Bowman. 2003b. Thiol-ene photopolymerization mechanism and rate limiting step changes for various vinyl functional group chemistries. Macromolecules. 36(21): 7964–7969.

Cui, H., M.J. Webber and S.I. Stupp. 2010. Self-assembly of peptide amphiphiles: from molecules to nanostructures to biomaterials. Biopolymers. 94(1): 1–18.

Dai, X.S., S.A. Knupp and Q.B. Xu. 2012. Patterning nanoparticles in a three-dimensional matrix using an electric-field-assisted gel transferring technique. Langmuir. 28(5): 2960–2964.

Dargaville, T.R., R. Forster, B.L. Farrugia, K. Kempe, L. Voorhaar, U.S. Schubert et al. 2012. Poly(2-oxazoline) hydrogel monoliths via thiol-ene coupling. Macromol. Rapid Commun. 33: 1695–1700.

Dargaville, T.R., B.G. Hollier, A. Shokoohmand and R. Hoogenboom. 2014. Poly(2-oxazoline) hydrogels as next generation three-dimensional cell supports. Cell Adhes. Migration. 8(2): 88–93.

Davis, M.E., J.P. M. Motion, D.A. Narmoneva, T. Takahashi, D. Hakuno, R.D. Kamm et al. 2005. Injectable self-assembling peptide nanofibers create intramyocardial microenvironments for endothelial cells. Circulation. 111(4): 442–450.

DeForest, C.A., B.D. Polizzotti and K. Anseth. 2009. Sequential click reactions for synthesizing and patterning three-dimensional cell microenvironments. Nat. Mater. 8(8): 659–664.

DeForest, C.A. and D.A. Tirrell. 2015. A photoreversible protein-patterning approach for guiding stem cell fate in three-dimensional gels. Nat. Mater. 14(5): 523–531.

Dondoni, A. 2008. The emergence of thiol-ene coupling as a click process for materials and bioorganic chemistry. Angew. Chem. Int. Ed. 47: 8995–8997.

Ellis-Behnke, R.G., Y.-X. Liang, S.-W. You, D.K.C. Tay, S. Zhang, K.-F. So et al. 2006. Nano neuro knitting: peptide nanofiber scaffold for brain repair and axon regeneration with functional return of vision. P. Natl. Acad. Sci. USA. 103(13): 5054–5059.

Eslami, M., N.E. Vrana, P. Zorlutuna, S. Sant, S. Jung, N. Masoumi et al. 2014. Fiber-reinforced hydrogel scaffolds for heart valve tissue engineering. J. Biomater. Appl. 29(3): 399–410.

Fairbanks, B.D., E.A. Sims, K.S. Anseth and C.N. Bowman. 2010. Reaction rates and mechanisms for radical, photoinitiated addition of thiols to alkynes, and implications for thiol-yne photopolymerizations and click reactions. Macromolecules. 43: 4113–4119.

Fan, V.H., K. Tamama, A. Au, R. Littrell, L.B. Richardson, J.W. Wright et al. 2007. Tethered epidermal growth factor provides a survival advantage to mesenchymal stem cells. Stem Cells (Dayton, Ohio). 25(5): 1241.

Farrugia, B.L., K. Kempe, U.S. Schubert, R. Hoogenboom and T.R. Dargaville. 2015. Poly(2-oxazoline) hydrogels for controlled fibroblast attachment. Biomacromolecules. 14: 2724–2732.

Fernández-Muiños, T., L. Recha-Sancho, P. López-Chicón, C. Castells-Sala, A. Mata and C.E. Semino. 2015. Bimolecular based heparin and self-assembling hydrogel for tissue engineering applications. Acta Biomaterialia. 16: 35–48.

Fichman, G. and E. Gazit. 2014. Self-assembly of short peptides to form hydrogels: design of building blocks, physical properties and technological applications. Acta Biomaterialia. 10(4): 1671–1682.

Freeman, R., J. Boekhoven, M.B. Dickerson, R.R. Naik and S.I. Stupp. 2015. Biopolymers and supramolecular polymers as biomaterials for biomedical applications. Mrs Bulletin. 40(12): 1089–1101.

Frith, J.E., D.J. Menzies, A.R. Cameron, P. Ghosh, D.L. Whitehead, S. Gronthos et al. 2014. Effects of bound versus soluble pentosan polysulphate in PEG/HA-based hydrogels tailored for intervertebral disc regeneration. Biomaterials. 35(4): 1150.

Fu, A., K. Gwon, M. Kim, G. Tae and J.A. Kornfield. 2015. Visible-light-initiated thiol-acrylate photopolymerization of heparin-based hydrogels. Biomacromolecules. 16: 497–506.

Fu, Y., K. Xu, X. Zheng, A.J. Giacomin, A.W. Mix and W.J. Kao. 2012. 3D cell entrapment in crosslinked thiolated gelatin-poly(ethylene glycol) diacrylate hydrogels. Biomaterials. 33: 48–58.

Fukuda, J., A. Khademhosseini, J. Yeh, G. Eng, J. Cheng, O.C. Farokhzad et al. 2006a. Micropatterned cell co-cultures using layer-by-layer deposition of extracellular matrix components. Biomaterials. 27(8): 1479–1486.

Fukuda, J., A. Khademhosseini, Y. Yeo, X. Yang, J. Yeh, G. Eng et al. 2006b. Micromolding of photocrosslinkable chitosan hydrogel for spheroid microarray and co-cultures. Biomaterials. 27(30): 5259–5267.

Gelain, F., D. Bottai, A. Vescovi and S. Zhang. 2006. Designer self-assembling peptide nanofiber scaffolds for adult mouse neural stem cell 3-dimensional cultures. PloS One. 1: e119.

Gelain, F., A. Horii and S. Zhang. 2007. Designer self-assembling peptide scaffolds for 3-D tissue cell cultures and regenerative medicine. Macromol. Biosci. 7(5): 544–551.

Gelain, F., D. Silva, A. Caprini, F. Taraballi, A. Natalello, O. Villa et al. 2011. BMHP1-derived self-assembling peptides: hierarchically assembled structures with self-healing propensity and potential for tissue engineering applications. ACS Nano. 5(3): 1845–59.

Gelain, F., D. Cigognini, A. Caprini, D. Silva, B. Colleoni, M. Donega et al. 2012. New bioactive motifs and their use in functionalized self-assembling peptides for NSC differentiation and neural tissue engineering. Nanoscale. 4(9): 2946–2957.

Gilbert, P.M., K.L. Havenstrite, K.E. Magnusson, A. Sacco, N.A. Leonardi, P. Kraft et al. 2010. Substrate elasticity regulates skeletal muscle stem cell self-renewal in culture. Science. 329(5995): 1078.

Gould, S.T., N.J. Darling and K.S. Anseth. 2012. Small peptide functionalized thiol-ene hydrogels as culture substrates for understanding valvular interstitial cell activation and *de novo* tissue deposition. Acta Biomater. 8: 3201–3209.

Gramlich, W.M., I.L. Kim and J.A. Burdick. 2013. Synthesis and orthogonal photopatterning of hyaluronic acid hydrogels with thiol-norbornene chemistry. Biomaterials. 34: 9803–9811.

Grube, S. and W. Oppermann. 2013. Inhomogeneity in hydrogels synthesized by thiol-ene polymerization. Macromolecules. 46: 1948–1955.

Guo, J., H. Su, Y. Zeng, Y.X. Liang, W.M. Wong, R.G. Ellis-Behnke et al. 2007. Reknitting the injured spinal cord by self-assembling peptide nanofiber scaffold. Nanomed.-Nanotechnol. 3(4): 311–321.

Guo, J., K.K.G. Leung, H. Su, Q. Yuan, L. Wang, T.H. Chu et al. 2009. Self-assembling peptide nanofiber scaffold promotes the reconstruction of acutely injured brain. Nanomedicine: Nanotechnology, Biology, and Medicine. 5(3): 345–351.

Gupta, N., B.F. Lin, L.M. Campos, M.D. Dimitriou, S.T. Hikita, N.D. Treat et al. 2010. A versatile approach to high-throughput microarrays using thiol-ene chemistry. Nat. Chem. (2): 138–145.

Guvendiren, M. and J.A. Burdick. 2010. The control of stem cell morphology and differentiation by hydrogel surface wrinkles. Biomaterials. 31(25): 6511–6518.

Hartgerink, J.D., E. Beniash and S.I. Stupp. 2001. Self-assembly and mineralization of peptide-amphiphile nanofibers. Science. 294(5547): 1684–8.

Heggli, M., N. Tirelli, A. Zisch and J.A. Hubbell. 2003. Michael-type addition as a tool for surface functionalization. Bioconjug. Chem. 14(5): 967–73.

Hensarling, R.M., V.A. Doughty, J.W. Chan and D.L. Patton. 2009. "Clicking" polymer brushes with thiol-yne chemistry: indoors and out. J. Am. Chem. Soc. 131(41): 14673.

Hermanson, G.T. 2008. Bioconjugate Techniques. 2nd ed. London: Academic.

Hern, D.L. and J.A. Hubbell. 1998. Incorporation of adhesion peptides into nonadhesive hydrogels useful for tissue resurfacing. J. Biomed. Mater. Res. 39(2): 266.

Ho, M.-H., D.-Mi. Wang, H.- Hsieh, H.-C. Liu, T.-Y. Hsien, J.-Y. Lai et al. 2005. Preparation and characterization of RGD-immobilized chitosan scaffolds. Biomaterials. 26(16): 3197.

Hoffmann, J.C. and J.L. West. 2013. Three-dimensional photolithographic micropatterning: a novel tool to probe the complexities of cell migration. Integr. Biol. 5(5): 817–827.

Holmes, T.C., S. de Lacalle, X. Su, G. Liu, A. Rich and S. Zhang. 2000. Extensive neurite outgrowth and active synapse formation on self-assembling peptide scaffolds. P. Natl. A. Sci. 97(12): 6728–6733.

Horii, A., X. Wang, F. Gelain and S. Zhang. 2007. Biological designer self-assembling peptide nanofiber scaffolds significantly enhance osteoblast proliferation, differentiation and 3-D migration. Plos One. 2(2): e190.

Hosseinkhani, H., M. Hosseinkhani, A. Khademhosseini and H. Kobayashi. 2007. Bone regeneration through controlled release of bone morphogenetic protein-2 from 3-D tissue engineered nano-scaffold. J. Control. Release. 117(3): 380–386.

Hoyle, C.E., T.Y. Lee and T. Roper. 2004. Thiol-enes: chemistry of the past with promise for the future. J. Polym. Sci., A: Polym. Chem. 42: 5301–5338.

Hoyle, C.E. and C.N. Bowman. 2010. Thiol-ene click chemistry. Angew. Chem. Int. Ed. 49: 1540–1573.

Inostroza-Brito, K.E., E. Collin, O. Siton-Mendelson, K.H. Smith, A. Monge-Marcet, D.S. Ferreira et al. 2015. Co-assembly, spatiotemporal control and morphogenesis of a hybrid protein-peptide system. Nat. Chem. 7(11): 897–904.

Jacob, J.T., J.R. Rochefort, J. Bi and B.M. Gebhardt. 2005. Corneal epithelial cell growth over tethered-protein/peptide surface-modified hydrogels. J. Biomed. Mater. Res. B. 72(1): 198.

Jiang, Y., J. Chen, C. Deng, E.J. Suuronen and Z. Zhong. 2014. Click hydrogels, microgels and nanogels: emerging platforms for drug delivery and tissue engineering. Biomaterials. 35: 4969–4985.

Jonkheijm, P., D. Weinrich, M. Kohn, H. Engelkamp, P.C.M. Christianen, J. Khuhlmann et al. 2008. Photochemical surface patterning by the thiol-ene reaction. Angew. Chem., Int. Ed. 47: 4421–4424.

Khetan, S., J.S. Katz and J.A. Burdick. 2009. Sequential crosslinking to control cellular spreading in 3-dimensional hydrogels. Soft Matter. 5: 1601–1606.

Khetan, S., M. Guvendiren, W.R. Legant, D.M. Cohen, C.S. Chen and J.A. Burdick. 2013. Degradation-mediated cellular traction directs stem cell fate in covalently crosslinked three-dimensional hydrogels. Nat. Mater. 12: 458–465.

Kim, J.E., S.H. Kim and Y. Jung. 2015. *In situ* chondrogenic differentiation of bone marrow stromal cells in bioactive self-assembled peptide gels. J. Biosci. Bioeng. 120(1): 91–98.

Kim, S.J., J. E. Kim, S.H. Kim, S.J. Kim, S.J. Jeon, S.H. Kim et al. 2016. Therapeutic effects of neuropeptide substance P coupled with self-assembled peptide nanofibers on the progression of osteoarthritis in a rat model. Biomaterials. 74: 119–130.

Kirschner, C.M. and K.S. Anseth. 2013. *In situ* control of cell substrate microtopographies using photolabile hydrogels. Small. 9(4): 578–584.

Kisiday, J., M. Jin, B. Kurz, H. Hung, C. Semino, S. Zhang et al. 2002. Self-assembling peptide hydrogel fosters chondrocyte extracellular matrix production and cell division: implications for cartilage tissue repair. P. Natl. A. Sci. 99(15): 9996–10001.

Koo, S.P.S, M.M. Stamenovic, R.A. Prasath, A.J. Inglis, F.E. Du Prez, C. Barner-Kowollik et al. 2010. Limitations of radical thiol-ene reactions for polymer-polymer conjugation. J. Polym. Sci., A: Polym. Chem. 48(8): 1699–1713.

Kopesky, P.W., E.J. Vanderploeg, J.S. Sandy, B. Kurz and A.J. Grodzinsky. 2010. Self-assembling peptide hydrogels modulate *in vitro* chondrogenesis of bovine bone marrow stromal cells. Tissue Eng. Pt. A. 16(2): 465–477.

Koutsopoulos, S. and S. Zhang. 2013. Long-term three-dimensional neural tissue cultures in functionalized self-assembling peptide hydrogels, matrigel and collagen I. Acta Biomaterialia. 9(2): 5162–5169.

Ladet, S., L. David and A. Domard. 2008. Multi-membrane hydrogels. Nature. 452(7183): 76–U6.

Lee, H.J., C. Yu, T. Chansakul, N.S. Hwang, S. Varghese, S.M. Yu et al. 2008. Enhanced chondrogenesis of mesenchymal stem cells in collagen mimetic peptide-mediated microenvironment. Tissue Eng. Pt. A. 14(11): 1843.

Lee, J.Y., J.E. Choo, Y.S. Choi, J.S. Suh, S.J. Lee, C.P. Chung et al. 2009. Osteoblastic differentiation of human bone marrow stromal cells in self-assembled BMP-2 receptor-binding peptide-amphiphiles. Biomaterials. 30(21): 3532–41.

Lee, S.C., I.K. Kwon and K. Park. 2013. Hydrogels for delivery of bioactive agents: a historical perspective. Adv. Drug Deliver. Rev. 65(1): 17–20.

Lee, S.S., E.L. Hsu, M. Mendoza, J. Ghodasra, M.S. Nickoli, A. Ashtekar et al. 2015a. Gel scaffolds of BMP-2-binding peptide amphiphile nanofibers for spinal arthrodesis. Adv. Healthc. Mater. 4(1): 131–41.

Lee, T.T., J.R. García, J.I. Paez, A. Singh, E.A. Phelps, S. Weis et al. 2015b. Light-triggered *in vivo* activation of adhesive peptides regulates cell adhesion, inflammation and vascularization of biomaterials. Nat. Mater. 14(3): 352.

Lin, Y.D., C.Y. Luo, Y.N. Hu, M.L. Yeh, Y.C. Hsueh, M.Y. Chang et al. 2012. Instructive nanofiber scaffolds with VEGF create a microenvironment for arteriogenesis and cardiac repair. Sci. Transl. Med. 4(146).

Liu, M.J., Y. Ishida, Y. Ebina, T. Sasaki, T. Hikima, M. Takata et al. 2015a. An anisotropic hydrogel with electrostatic repulsion between cofacially aligned nanosheets. Nature. 517(7532): 68–72.

Liu, X., B. Pi, H. Wang and X.-M. Wang. 2015b. Self-assembling peptide nanofiber hydrogels for central nervous system regeneration. Front Mater. Sci. 9(1): 1–13.

Lowe, S.B., V.T.G. Tan, A.H. Soeriyadi, T.P. Davis and J.J. Gooding. 2014. Synthesis and high-throughput processing of polymeric hydrogels for 3D cell culture. Bioconj. Chem. 25: 1581–1601.

Luo, Y. and M.S. Shoichet. 2004. A photolabile hydrogel for guided three-dimensional cell growth and migration. Nat. Mater. 3(4): 249–253.

Lutolf, M.P., J.L. Lauer-Fields, H.G. Schmoekel, A.T. Metters, F.E. Weber, G.B. Fields et al. 2003. Synthetic matrix metalloproteinase-sensitive hydrogels for the conduction of tissue regeneration: engineering cell-invasion characteristics. P. Natl. A. Sci. USA. 100(9): 5413.

Mann, B.K., A.S. Gobin, A.T. Tsai, R.H. Schmedlen and J.L. West. 2001. Smooth muscle cell growth in photopolymerized hydrogels with cell adhesive and proteolytically degradable domains: synthetic ECM analogs for tissue engineering. Biomaterials. 22(22): 3045.

Marklein, R.A. and J.A. Burdick. 2010. Spatially controlled hydrogel mechanics to modulate stem cell interactions. Soft Matter. 6: 136–143.

Martino, M.M., F. Tortelli, M. Mochizuki, S. Traub, D. Ben-David, G.A. Kuhn et al. 2011. Engineering the growth factor microenvironment with fibronectin domains to promote wound and bone tissue healing. Sci. Transl. Med. 3(100).

Martino, M.M., P.S. Briquez, A. Ranga, M.P. Lutolf and J.A. Hubbell. 2013. Heparin-binding domain of fibrin(ogen) binds growth factors and promotes tissue repair when incorporated within a synthetic matrix. P. Natl. A. Sci. USA. 110(12): 4563.

Mata, A., L. Hsu, R. Capito, C. Aparicio, K. Henrikson and S.I. Stupp. 2009. Micropatterning of bioactive self-assembling gels. Soft Matter. 5(6): 1228–1236.

Mata, A., Y. Geng, K.J. Henrikson, C. Aparicio, S.R. Stock, R.L. Satcher et al. 2010. Bone regeneration mediated by biomimetic mineralization of a nanofiber matrix. Biomaterials. 31(23): 6004–6012.

Matson, J.B., R.H. Zha and S.I. Stupp. 2011. Peptide self-assembly for crafting functional biological materials. Curr. Opin. Solid. St. M. 15(6): 225–235.

Maude, S., E. Ingham and A. Aggeli. 2013. Biomimetic self-assembling peptides as scaffolds for soft tissue engineering. Nanomedicine (Lond.). 8(5): 823–47.

Mehta, G., C.M. Williams, L. Alvarez, M. Lesniewski, R.D. Kamm and L.G. Griffith. 2010. Synergistic effects of tethered growth factors and adhesion ligands on DNA synthesis and function of primary hepatocytes cultured on soft synthetic hydrogels. Biomaterials. 31(17): 4657.

Mendes, A.C., E.T. Baran, R.L. Reis and H.S. Azevedo. 2013a. Self-assembly in nature: using the principles of nature to create complex nanobiomaterials. Wiley Interdiscip. Rev. Nanomed. Nanobiotechnol. 5(6): 582–612.

Mendes, A.C., K.H. Smith, E. Tejeda-Montes, E. Engel, R.L. Reis, H.S. Azevedo et al. 2013b. Co-assembled and microfabricated bioactive membranes. Adv. Funct. Mater. 23(4): 430–438.

Mergy, J., A. Fournier, E. Hachet and R. Auzely-Velty. 2012. Modification of polysaccharides via thiol-ene chemistry: a versatile route to functional biomaterials. J. Polym. Sci., A: Polym. Chem. 50: 4019–4028.

Miller, R.E., A.J. Grodzinsky, E.J. Vanderploeg, C. Lee, J.D. Ferris, M.F. Barrett et al. 2010. Effect of self-assembling peptide, chondrogenic factors, and bone marrow-derived stromal cells on osteochondral repair. Osteoarthr. Cartilage. 18(12): 1608–1619.

Misawa, H., N. Kobayashi, A. Soto-Gutierrez, Y. Chen, A. Yoshida, J.D. Rivas-Carrillo et al. 2006. PuraMatrix facilitates bone regeneration in bone defects of calvaria in mice. Cell Transplant. 15(10): 903–10.

Mortisen, D., M. Peroglio, M. Alini and D. Eglin. 2010. Tailoring thermoreversible hyaluronan hydrogels by "click" chemistry and raft polymerization for cell and drug therapy. Biomacromolecules. 11(5): 1261–1272.

Narmoneva, D.A., R. Vukmirovic, M.E. Davis, R.D. Kamm and R.T. Lee. 2004. Endothelial cells promote cardiac myocyte survival and spatial reorganization. Circulation. 110(8): 962–968.

Northrop, B.H. and R.N. Coffey. 2012. Thiol-ene click chemistry: computational and kinetic analysis of the influence of alkene functionality. J. Am. Chem. Soc. 134: 13804–13817.

Nuttelman, C.R., M.C. Tripodi and K.S. Anseth. 2005. Synthetic hydrogel niches that promote hMSC viability. Matrix Biol. 24(3): 208.

Orsi, G., M. Fagnano, C. De Maria, F. Montemurro and G. Vozzi. 2014. A new 3D concentration gradient maker and its application in building hydrogels with a 3D stiffness gradient. J. Tissue Eng. Regen. Med.

Palmgren, B., Y. Jiao, E. Novozhilova, S.I. Stupp and P. Olivius. 2012. Survival, migration and differentiation of mouse tau-GFP embryonic stem cells transplanted into the rat auditory nerve. Exp. Neurol. 235(2): 599–609.

Peppas, N.A., J.Z. Hilt, A. Khademhosseini and R. Langer. 2006. Hydrogels in biology and medicine: from molecular principles to bionanotechnology. Adv. Mater. 18(11): 1345–1360.

Perez-Castillejos, R. 2010. Replication of the 3D architecture of tissues. Mater. Today. 13(1-2): 32–41.

Petrie, T.A., J.R. Capadona, C.D. Reyes and A.J. Garcia. 2006. Integrin specificity and enhanced cellular activities associated with surfaces presenting a recombinant fibronectin fragment compared to RGD supports. Biomaterials. 27(31): 5459.

Petrie, T.A., J.E. Raynor, C.D. Reyes, K.L. Burns, D.M. Collard and A.J. Garcia. 2008. The effect of integrin-specific bioactive coatings on tissue healing and implant osseointegration. Biomaterials. 29(19): 2849.

Phelps, E.A., N.O. Enemchukwu, J.C. Fiore, N. Murthy, T.A. Sulchek, T.H. Barker et al. 2012. Maleimide cross-linked bioactive PEG hydrogel exhibits improved reaction kinetics and cross-linking for cell encapsulation and *in situ* delivery. Adv. Mater. (Deerfield Beach, Fla.). 24(1): 64.

Platt, M.O., A.J. Roman, A. Wells, D.A. Lauffenburger and L.G. Griffith. 2009. Sustained epidermal growth factor receptor levels and activation by tethered ligand binding enhances osteogenic differentiation of multi-potent marrow stromal cells. J. Cell Physiol. 221(2): 306.

Porel, M. and C.A. Alabi. 2014. Sequence-defined polymers via orthogonal allyl acrylamide building blocks. J. Am. Chem. Soc. 136: 13162–13165.

Reddy, S.K., N.B. Cramer and C.N. Bowman. 2006. Thiol-vinyl mechanisms. 1. Termination and propagation kinetics in thiol-ene pohotpolymerizations. Macromolecules. 39: 3673–3680.

Reyes, C.D. and A.J. García. 2003. Engineering integrin-specific surfaces with a triple-helical collagen-mimetic peptide. J. Biomed. Mater. Res. A. 65(4): 511.

Roper, T., C.A. Guymon, E.S. Jonsson and C.E. Hoyle. 2004. Influence of the alkene structure on the mechanism and kinetics of thiol-alkene photopolymerizations with real-time infrared spectroscopy. J. Polym. Sci., A: Polym. Chem. 42: 6283–6298.

Rostovtsev, V.V., L.G. Green, V.V. Fokin and K.B. Sharpless. 2002. A stepwise huisgen cycloaddition process: copper(I)-catalyzed regioselective "ligation" of azides and terminal alkynes. Angew. Chem. Int. Ed. Engl. 41(14): 2596.

Rowley, J.A., G. Madlambayan and D.J. Mooney. 1999. Alginate hydrogels as synthetic extracellular matrix materials. Biomaterials. 20(1): 45.

Rubert Perez, C.M., N. Stephanopoulos, S. Sur, S.S. Lee, C. Newcomb and S.I. Stupp. 2015. The powerful functions of peptide-based bioactive matrices for regenerative medicine. Ann. Biomed. Eng. 43(3): 501–14.

Rydholm, A.E., C.N. Bowman and K. Anseth. 2005. Degradable thiol-acrylate photopolymers: polymerization and degradation behavior of an *in situ* forming biomaterial. Biomaterials. 26: 4495–4506.

Salinas, C.N. and K. Anseth. 2008. Mixed mode thiol-acrylate photopolymerizations for the synthesis of PEG-peptide hydrogels. Macromolecules. 41: 6019–6026.

Salinas, C.N. and K.S. Anseth. 2008. The influence of the RGD peptide motif and its contextual presentation in PEG gels on human mesenchymal stem cell viability. J. Tissue Eng. Regen. M. 2(5): 296.

Schenk, V., E. Rossegger, C. Ebner, F. Bangerl, K. Reichmann, B. Hoffmann et al. 2014. RGD-functionalization of poly(2-oxazoline)-based networks for enhanced adhesion to cancer cells. Polymers. 6: 264–279.

Schmedlen, R.H., K.S. Masters and J.L. West. 2002. Photocrosslinkable polyvinyl alcohol hydrogels that can be modified with cell adhesion peptides for use in tissue engineering. Biomaterials. 23(22): 4325.

Semino, C.E. 2008. Self-assembling peptides: from bio-inspired materials to bone regeneration. J. Dent. Res. 87(7): 606–616.

Shah, R.N., N.A. Shah, M.M. Del Rosario Lim, C. Hsieh, G. Nuber and S.I. Stupp. 2010. Supramolecular design of self-assembling nanofibers for cartilage regeneration. P. Natl. Acad. Sci. USA. 107(8): 3293–8.

Shin, H., S. Jo and A.G. Mikos. 2002. Modulation of marrow stromal osteoblast adhesion on biomimetic oligo poly(ethylene glycol) fumarate hydrogels modified with Arg-Gly-Asp peptides and a poly(ethyleneglycol) spacer. J. Biomed. Mater. Res. 61(2): 169.

Shu, X.Z., K. Ghosh, Y. Liu, F.S. Palumbo, Y. Luo, R.A. Clark et al. 2004. Attachment and spreading of fibroblasts on an RGD peptide-modified injectable hyaluronan hydrogel. J. Biomed. Mater. Res. A. 68(2): 365.

Silva, G.A., C. Czeisler, K.L. Niece, E. Beniash, D.A. Harrington, J.A. Kessler et al. 2004. Selective differentiation of neural progenitor cells by high-epitope density nanofibers. Science. 303(5662): 1352–1355.

Smith, K.H., E. Tejeda-Montes, M. Poch and A. Mata. 2011. Integrating top-down and self-assembly in the fabrication of peptide and protein-based biomedical materials. Chem. Soc. Rev. 40(9): 4563–4577.

Stoppel, W.L., D.J. Hu, I.J. Domian, D.L. Kaplan and L.D. Black. 2015. Anisotropic silk biomaterials containing cardiac extracellular matrix for cardiac tissue engineering. Biomed. Mater. 10(3).

Studart, A.R. 2015. Biologically inspired dynamic material systems. Angew. Chem. Int. Edit. 54(11): 3400–3416.

Tejeda-Montes, E., K.H. Smith, M. Poch, M.J. Lopez-Bosque, L. Martin, M. Alonso et al. 2012. Engineering membrane scaffolds with both physical and biomolecular signaling. Acta Biomaterialia. 8(3): 998–1009.

Tejeda-Montes, E., K.H. Smith, E. Rebollo, R. Gomez, M. Alonso, J.C. Rodriguez-Cabello et al. 2014. Bioactive membranes for bone regeneration applications: effect of physical and biomolecular signals on mesenchymal stem cell behavior. Acta Biomaterialia. 10(1): 134–141.

Tibbitt, M.W., A.M. Kloxin, L.A. Sawicki and K. Anseth. 2013. Mechanical properties and degradation of chain and step-polymerized photodegradable hydrogels. Macromolecules. 46: 2785–2792.

Tibbitt, M.W., C.B. Rodell, J.A. Burdick and K.S. Anseth. 2015. Progress in material design for biomedical applications. P. Natl. Acad. Sci. USA. 112(47): 14444–14451.

Tongers, J., M.J. Webber, E.E. Vaughan, E. Sleep, M.-A. Renault, J.G. Roncalli et al. 2014. Enhanced potency of cell-based therapy for ischemic tissue repair using an injectable bioactive epitope presenting nanofiber support matrix. J. Mol. Cell Cardiol. 74: 231–239.

Trmcic-Cvitas, J., E. Hasan, M. Ramstedt, X. Li, M.A. Cooper, C. Abell et al. 2009. Biofunctionalized protein resistant oligo(ethylene glycol)-derived polymer brushes as selective immobilization and sensing platforms. Biomacromolecules. 10(10): 2885.

Tysseling-Mattiace, V.M., V. Sahni, K.L. Niece, D. Birch, C. Czeisler, M.G. Fehlings et al. 2008. Self-assembling nanofibers inhibit glial scar formation and promote axon elongation after spinal cord injury. J. Neurosci. 28(14): 3814–3823.

Tysseling, V.M., V. Sahni, E.T. Pashuck, D. Birch, A. Herbert, C. Czeisler et al. 2010. Self-assembling peptide amphiphile promotes plasticity of serotonergic fibers following spinal cord injury. J. Neurosci. Res. 88(14): 3161–3170.

Utech, S. and A.R. Boccaccini. 2016. A review of hydrogel-based composites for biomedical applications: enhancement of hydrogel properties by addition of rigid inorganic fillers. J. Mater. Sci. 51(1): 271–310.

Uygun, M., M.A. Tasdelen and Y. Yagci. 2010. Influence of type of initiation on thiol-ene "click" chemistry. Macromol. Chem. Phys. 211: 103–110.

Varghese, S., N.S. Hwang, A.C. Canver, P. Theprungsirikul, D.W. Lin and J. Elisseeff. 2008. Chondroitin sulfate based niches for chondrogenic differentiation of mesenchymal stem cells. Matrix Biol. 27(1): 12.

Verhulsel, M., M. Vignes, S. Descroix, L. Malaquin, D.M. Vignjevic and J.L. Viovy. 2014. A review of microfabrication and hydrogel engineering for micro-organs on chips. Biomaterials. 35(6): 1816–1832.

Walker, K.J. and S.V. Madihally. 2015. Anisotropic temperature sensitive chitosan-based injectable hydrogels mimicking cartilage matrix. J. Biomed. Mater. Res. B. 103(6): 1149–1160.

Wang, L., Y.B. Wu, B.L. Guo and P.X. Ma. 2015. Nanofiber yarn/hydrogel core-shell scaffolds mimicking native skeletal muscle tissue for guiding 3D myoblast alignment, elongation, and differentiation. Acs Nano. 9(9): 9167–9179.

Watarai, A., L. Schirmer, S. Thönes, U. Freudenberg, C. Werner, J.C. Simon et al. 2015. TGFβ functionalized starPEG-heparin hydrogels modulate human dermal fibroblast growth and differentiation. Acta Biomaterialia. 25: 65.

Webber, M.J., X. Han, S.N. Prasanna Murthy, K. Rajangam, S.I. Stupp and J.W. Lomasncy. 2010a. Capturing the stem cell paracrine effect using heparin-presenting nanofibres to treat cardiovascular diseases. J. Tissue Eng. Regen. M. 4(8): 600–610.

Webber, M.J., J. Tongers, M.A. Renault, J.G. Roncalli, D.W. Losordo and S.I. Stupp. 2010b. Development of bioactive peptide amphiphiles for therapeutic cell delivery. Acta Biomaterialia. 6(1): 3–11.

Webber, M.J., E.A. Appel, E.W. Meijer and R. Langer. 2016. Supramolecular biomaterials. Nat. Mater. 15(1): 13–26.

Whitesides, G.M. 2005. Nanoscience, nanotechnology, and chemistry. Small. 1(2): 172–179.

Woolfson, D.N. 2010. Building fibrous biomaterials from α-helical and collagen-like coiled-coil peptides. J. Pept. Sci. 94(1): 118–127.

Xia, Y.N. and G.M. Whitesides. 1998. Soft lithography. Annu. Rev. Mater. Sci. 28: 153–184.

Xu, J. and C. Boyer. 2015. Visible light photocatalytic thiol-ene reaction: an elegant approach for fast polymer postfunctionalization and step-growth polymerization. Macromolecules. 48: 520–529.

Yang, F., C.G. Williams, D.-A. Wang, H. Lee, P.N. Manson and J. Elisseeff. 2005. The effect of incorporating RGD adhesive peptide in polyethylene glycol diacrylate hydrogel on osteogenesis of bone marrow stromal cells. Biomaterials. 26(30): 5991.

Yu, T.T. and M.S. Shoichet. 2005. Guided cell adhesion and outgrowth in peptide-modified channels for neural tissue engineering. Biomaterials. 26(13): 1507.

Zha, R.H., Y.S. Velichko, R. Bitton and S.I. Stupp. 2016. Molecular design for growth of supramolecular membranes with hierarchical structure. Soft Matter. 12(5): 1401–1410.

Zhang, S.G. 2003. Fabrication of novel biomaterials through molecular self-assembly. Nat. Biotechnol. 21(10): 1171–1178.

Zhang, S.M., M.A. Greenfield, A. Mata, L.C. Palmer, R. Bitton, J.R. Mantei et al. 2010. A self-assembly pathway to aligned monodomain gels. Nat. Mater. 9(7): 594–601.

Zhu, B., B. Jiang, Z. Na and S.Q. Yao. 2015. Controlled proliferation and screening of mammalian cells on a hydrogel-functionalized small molecule microarray. Chem. Commun. (Cambridge, England). 51(52): 10431.

Zisch, A.H., M.P. Lutolf, M. Ehrbar, G.P. Raeber, S.C. Rizzi, N. Davies et al. 2003. Cell-demanded release of VEGF from synthetic, biointeractive cell ingrowth matrices for vascularized tissue growth. FASEB J: Official Publication of the Federation of American Societies for Experimental Biology. 17(15): 2260.

CHAPTER 18

Synthetic Hydrogels for 3D Cell Culture

Chien-Chi Lin

Introduction

Using two-dimensional (2D) tissue-culture dishes, *in vitro* cell/tissue culture has become a common practice in biomedical laboratories worldwide. Through adding defined supplements (i.e., growth factors, carbohydrates, lipids, or other soluble nutrients) in cell culture media, one can readily examine the effects of soluble biochemical cues on cell behaviors. However, evidence and intuition suggest that 2D cell cultures are less physiologically relevant since cells plated on a rigid 2D surface do not receive proper environmental stimuli that are presented from a three-dimensional (3D) extracellular matrix (ECM) (Cushing and Anseth 2007; Tibbitt and Anseth 2009). Since the early 21st century, there has been a paradigm shift in cell culture *in vitro*, where 3D culture techniques are being developed to overcome the shortfalls of conventional 2D methods. The advancements in 3D cell culture have benefited modern biomedical sciences, molecular and cellular biology, cancer cell biology, regenerative medicine, and tissue engineering. For example, matrices derived from animal ECM (e.g., Matrigel®, gelatin, and collagen gels) are widely used for 3D cell culture by biomedical researchers (Benton et al. 2014). The easy preparation of these animal-derived matrices has allowed researchers to verify 2D cell culture results in 3D, a step closer to mimicking the *in vivo* microenvironment. However, these 'natural' matrices are often mechanically weak when comparing with the mechanics of many tissues *in vivo*. Furthermore, these matrices often contain batch-dependent properties, including the compositions of matrix proteins and residual growth factors. Hence, they might not be ideal for studying molecular pathways elicited by mechanical stimuli, cell-matrix interactions, and growth factor signaling.

Department of Biomedical Engineering, Indiana University-Purdue University Indianapolis, Indianapolis, IN. USA, 723 W. Michigan St. SL220K, Indianapolis, IN. USA 46202.
E-mail: lincc@iupui.edu

A variety of biomaterial-based 3D cell culture platforms have been developed to circumvent the disadvantages associated with animal-derived 3D matrices (Tibbitt and Anseth 2009; DeForest and Anseth 2012; Liu et al. 2015). For example, polymeric scaffolds can be fabricated to have porous structures for 'housing' cells and permitting their proliferation, migration, and other cellular activities (Elbert 2011). Solid and porous scaffolds can be fabricated prior to cell seeding, thus allowing a variety of materials to be used. These scaffolds are typically fabricated to have larger pore sizes, usually on the order of tens of micrometer or sub-millimeter to facilitate uniform cell seeding. Scaffold with a larger pore size is ideal for cell seeding, but the trade-off is weaker mechanical properties. It also cannot truly recapitulate a 3D extracellular microenvironment where cells are often in close contact with their surrounding matrix. Additionally, creating a porous scaffold with interconnected pores is necessary but challenging. An easier route to creating interconnecting space in a polymeric scaffold is to use fibrous materials (Stephens-Altus et al. 2011). Fibrous scaffolds are ideal for many tissue engineering applications because they mimic the fibrous architectures of many native tissues, especially those rich in fibrous collagens (Wade et al. 2015).

Another attractive class of biomaterial suitable for 3D cell culture is semi-synthetic biomimetic hydrogels (DeForest and Anseth 2012; Lin et al. 2015). These crosslinked and water-imbibing polymeric network are increasingly used for modeling diseases *in vitro* and for regenerative medicine applications. Hydrogels are particularly suitable for investigating the influence of extracellular milieu on cell fate because the components of a biomimetic hydrogel can be precisely engineered. The mesh size of hydrogels is on the order of tens of micrometers, a scale much smaller than the size of a cell but larger than most of the growth factors, cytokines, chemokines. Hence, the accessibility of encapsulated cells to these small molecular weight proteins are not significantly hindered (Lin and Metters 2006). The high water content and good permeability of a hydrogel allow facile nutrient-waste exchange, while the crosslinked polymeric network gives rise to tunable elasticity and easy tethering of bioactive motifs for supporting cell survival and function in 3D (Lin and Anseth 2009). In the past few decades, the field of biomaterials science and engineering has witnessed drastic improvement in hydrogel-based 3D cell culture, which is the focus of this chapter.

Design Criteria in Preparing Hydrogels for 3D Cell Culture

For all biomimetic hydrogels intended for cell culture application, the most important design criterion is that the components (e.g., macromers, crosslinkers, initiators, catalysts, functional motifs, etc.) used to prepare cell-laden hydrogels must be non-cytotoxic. Furthermore, the crosslinking conditions must be mild for maintaining viability and phenotype of the cells. Ideally, these hydrogels should present functional moieties found in the native ECM for sustaining long-term cell function or for guiding cell fate processes. These preferential properties include, but not limited to, permitting facile transport of biomolecules (e.g., sugars, lipids, polysaccharides, proteins, and cellular metabolites), matching matrix mechanics to native tissues, sequestration and liberation of bioactive growth factors, as well as providing cell-matrix interactions through ligand-receptor binding and protease-medicated matrix cleavage (Drury and

Mooney 2003). Depending on the applications, however, not all of the above criteria must be simultaneously fulfilled within a particular hydrogel.

Transport properties

As the survival and function of cells rely largely on the availability of essential nutrients and timely removal of metabolic wastes, the transport property of cell-laden hydrogels is of the utmost importance. Although most cell-laden hydrogels contain large quantity of water, slight variation of polymer crosslinking density affects largely the diffusivity of large molecules (proteins, antibodies, polysaccharides, etc.) (Lin and Anseth 2009). Diffusion is the most common means of molecular transport within a cell-laden hydrogel. Thus, the transport property of a cell-laden hydrogel can be evaluated by the diffusivity of the molecule of interest. In a highly swollen hydrogel with no apparent intermolecular interactions between the molecule and the polymeric network, diffusivity of any molecule is positively correlated to the mesh size of the hydrogel and negatively correlated to the hydrodynamic radius of the molecule (Lin and Metters 2006). To increase molecular diffusivity within a cell-laden hydrogel, one can decrease the crosslinking density of the hydrogel. Such approach, however, leads to weakening of the cell-laden matrix. Hydrogels with independently controllable molecular transport and matrix stiffness should be highly valuable in both fundamental and applied research. These advanced hydrogel materials are often made of heterogeneous components, including composites, double-networks, or materials with hierarchical structures. Under some circumstances, one may wish to retard the transport of certain molecules, such as growth factors, cytokines, or chemokines. Adjusting up the network crosslinking is highly effective in reducing molecular transport. However, hydrogel crosslinking density is often positively proportional to the stiffness of the hydrogel (Anseth et al. 2002). Care must be taken if altering stiffness would lead to unexpected complications in data interpretation. Increasing efforts have been dedicated to developing 'affinity hydrogel' where the rate-limiting step of protein diffusion is governed by the engineered intermolecular interactions, rather than simple diffusion (Pratt et al. 2004; Lin and Anseth 2009; Impellitteri et al. 2012; Belair et al. 2014; Lin et al. 2015).

Depot for growth factors

Native ECM is rich in glycosaminoglycans (GAGs) that interact with biomacromolecules through non-specific electrostatic interactions. As such, ECM serves as a depot for storing and supplying growth factors to the cells. When hydrogels are used for 3D cell culture, the administration of solution growth factor to the encapsulated cells can be achieved simply by media supplement. However, this simple approach may not recapitulate the dynamic and complex growth factor availability *in vivo*. Designing biomimetic hydrogels with highly tunable delivery of soluble cues is not a trivial task, given that most hydrogels are highly swollen with high permeability. Various strategies have been integrated into the crosslinking of cell-laden hydrogels in an attempt to provide sustainable delivery of soluble cues. Early work by Hubbell and Sakiyama showed that heparin could be incorporated in fibrin-based hydrogels for sequestering growth factors and prolonging their release *in vitro* and *in vivo* (Hoyle and Bowman 2010; Daniele et al. 2014; Jiang et al. 2014). To this date, heparin is still one of the most commonly used molecules to regulate local availability of growth factors for hydrogel-encapsulated cells. In addition to heparin, 'affinity' peptides (Willerth et al. 2007; Lin and Anseth 2009; Lin et al. 2010; Impellitteri et al. 2012; Belair et al. 2014), aptamers (Altunbas and Pochan 2012; Su et al. 2014; Lau and Kiick 2015), or other ligands can be immobilized in the hydrogel network for binding to and releasing unmodified soluble factors. The availability of soluble factors from an affinity depot is governed by the equilibrium binding between the soluble factors to their immobilized ligands. In other words, only the un-bound factors can be released from the hydrogel network and become available for cellular recognition. These affinity-based release strategies are highly appropriate when chemical modification of proteins/growth factors is not desirable. If chemical modification of soluble factor does not adversely affect its bioactivity, a 'pro-drug' approach can be used (MacEwan and Chilkoti 2010; Yang et al. 2012; Zhang et al. 2015). In such scenario, molecules to be delivered are initially tethered onto the polymeric network through degradable linkers and molecular delivery happens only when the linker is degraded. In recent years, linkers that can be degraded through different mechanisms (e.g., hydrolysis, proteolysis, photolysis, redox, etc.) have been successfully designed and implemented for drug delivery *in vitro* and *in vivo*.

Cell-matrix interactions

Cells process signals coming from their surrounding matrix to determine their fate in maintaining quiescence, proliferation, migration, differentiation, or apoptosis. One of the biggest challenges in designing biomimetic hydrogels is to create one that can emulate appropriate cell signaling motifs that relay signals to cells at appropriate time and location. The presentation of receptor-binding ligands (e.g., Arginine-Glycine-Aspartic acid (RGD) peptide, often as network-immobilized pendant motifs) induces receptor-mediated intracellular signaling important in maintaining or guiding cell viability and function. Pioneering work by Bissell showed that integrin signaling affects cell motility and proliferation in 3D (Annabi et al. 2013; Lampe et al. 2013; Wang et al. 2014). In the past few decades, numerous integrin-signaling motifs have been identified and incorporated in cell-laden hydrogels to affect cell fate processes. Integrin-binding ligands (e.g., RGD) can be clustered through chemical conjugation to facilitate the clustering of integrins and the formation of focal adhesions that subsequently affect cell fate (Hern and Hubbell 1998). One criterion to note is that the relation between the concentration of integrin-binding ligand and corresponding cellular response is not necessary linear. Indeed, numerous reports have shown that cell migration is not apparent or even inhibited at both low and high concentrations of integrin-binding ligand (Schwartz et al. 2010). In this regard, design of experiments (DOE) has used to systematically determine the relationship between the concentration of integrin-binding ligands and related cellular fate (Li et al. 2013; McGann et al. 2016). Modern bioconjugation chemistries offer researchers further exquisite control in presenting integrin-signaling ligands in a spatial-temporally controllable manner for guiding cell migration in 3D (Lin et al. 2015). In addition to integrin-signaling motifs, protease-sensitive substrates (e.g., matrix metalloproteinases (MMPs) cleavable peptides, often serve as gel crosslinker) also dictate how cells behave in 3D (West and Hubbell 1999; Lutolf et al. 2003a; Lutolf et al. 2003b; Lutolf and Hubbell 2005). This is not surprising because without matrix degradation cells simply cannot migrate. While matrix degradation can be designed *a priori* by the experimenter (i.e., through integrating hydrolytic or photolytic degradable linkers in the gel network), cell-mediated matrix cleavage often is more decisive in cell fate determination, including migration, extension of cellular processes, and proliferation (also see section below). The overarching goal of creating biomimetic hydrogels is to recapitulate local cell-matrix interactions for improving the outcome of global tissue regeneration and/ or to understand fundamental mechanisms by which specific extracellular signals influence cell fate determination.

Matrix mechanics

Matrix mechanics (e.g., stiffness, elasticity, modulus, toughness, stress relaxation, etc.) affects cell fate processes by regulating intracellular tension and signaling (Rehfeldt et al. 2007; Sen et al. 2009). Emerging work has demonstrated that matrix mechanics influences cell spreading, proliferation, and differentiation. Hydrogels are ideal matrices for this type of study as the mechanical properties of these water-swollen matrices can be easily and sometimes independently tuned to mimic native tissue elasticity and biofunctionality. Seminal work by Engler and Discher demonstrated that, even when exposed to identical culture media supplements, the fate of mesenchymal stem cells (MSCs) plated on the surface of polyacrylamide hydrogels was dictated by the stiffness of the underneath substrates (Engler et al. 2006). Anseth and colleagues later showed that 'mechanical dosing' effect should be taken into consideration when designing experiments for MSC culture and differentiation (Yang et al. 2014). Specifically, when cultured on stiff substrate for expended period of time, the differentiation of MSCs is biased toward osteogenic lineage. Stem cell fate in 3D, however, is not exclusively dependent on matrix stiffness and can be complicated by the intricate cell-matrix interactions that include integrin receptor activation and matrix cleavage. For example, Burdick and colleagues showed that, when MSCs were encapsulated in inert hydrogels without cell-mediated matrix cleavage, the differentiation of MSCs was biased toward adipogenic lineage even within a stiff microenvironment (Khetan et al. 2013). On the other hand, when cell-mediated matrix degradation is allowed, osteogenic differentiation potential was restored. In addition to the hydrogel's initial stiffness, another important but less studied aspect of matrix mechanic on cell fate processes in 3D is viscoelasticity. Natural tissues are viscoelastic with noticeable stress relaxation, whereas most biomimetic hydrogels for purely elastic that does not recapitulate the viscoelastic property of the native ECM. In this aspect, Mooney et al. recently show that the spreading, proliferation, and osteogenic differentiation of MSCs are promoted in hydrogels with faster stress relaxation (Chaudhuri et al. 2015). More importantly, the effects of stress relaxation on MSC fate are mediated by actomyosin contractility and mechanical clustering of adhesion ligands.

Synthetic Hydrogel Materials Suitable for 3D Cell Culture

Synthetic polymers for crosslinking of cell-laden hydrogels

Many hydrophilic synthetic polymers and co-polymers are utilized as backbone of cell-laden hydrogels for 3D cell culture. Synthetic hydrogels can be prepared from small molecular weight monomers (e.g., acrylamide, N-isopropylacrylamide, N-vinylpyrrolidone, hydroxyethyl methacrylate, etc.) or crosslinked from high molecular weight macromers (e.g., poly(ethylene glycol) (PEG), poly(vinyl alcohol) (PVA), etc.) or their derivatives (e.g., PEG-diacrylate, PEG-vinylsulfone, PEG-norbornene, thiolated-PVA, tyramine-PVA, etc.). When polymerized from small molecular weight monomers, extensive washes post-gelation are required to remove residual unreactive monomers and initiators that might be harmful for the cells. *In situ* cell encapsulation is less likely to be compatible with hydrogels polymerized from small molecular weight monomers, although these gels can be made with highly controllable properties, such as crosslinking density, degradability, and even porosity (when porogens are used). On the other hand, hydrogels prepared from polymerizable hydrophilic macromers often are more compatible for *in situ* cell encapsulation, given that all components used for hydrogel crosslinking are cytocompatible. Regardless of the route of hydrogel preparation, synthetic polymers do not contain bioactive motifs critical for cell survival, proliferation, and morphogenesis. Therefore, major research efforts in preparing synthetic hydrogels are to conjugate or co-polymerize biomimetic ligands for improving cell-material interactions (DeForest and Anseth 2012).

Radical-mediated chain- and mixed-mode polymerizations

The most commonly used method to prepared hydrogels for 3D cell culture is through radical-mediated chain-growth polymerization of functionalized macromers (e.g., acrylated or methacrylated PEGs). Immobilization of pendant ligand is easily achieved through co-polymerization of acrylated or methacrylated peptides/proteins in the crosslinked polymer network. Hubbell and colleagues pioneered the field by using N-hydroxysuccinimidyl (NHS)-activated esters (with or without a PEG spacer) to immobilize acrylated integrin-binding peptides to the otherwise inert PEGDA hydrogels (West and Hubbell 1995; Hern and Hubbell 1998; West and Hubbell 1999). This approach has become a popular method of functionalizing PEG hydrogels with bioactive motifs. Even though this approach is simple, it may not be ideal for some applications due to the fact that the pendant peptides are linked to hydrophobic poly(acrylate) or poly(methacrylate) kinetic chains, resulting in decreased accessibility of the peptides/proteins to the cells (Lin and Anseth 2009). Furthermore, the immobilization efficiencies (i.e., percentage of immobilized peptides/proteins) of (meth)acrylated pendant peptides are relatively low (~60%) (Elbert and Hubbell 2001; Hao and Lin 2014), which means that the non-crosslinked peptides may bind to cell surface receptor and act as soluble agonist or antagonist.

Acrylated PEGs are a unique class of macromer in that they are crosslinkable through radical-mediated chain-growth or mixed-mode polymerization (Salinas and Anseth 2008; Hao and Lin 2014; Hao et al. 2014; Lin et al. 2015). The latter describes a polymerization mechanism that combines the features of both chain- and step-growth polymerizations. When thiol-containing macromers/monomers are added to the pre-polymer solution, thiyl radicals generated by primary radicals (i.e., photoinitiator fragments) are responsible for initiating radical propagation that involves thiol-acrylate addition and carbonyl radical generation. The later can participate in further chain-growth polymerization or to abstract protons from nearby thiols. The alternate step-and-chain-growth polymerization leads to a crosslinked hydrogel network with heterogeneous crosslinks in which some are non-degradable (i.e., polyacrylate kinetic chains) but some are labile through hydrolysis of thiol-ether ester bonds (Hao and Lin 2014). The degradability of the hydrogel is mainly determined by the ratio of thiol-to-acrylate in the pre-polymer solution. This polymerization mechanism allows one to easily immobilized thiolated peptides or proteins in the hydrogels with high immobilization efficiency (80–90%) (Hao and Lin 2014). When bioactive peptides are used, cysteines or additional spacers can be readily added during solid phase peptide synthesis, hence eliminating post-synthesis modification. Mixed-mode polymerization of hydrogels can also be initiated by visible light (400–700 nm), arguably a more cytocompatible light source. Lin and colleagues developed visible light initiated mixed-mode thiol-acrylate photopolymerization for fabricating cell-laden hydrogels that are labile by means of both hydrolysis and proteolysis (Hao and Lin 2014; Hao et al. 2014). One of the differences between visible light initiated thiol-acrylate photopolymerization and chain-growth polymerization of acrylated macromer is that no amine-based co-initiated is needed for the former, which may be more favorable for some cell encapsulation studies. Furthermore, visible light initiated thiol-acrylate photopolymerization yields networks that are labile hydrolytically without the need of using degradable macromers.

Step-growth polymerizations

Chemically crosslinked hydrogels can be prepared from step-growth polymerization, including radical-mediated and orthogonal 'click' reactions. Differing from chain-growth and mixed-mode polymerized network, step-growth hydrogels possess more homogeneous network structure and better mechanical properties. In particular, PEG-based multi-arm macromers are routinely functionalized with alkene or alkyne moieties for orthogonal thiol-ene or thiol-yne polymerizations (Hoyle and Bowman 2010; Jiang et al. 2014). These radical-mediated thiol-ene/yne hydrogels are increasingly used for in situ cell encapsulation. This type of gelation often requires using long-wavelength ultraviolet (UV) light and cleavage-type photoinitiators to initiate gelation. For example, Anseth and colleagues developed a thiol-norbornene photo-click hydrogel system (Fairbanks et al. 2009). The thiol-norbornene hydrogels are attractive in that the polymerization is extremely efficient (a few seconds of gel points) owing to the non-oxygen-inhibiting nature of thiol-norbornene reaction (Shih and Lin 2012). This reaction is also highly cytocompatible, even for radical sensitive pancreatic beta cells (Lin et al. 2011). Others have also developed dual network formed by simultaneous thiol-ene and thiol-yne polymerizations (Daniele et al. 2014). Thiol-norbornene reaction can also be initiated by visible light (400–700 nm) irradiation following a similar initiation mechanism except that a type-II photoinitiator (e.g., eosin-Y) is used to created thiyl radicals from thiol-containing crosslinkers (Shih et al. 2013; Shih and Lin 2013; Fraser et al. 2014). The use of visible light eliminates the biosafety concerns of UV light, which some argue that it might cause cellular damages or genetic mutation. Light and radical mediated step-growth polymerizations are beneficial in that the gelation kinetics and bioconjugation can be achieved and controlled spatiotemporally. This feature is extremely useful when studying cell fate process under the influence of dynamic microenvironmental cues.

Another increasingly explored step-growth polymerization is the 'Click' chemistry, which is used to describe highly efficient and quantitative reactions between mutually reactive functional groups (Hoyle and Bowman 2010). Hubbell et al. established click-based hydrogels using functional PEG macromers (e.g., PEG-acrylate or PEG-vinylsulfone) and bis-cysteine containing MMP-sensitive peptide sequence (Lutolf and Hubbell 2003; Lutolf et al. 2003; Lutolf et al. 2003a). Methacrylate, acrylate, and maleimide-terminated macromers can also be used to crosslink with bis-cysteine peptides for forming cell-laden biomimetic hydrogels. Other notable click chemistries developed in recent years include native chemical ligation (Hu et al. 2009; Su et al. 2010; Jung et al. 2013; Strehin et al. 2013), oxime click chemistry (Grover et al. 2012; Grover et al. 2013; Lin et al. 2013), azide-alkyne addition (Polizzotti et al. 2008; DeForest et al. 2009), Diels-Alder reaction (Koehler et al. 2013, Jiang et al. 2014) and tetrazine-norbornene chemistry (Alge et al. 2013; Zhang et al. 2014). Similar to the Michael-type conjugation reaction, the reactions of these orthogonal click chemistries are independent of light irradiation nor do they generate propagating radicals during gel crosslinking. Furthermore, the gelation process is amenable to create 'injectable hydrogel', which is highly valuable for translational and clinically relevant applications.

Engineered polypeptides

Genetic engineering is a powerful tool for creating 'designer' peptides with modular properties. The design of these engineered peptides are often inspired by the structures of natural macromolecules, such as elastin and resilin (Su et al. 2014; Lau and Kiick 2015). Elastin is one of the major structural proteins found in many native tissues, including tendons, ligaments, and blood vessels. The elastic nature of elastin stems from the extensive crosslinks of the protein, as well as the canonical peptide sequence VPGXG repeat where X represents any natural amino acid other than proline (Annabi et al. 2013; Lampe et al. 2013; Wang et al. 2014; Lau and Kiick 2015; Zhang et al. 2015). Various elastin-like polypeptides (ELPs) have been designed and produced recombinantly for forming biosynthetic scaffolds suitable for 3D cell culture (MacEwan and Chilkoti 2010; Altunbas and Pochan 2012). The sequence of ELPs can be designed such that the resulting polypeptides can be readily crosslinked, either physically or chemically, and with preferential and predictable properties (e.g., extensibility, elasticity, and tensile strength). In addition, cell adhesive ligands (e.g., RGD peptide) can be easily incorporated either within the ELP peptide sequence or modified post-gelation through thiol-maleimide Michael-type addition.

Resilin, a structural protein found in insects, is another example of engineered polypeptide gaining increasing attention in biosynthetic scaffold for 3D cell culture (Li et al. 2013; Su et al. 2014). Resilin, as suggested by its name, has excellent resilience and energy storage capabilities, which allow it to recover from high-strain cyclic loading with no hysteresis. Polypeptide constructs containing resilin consensus sequence (e.g., GGRPSDSYGAPGGGN) have been produced from Drosophila CG15920 gene via recombinant DNA techniques (Su et al. 2014). These resilin-like polypeptides (RLPs) have been used to fabricate 3D hydrogels by means of temperature-induced transition or chemical crosslinking. Similar to the incorporation of cell-responsive motifs in ELPs, the biological functionality of RLPs can be improved through incorporating cell adhesive or protease sensitive sequences in the peptide backbone. Other functional peptide sequences, such as RGD, have also been designed into RLPs for improving differentiation of human mesenchymal stem cells (hMSCs) (Renner et al. 2012; McGann et al. 2016a; McGann et al. 2016b).

Small molecular weight hydrogelators

Supramolecular assembly describes the association of molecules by means of hydrogen bonding, metal chelation, van der Waals forces, hydrophobic interaction, π-π stacking, or other non-covalent and directional bindings (Nagarkar and Schneider 2008). This attractive class of macromolecular chemistry has found numerous applications in non-covalent surface modification, affinity-based drug delivery, imaging and diagnostic applications, and more recently hydrogel synthesis and fabrication (Liebmann et al. 2007; Das et al. 2009; Shao and Parquette 2010). Two types of supramolecular hydrogels are suitable for 3D cell culture: namely hydrogels fabricated from small molecular weight 'hydrogelator' and those prepared from macromolecular host-guest interactions (see section below). In addition to the gelation mechanisms, these two classes of supramolecular hydrogels also differ in cell loading method. In small molecular hydrogelator (e.g., aromatic Fmoc-linked or alkyl group oligopeptides), hydrogels are formed due to π-π stacking of the hydrophobic aromatic Fmoc groups or hydrophobic interactions between the alkyl chains (Fleming and Ulijn 2014). Due to the hydrophobicity of the constituent molecules, the precursor solutions are often prepared using solvents (e.g., dimethyl sulfoxide, DMSO). Upon dilution using aqueous buffer, the hydrophobic interactions between Fmoc or alkyl groups yield nanoscale molecular assembly that can further entangle to form hydrogels with higher order fibrillar structures and interconnected pores. Due to the use of organic solvents during gelation, cells are loaded to the Fmoc-peptide hydrogels post-gelation. Cell adhesive peptides can be readily incorporated in the form of Fmoc-linked peptide (e.g., Fmoc-RGD) (Zhou et al. 2009; Zhou et al. 2014; Zanuy et al. 2016). When Fmoc-peptide hydrogels are utilized for 3D cell culture, care must be taken in terms of residual solvents. Another concern is that the assembly of these small molecular weight gelators often leads to kinetically trapped aggregates. Nonetheless, this form of supramolecular hydrogel can be controlled to produce nanoscale fibrillar structure, which resembles fibrillar structure found in native ECM.

Biomimetic Hydrogels for Supporting Cell Fate Processes

Hydrogels prepared from natural materials (e.g., collagen, gelatin, hyaluronic acid, etc.) inherently contain bioactive motifs that can support certain aspects of cell fate processes. While not containing cell-signaling motifs, hydrogels prepared from purely synthetic polymers (e.g., PEG, PVA, etc.) can sometimes support the survival and even proliferation of certain cells (Lin et al. 2011). These passive matrices do not interact with the cells, necessitating the incorporation of artificial bioactive motifs for supporting complex cell fate processes. Much of the knowledge regarding biomimetic motifs comes from our ever-increasing understanding of the compositions of extracellular matrix proteins (Lutolf and Hubbell 2005; Martino et al. 2014). The presentations of ECM proteins/signals in a cell's native microenvironment are far from static because ECM proteins (e.g., fibrin, fibronectin, laminin, collagen, etc.) are secreted by cells residing within the regenerating niche or recruited from neighboring tissue. The arrival of different types of cells at different time scales during tissue morphogenesis or regeneration explains the dynamic nature of these cell-secreted ECM motifs.

To mimic a natural cell niche, it has become a common practice to tether individual biomimetic motifs into synthetic hydrogels. This approach allows for studying receptor-mediated intracellular signaling. Since most of the cell fate processes are elicited by receptor-mediated intracellular signaling events, hydrogels contain ECM motifs are useful in not only providing a 3D culture context, but also in studying ligand-mediated receptor activation. In addition to full-length ECM proteins, integrin receptor activation can also be induced by short peptides derived from ECM proteins. The most ubiquitous integrin-binding peptide is the tri-peptide RGD, which represent the smallest peptide sequence for activating integrins. Although RGD was first discovered from fibronectin, it is also found in the peptide sequence of numerous matrix proteins, including fibrin, osteopontin, TGFβ-latent protein. Other receptor binding peptides/proteins (e.g., laminin-derived peptides (Raza et al. 2013; Bal et al. 2014; Lam et al. 2015), stromal cell derived factor 1 (SDF-1) (Cuchiara et al. 2013), Notch ligands (Dishowitz et al. 2014), etc.) have also been increasingly used to study stem cell differentiation, and for promoting tissue regeneration.

In addition to mimicking cell-matrix interactions through conjugating matrix proteins or peptides in the crosslinked hydrogels, increasing efforts have been devoted to recapitulating aspects of cell-cell interactions in biomimetic matrices. For example, Lin and Anseth identified cell density as a crucial factor governing pancreatic β-cell survival and function in chain-polymerized PEGDA hydrogels (Lin and Anseth 2011). They further integrated cell-cell communication mimicry motifs in the cell-laden hydrogels through co-polymerizing thiolated recombinant Ephrin and Eph, a pair of cell surface receptor/ligand important in regulating β-cell viability and insulin secretion. The immobilized Ephrin/Eph motifs provided additional cell-signaling motifs in the otherwise inert PEG gel network to support the survival and function of MIN6 β-cell even when they were encapsulated at low cell density.

The development of biomimetic hydrogels for 3D cell culture has also benefited significantly from recent development in advanced biofabrication, such as 3D bioprinting and gradient biomaterials. Various forms of 3D bioprinting are increasingly being developed and are ideal for creating cell culture matrices with 3D micro-, macro, and meso-scale structures. On the other hand, hydrogels with gradient biochemical or biophysical cues are designed through bioconjugation or degradation chemistries (Rice et al. 2013). These matrices are capable of mimicking the spatial presentation of bioactive motifs (e.g., morphogens) or matrix stiffness (e.g., during tissue fibrosis or tumor development).

Dynamic Hydrogels for Tuning Cell Fate

The dynamic presentation of biochemical and biophysical cues during tissue development and regeneration has been well recognized for decades. However, the design of hydrogel matrices capable of recapitulating dynamic nature of ECM has not begun until the early 2000s. Hydrogels with properties that can be dynamically tuned are not only useful in fundamental understanding of matrix turnover and cell-matrix interactions, but also important in promoting tissue regeneration (DeForest and Anseth 2012). A seminal work from the Shoichet group demonstrated the utility of a dynamic hydrogel system, which is based on agarose and nitrobenzyl-protected cysteine, on guiding cell growth and migration in 3D (Luo and Shoichet 2004a; Luo and Shoichet 2004b). The removal of nitrobenzyl group upon UV exposure exposes free sulfhydryl group for patterning biomolecules through thiol-maleimide reaction. The Anseth group developed patternable step-growth PEG-based hydrogels using thiol-norbornene photo-click reaction (Fairbanks et al. 2009). The orthogonal reactivity between norbornene (terminal group on multi-arm PEG) and thiol (cysteine-containing peptide linkers) permits post-gelation matrix modification in the presence of cells, given that the hydrogel is prepared with a stoichiometrically imbalanced norbornene group.

Adaptable hydrogels with reversibility for supporting cell fate

Conventional hydrogels for 3D cell culture are often composed of polymers crosslinked by covalent bonds that exhibit purely elastic properties. These elastic hydrogels are excellent artificial tissue mimics for recapitulating aspects of native ECM, including elasticity, permeability, and presentations of bioactive motifs. However, purely elastic hydrogels do not capture the viscoelastic and stress-relaxation properties of native tissues, which may play a significant role in cell fate processes and tissue development. Recent efforts have addressed this through developing advanced hydrogels with reversible crosslinks that can be reformed after breaking up by local cellular processes (McKinnon et al. 2014a; McKinnon et al. 2014b; Wang and Heilshorn 2015). This section describes hydrogels formed by, or consists of, reversible or adaptable crosslinks: the linkages that can be broken upon forces, and be re-formed upon the removal of the forces. This new class of reversible/adaptable hydrogels is highly desirable for studies concerning the influence of matrix viscoelastic properties on cell behavior, including migration, mechanosensing, differentiation, and other more complicated cell fate processes.

Physical hydrogels composed of macromolecular self-assembly

Entropy-driven hydrophobic interaction is an effective way of creating stable bonds linking polymer chains into crosslinked hydrogels. A variety of hydrophobic interactions, such as coiled-coil peptides and amphiphilic block copolymers, have been explored in cell-compatible hydrogel fabrication (Banta et al. 2010; Woolfson 2010). The coiled-coil domain is a left-handed superhelix composed of two or more right-handed α-helices. Its signature amino acid sequence typically contains repeat units of (*abcdefg*) with *a* and *d* being hydrophobic residues and the rest are polar residues. The hydrophobic residues are line up to form the hydrophobic core, which undergoes conformational changes upon applying external stimuli (e.g., temperature, pH, ionic strength, etc.). When the coiled-coil domain is incorporated in hydrogel design, external stimuli cause microscopic protein conformational changes that also lead to changes in macroscopic material properties. For example, Wang et al. combined the coiled-coil protein domains and metal ion chelation to synthesize thermal-responsive hydrogels (Wang et al. 1999). Genetically engineered coiled-coil proteins with a hexa-histidine (6xHis) tag are assembled on a linear copolymer composed of N-(2-hydroxypropyl)-methacrylamide (HPMA) and metal-chelaing (N',N'-dicarboxymethylaminopropyl)-methacrylamide (DAMA), the later serves as a pendant metal-chelating ligand (i.e., iminodiacetate, IDA) for chelating with Ni^{2+} and the His-tagged coiled-coil protein. Due to temperature-induced cooperative conformational transition in the coiled-coil protein domain, these hybrid hydrogels collapse (i.e., decreased swelling) at an elevated temperature (mid-point transition temperature of 39°C).

While the aforementioned coiled-coil protein hydrogel was not used in cell encapsulation or cell culture, it paved the way for later studies in such endeavor. In one recent example, coiled-coil domains with free terminal cysteine were engineered and used to form self-assembled multifunctional thiols, which react with vinylsulfone-conjugated PEG through Michael-addition (Liu et al. 2011). The resulting hydrogels are composed of both physical coiled-coil association and chemical thiol-vinylsulfone crosslinks. The system is compatible for cell encapsulation and the dynamic nature of the coiled-coil association is believed to serve as open paths for cell migration and higher order morphogenesis (e.g., epithelial cyst formation) in 3D. Similar coiled-coil protein domains have also being conjugated to synthetic polymers for forming shear-thinning and temperature-responsive hydrogels (Glassman et al. 2013).

Physical hydrogels formed by host-guest interactions

Supramolecular 'host-guest' interactions have been exploited to form hydrogels capable of 'self-healing' due to their reversible binding nature (Webber et al. 2015). However, most of the early work on host-guest hydrogels employed organic solvents for dissolution of the hydrophobic macromers. Recently, researchers have begun to design host-guest hydrogels suitable for cell encapsulation. Host and guest molecules that non-covalently interact with each other are separately conjugated to multi-functional polymers (e.g., polyvinyl alcohol, hyaluronan, gelatin, etc.) and are assembled into gels upon mixing the host macromers with multifunctional guest crosslinkers (Highley et al. 2015; Mealy et al. 2015; Rodell et al. 2015a; Rodell et al. 2015b). Many of these host-guest supramolecular hydrogels can be conjugated on water-soluble macromers, thus permitting *in situ* cell encapsulation. These hydrogels, similar to covalently crosslinked mesh-like hydrogels, do not possess fibrillar or porous structures. However, this system offers 'injectability' and the supramolecular macromers are increasingly being used as 'building blocks' to fabricate cell-compatible hydrogels.

The gelation and stability of physical hydrogels formed by host-guest interactions are governed by the principles of thermodynamics and the kinetics of the affinity binding. The equilibrium binding strengths between the host and guest molecules are determined by the equilibrium dissociation constant (K_D, unit: M), which is the ratio of dissociation (or reverse) rate constant (k_{off} or k_{-1}, unit: sec^{-1}) and association (or forward) rate constant (k_{on} or k_1, unit: $sec^{-1}M^{-1}$). In the formation of supramolecular host-guest hydrogels, it is essential to use multifunctional macromers for both the host and the guest macromers, which increase both the speed of gelation and the stability of the resulting gels in an aqueous environment. The thermodynamic equilibrium of the host-guest binding is determined by the binding affinity, as well as the concentrations and the stoichiometric ratio of the host and guest moieties. Delicate adjustment of the various parameters related to host-guest affinity binding is essential in maintaining a stable hydrogels while allowing cell-mediated reversible bond dissociation.

One example of 'host' molecule is amphiphilic cyclodextrins (CD, including α-CD, β-CD, and γ-CD), whose inner hydrophobic cavity is capable of binding with hydrophobic bulky molecules, such as adamantane, azobenzene, ferrocene, and stilbene (Appel et al. 2010; Appel et al. 2012a; Appel et al. 2012b; Webber et al. 2015). Various forms of functionalized CD have been synthesized for creating matrices for in biomaterials, drug delivery, and tissue engineering applications. For example, the Burdick group developed CD and adamantane (Ad) conjugated hyaluronic acid (HA) for forming shear-thinning hydrogels suitable for cell encapsulation (Rodell et al. 2015a; Rodell et al. 2015b). The association between CD and Ad led to gelation but the complexes disassembled upon applying shear force, which leads to gel-sol transition. Upon removing the shear force, the host-guest interaction re-establishes and the hydrogel re-forms. Similar gelling principles are used to create supramolecular hydrogels based on macrocyclic oligomer cucurbit[8]uril and its corresponding guest molecules fabricated in the form of pendant linear macromers (Appel et al. 2010; Appel et al. 2012a; Appel et al. 2012b). Alternatively, transient protein-protein or protein-peptide interactions are exploited for forming affinity-based supramolecular hydrogels (Lu et al. 2012). For example, two-component hydrogels formed by multivalent binding of WW domains and proline-rich peptides have been developed for cell encapsulation (Wong Po Foo et al. 2009; Parisi-Amon et al. 2013).

Covalently crosslinked hydrogels with reversible crosslinks

Covalently adaptable hydrogels describe a class of hydrogels formed by reversible linkage (Wang and Heilshorn 2015). The reactions between the complementary reactive motifs form metastable bonds that can be broken and reformed under certain environmental conditions (e.g., temperature, stress, etc.). Unlike hydrogels crosslinked by pure covalent bonds, these materials typically exhibit viscoelastic properties similar to that found in native tissues (McKinnon et al. 2014a; McKinnon et al. 2014b;

Chaudhuri et al. 2015). Therefore, covalently adaptable hydrogels are ideal for studying the influence of matrix viscoelasticity on cell fate processes. For example, Mooney and colleagues utilized alginate hydrogels exhibiting stress-relaxation, a property unique to viscoelastic material, to study spreading and differentiation of mesenchymal stem cells (Chaudhuri et al. 2015). In addition to immobilizing pendant ligand in the presence of cells, one may wish to 'exchange' the ligands to truly recapitulate a dynamic developmental process during tissue morphogenesis. In this regard, an addition-fragmentation-chain transfer reaction was developed to allow controlled and reversible exchange of biochemical ligands within an allyl sulfide functionalized PEG hydrogel (Gandavarapu et al. 2014). This approach allows user-defined introduction of immobilized ligands during cell culture, which may be highly useful in understanding the influence of temporal presentation of selective ligands on tissue development.

Conclusion

In summary, synthetic hydrogels have emerged as a class of powerful and diverse cell culture platform for studying cell biology and for promoting tissue regeneration. In most applications, bioactive motifs are integrated in the design of biomimetic hydrogels for enhancing the utility of the otherwise inert hydrogels. In addition to immobilized ligands, increasing efforts are devoted to understanding the influence of static and dynamic matrix mechanics on cell fate processes in 3D. These efforts have led to the increased recognition of the importance of hydrogels for 3D cell culture, both in basic biological sciences and translation applications. As the design and development of biosynthetic hydrogels continue to improve, it is anticipated that biosynthetic hydrogels will become highly desirable for cellular and molecular biology research, tissue engineering and regenerative medicine, as well as *in vitro* disease models for drug screening and testing.

References

Alge, D.L., M.A. Azagarsamy, D.F. Donohue and K.S. Anseth. 2013. Synthetically tractable click hydrogels for three-dimensional cell culture formed using tetrazine-norbornene chemistry. Biomacromolecules. 14: 949–953.

Altunbas, A. and D.J. Pochan. 2012. Peptide-based and polypeptide-based hydrogels for drug delivery and tissue engineering. Top Curr. Chem. 310: 135–167.

Annabi, N., S.M. Mithieux, G. Camci-Unal, M.R. Dokmeci, A.S. Weiss and A. Khademhosseini. 2013. Elastomeric Recombinant Protein-based Biomaterials. Biochem. Eng. J. 77: 110–118.

Anseth, K.S., A.T. Metters, S.J. Bryant, P.J. Martens, J.H. Elisseeff and C.N. Bowman 2002. *In situ* forming degradable networks and their application in tissue engineering and drug delivery. J. Control. Release. 78: 199–209.

Appel, E.A., F. Biedermann, U. Rauwald, S.T. Jones, J.M. Zayed and O.A. Scherman. 2010. Supramolecular cross-linked networks via host-guest complexation with cucurbit 8 uril. Journal of the American Chemical Society. 132: 14251–14260.

Appel, E.A., X.J. Loh, S.T. Jones, F. Biedermann, C.A. Dreiss and O.A. Scherman. 2012a. Ultrahigh-water-content supramolecular hydrogels exhibiting multistimuli responsiveness. Journal of the American Chemical Society. 134: 11767–11773.

Appel, E.A., X.J. Loh, S.T. Jones, C.A. Dreiss and O.A. Scherman. 2012b. Sustained release of proteins from high water content supramolecular polymer hydrogels. Biomaterials. 33: 4646–4652.

Bal, T., C. Nazli, A. Okcu, G. Duruksu, E. Karaoz and S. Kizilel. 2014. Mesenchymal stem cells and ligand incorporation in biomimetic poly(ethylene glycol) hydrogels significantly improve insulin secretion from pancreatic islets. J. Tissue Eng. Regen. Med.

Banta, S., I.R. Wheeldon and M. Blenner. 2010. Protein engineering in the development of functional hydrogels. Annu. Rev. Biomed. Eng. 12: 167–186.

Belair, D.G., A.S. Khalil, M.J. Miller and W.L. Murphy. 2014. Serum-dependence of affinity-mediated vegf release from biomimetic microspheres. Biomacromolecules. 15: 2038–2048.

Benton, G., I. Arnaoutova, J. George, H.K. Kleinman and J. Koblinski. 2014. Matrigel: from discovery and ECM mimicry to assays and models for cancer research. Adv. Drug Deliv. Rev. 79-80: 3–18.

Chaudhuri, O., L. Gu, D. Klumpers, M. Darnell, S.A. Bencherif, J.C. Weaver et al. 2015. Hydrogels with tunable stress relaxation regulate stem cell fate and activity. Nat. Mater.

Cuchiara, M.L., K.L. Horter, O.A. Banda and J.L. West. 2013. Covalent immobilization of stem cell factor and stromal derived factor 1alpha for *in vitro* culture of hematopoietic progenitor cells. Acta Biomater. 9: 9258–9269.

Cushing, M.C. and K.S. Anseth. 2007. Hydrogel cell cultures. Science. 316: 1133–1134.

Daniele, M.A., A.A. Adams, J. Naciri, S.H. North and F.S. Ligler. 2014. Interpenetrating networks based on gelatin methacrylamide and PEG formed using concurrent thiol click chemistries for hydrogel tissue engineering scaffolds. Biomaterials. 35: 1845–1856.

Das, A.K., A.R. Hirsth and R.V. Ulijn. 2009. Evolving nanomaterials using enzyme-driven dynamic peptide libraries (eDPL). Faraday Discuss. 143: 293–303; discussion 359–272.

DeForest, C.A., B.D. Polizzotti and K.S. Anseth. 2009. Sequential click reactions for synthesizing and patterning three-dimensional cell microenvironments. Nat. Mater. 8: 659–664.

DeForest, C.A. and K.S. Anseth. 2012. Advances in bioactive hydrogels to probe and direct cell fate. Annu. Rev. Chem. Biomol. Eng. 3: 421–444.

Dishowitz, M.I., F. Zhu, H.G. Sundararaghavan, J.L. Ifkovits, J.A. Burdick and K.D. Hankenson. 2014. Jagged1 immobilization to an osteoconductive polymer activates the notch signaling pathway and induces osteogenesis. J. Biomed. Mater. Res. A. 102: 1558–1567.

Drury, J.L. and D.J. Mooney. 2003. Hydrogels for tissue engineering: scaffold design variables and applications. Biomaterials. 24: 4337–4351.

Elbert, D.L. and J.A. Hubbell. 2001. Conjugate addition reactions combined with free-radical cross-linking for the design of materials for tissue engineering. Biomacromolecules. 2: 430–441.

Elbert, D.L. 2011. Liquid-liquid two-phase systems for the production of porous hydrogels and hydrogel microspheres for biomedical applications: a tutorial review. Acta Biomater. 7: 31–56.

Engler, A.J., S. Sen, H.L. Sweeney and D.E. Discher. 2006. Matrix elasticity directs stem cell lineage specification. Cell. 126: 677–689.

Fairbanks, B.D., M.P. Schwartz, A.E. Halevi, C.R. Nuttelman, C.N. Bowman and K.S. Anseth. 2009. A versatile synthetic extracellular matrix mimic via thiol-norbornene photopolymerization. Adv. Mater. 21: 5005–+.

Fleming, S. and R.V. Ulijn. 2014. Design of nanostructures based on aromatic peptide amphiphiles. Chem. Soc. Rev. 43: 8150–8177.

Fraser, A.K., C.S. Ki and C.C. Lin. 2014. PEG-based microgels formed by visible-light-mediated thiol-ene photo-click reactions. Macromol. Chem. Phys. 215: 507–515.

Gandavarapu, N.R., M.A. Azagarsamy and K.S. Anseth. 2014. Photo-click living strategy for controlled, reversible exchange of biochemical ligands. Adv. Mater. 26: 2521–2526.

Glassman, M.J., J. Chan and B.D. Olsen. 2013. Reinforcement of shear thinning protein hydrogels by responsive block copolymer self-assembly. Adv. Funct. Mater. 23: 1182–1193.

Grover, G.N., J. Lam, T.H. Nguyen, T. Segura and H.D. Maynard. 2012. Biocompatible hydrogels by oxime click chemistry. Biomacromolecules. 13: 3013–3017.

Grover, G.N., R.L. Braden and K.L. Christman. 2013. Oxime cross-linked injectable hydrogels for catheter delivery. Adv. Mater. 25: 2937–2942.

Hao, Y. and C.-C. Lin. 2014. Degradable thiol-acrylate hydrogels as tunable matrices for three-dimensional hepatic culture. Journal of Biomedical Materials Research Part A. 102: 3813–3827.

Hao, Y.T., H. Shih, Z. Munoz, A. Kemp and C.C. Lin. 2014. Visible light cured thiol-vinyl hydrogels with tunable degradation for 3D cell culture. Acta Biomaterialia. 10: 104–114.

Hern, D.L. and J.A. Hubbell. 1998. Incorporation of adhesion peptides into nonadhesive hydrogels useful for tissue resurfacing. Journal of Biomedical Materials Research. 39: 266–276.

Highley, C.B., C.B. Rodell and J.A. Burdick. 2015. Direct 3D printing of shear-thinning hydrogels into self-healing hydrogels. Adv. Mater. 27: 5075–5079.

Hoyle, C.E. and C.N. Bowman. 2010. Thiol-ene click chemistry. Angew. Chem. Int. Ed. Engl. 49: 1540–1573.

Hu, B.H., J. Su and P.B. Messersmith. 2009. Hydrogels cross-linked by native chemical ligation. Biomacromolecules. 10: 2194–2200.

Impellitteri, N.A., M.W. Toepke, S.K. Levengood and W.L. Murphy. 2012. Specific VEGF sequestering and release using peptide-functionalized hydrogel microspheres. Biomaterials. 33: 3475–3484.

Jiang, Y., J. Chen, C. Deng, E.J. Suuronen and Z. Zhong. 2014. Click hydrogels, microgels and nanogels: emerging platforms for drug delivery and tissue engineering. Biomaterials. 35: 4969–4985.

Jung, J.P., A.J. Sprangers, J.R. Byce, J. Su, J.M. Squirrell, P.B. Messersmith et al. 2013. ECM-incorporated hydrogels cross-linked via native chemical ligation to engineer stem cell microenvironments. Biomacromolecules. 14: 3102–3111.

Khetan, S., M. Guvendiren, W.R. Legant, D.M. Cohen, C.S. Chen and J.A. Burdick. 2013. Degradation-mediated cellular traction directs stem cell fate in covalently crosslinked three-dimensional hydrogels. Nature Materials. 12: 458–465.

Koehler, K.C., D.L. Alge, K.S. Anseth and C.N. Bowman. 2013. A diels-alder modulated approach to control and sustain the release of dexamethasone and induce osteogenic differentiation of human mesenchymal stem cells. Biomaterials. 34: 4150–4158.

Lam, J., S.T. Carmichael, W.E. Lowry and T. Segura. 2015. Hydrogel design of experiments methodology to optimize hydrogel for iPSC-NPC culture. Adv. Healthc. Mater. 4: 534–539.

Lampe, K.J., A.L. Antaris and S.C. Heilshorn. 2013. Design of three-dimensional engineered protein hydrogels for tailored control of neurite growth. Acta Biomater. 9: 5590–5599.

Lau, H.K. and K.L. Kiick. 2015. Opportunities for multicomponent hybrid hydrogels in biomedical applications. Biomacromolecules. 16: 28–42.

Li, L., Z. Tong, X. Jia and K.L. Kiick. 2013. Resilin-like polypeptide hydrogels engineered for versatile biological functions. Soft Matter. 9: 665–673.

Liebmann, T., S. Rydholm, V. Akpe and H. Brismar. 2007. Self-assembling Fmoc dipeptide hydrogel for *in situ* 3D cell culturing. BMC Biotechnol. 7: 88.

Lin, C.-C. and K.S. Anseth. 2009. Controlling affinity binding with peptide-functionalized poly(ethylene glycol) hydrogels. Advanced Functional Materials. 19: 2325–2331.

Lin, C.-C., P.D. Boyer, A.A. Aimetti and K.S. Anseth. 2010. Regulating MCP-1 diffusion in affinity hydrogels for enhancing immuno-isolation. Journal of Controlled Release. 142: 384–391.

Lin, C.-C., C.S. Ki and H. Shih. 2015. Thiol-norbornene photoclick hydrogels for tissue engineering applications. Journal of Applied Polymer Science. 132.

Lin, C.C. and A.T. Metters. 2006. Hydrogels in controlled release formulations: network design and mathematical modeling. Adv. Drug Deliver. Rev. 58: 1379–1408.

Lin, C.C. and K.S. Anseth. 2009. PEG hydrogels for the controlled release of biomolecules in regenerative medicine. Pharma. Res. 26: 631–643.

Lin, C.C. and K.S. Anseth. 2011. Cell-cell communication mimicry with poly(ethylene glycol) hydrogels for enhancing beta-cell function. Proc. Natl. Acad. Sci USA. 108: 6380–6385.

Lin, C.C., A. Raza and H. Shih. 2011. PEG hydrogels formed by thiol-ene photo-click chemistry and their effect on the formation and recovery of insulin-secreting cell spheroids. Biomaterials. 32: 9685–9695.

Lin, F., J.Y. Yu, W. Tang, J.K. Zheng, A. Defante, K. Guo et al. 2013. Peptide-functionalized oxime hydrogels with tunable mechanical properties and gelation behavior. Biomacromolecules. 14: 3749–3758.

Lin, T.Y., J.C. Bragg and C.C. Lin. 2015. Designing visible light-cured thiol-acrylate hydrogels for studying the HIPPO pathway activation in hepatocellular carcinoma cells. Macromol. Biosci.

Liu, S., K.T. Dicker and X. Jia. 2015. Modular and orthogonal synthesis of hybrid polymers and networks. Chemical Communications (Cambridge, England). 51: 5218–5237.

Liu, Y., B. Liu, J.J. Riesberg and W. Shen. 2011. *In situ* forming physical hydrogels for three-dimensional tissue morphogenesis. Macromol. Biosci. 11: 1325–1330.

Lu, H.D., M.B. Charati, I.L. Kim and J.A. Burdick. 2012. Injectable shear-thinning hydrogels engineered with a self-assembling dock-and-Lock mechanism. Biomaterials. 33: 2145–2153.

Luo, Y. and M.S. Shoichet. 2004a. Light-activated immobilization of biomolecules to agarose hydrogels for controlled cellular response. Biomacromolecules. 5: 2315–2323.

Luo, Y. and M.S. Shoichet. 2004b. A photolabile hydrogel for guided three-dimensional cell growth and migration. Nature Materials. 3: 249–253.

Lutolf, M.P. and J.A. Hubbell. 2003. Synthesis and physicochemical characterization of end-linked poly(ethylene glycol)-co-peptide hydrogels formed by Michael-type addition. Biomacromolecules. 4: 713–722.

Lutolf, M.P., J.L. Lauer-Fields, H.G. Schmoekel, A.T. Metters, F.E. Weber, G.B. Fields et al. 2003a. Synthetic matrix metalloproteinase-sensitive hydrogels for the conduction of tissue regeneration: engineering cell-invasion characteristics. Proc. Natl. Acad. Sci. USA. 100: 5413–5418.

Lutolf, M.P., G.P. Raeber, A.H. Zisch, N. Tirelli and J.A. Hubbell. 2003b. Cell-responsive synthetic hydrogels. Adv. Mater. 15: 888–+.

Lutolf, M.P. and J.A. Hubbell. 2005. Synthetic biomaterials as instructive extracellular microenvironments for morphogenesis in tissue engineering. Nature Biotechnology. 23: 47–55.

MacEwan, S.R. and A. Chilkoti. 2010. Elastin-like polypeptides: biomedical applications of tunable biopolymers. Biopolymers. 94: 60–77.

Martino, M.M., P.S. Briquez, E. Guc, F. Tortelli, W.W. Kilarski, S. Metzger et al. 2014. Growth factors engineered for super-affinity to the extracellular matrix enhance tissue healing. Science. 343: 885–888.

McGann, C.L., R.E. Akins and K.L. Kiick. 2016a. Resilin-PEG hybrid hydrogels yield degradable elastomeric scaffolds with heterogeneous microstructure. Biomacromolecules. 17: 128–140.

McGann, C.L., R.E. Dumm, A.K. Jurusik, I. Sidhu and K.L. Kiick. 2016b. Thiol-ene photocrosslinking of cytocompatible resilin-like polypeptide-PEG hydrogels. Macromol. Biosci. 16: 129–138.

McKinnon, D.D., D.W. Domaille, T.E. Brown, K.A. Kyburz, E. Kiyotake, J.N. Cha et al. 2014a. Measuring cellular forces using bis-aliphatic hydrazone crosslinked stress-relaxing hydrogels. Soft Matter. 10: 9230–9236.

McKinnon, D.D., D.W. Domaille, J.N. Cha and K.S. Anseth. 2014b. Biophysically defined and cytocompatible covalently adaptable networks as viscoelastic 3d cell culture systems. Advanced Materials. 26: 865–872.

Mealy, J.E., C.B. Rodell and J.A. Burdick. 2015. Sustained small molecule delivery from injectable hyaluronic acid hydrogels through host-guest mediated retention. J. Mater. Chem. B. Mater. Biol. Med. 3: 8010–8019.

Nagarkar, R.P. and J.P. Schneider. 2008. Synthesis and primary characterization of self-assembled peptide-based hydrogels. Methods Mol. Biol. 474: 61–77.

Parisi-Amon, A., W. Mulyasasmita, C. Chung and S.C. Heilshorn. 2013. Protein-engineered injectable hydrogel to improve retention of transplanted adipose-derived stem cells. Adv. Healthc. Mater. 2: 428–432.

Polizzotti, B.D., B.D. Fairbanks and K.S. Anseth. 2008. Three-dimensional biochemical patterning of click-based composite hydrogels via thiolene photopolymerization. Biomacromolecules. 9: 1084–1087.

Pratt, A.B., F.E. Weber, H.G. Schmoekel, R. Muller and J.A. Hubbell. 2004. Synthetic extracellular matrices for *in situ* tissue engineering. Biotechnol. Bioeng. 86: 27–36.

Raza, A., C.S. Ki and C.C. Lin. 2013. The influence of matrix properties on growth and morphogenesis of human pancreatic ductal epithelial cells in 3D. Biomaterials. 34: 5117–5127.

Rehfeldt, F., A.J. Engler, A. Eckhardt, F. Ahmed and D.E. Discher. 2007. Cell responses to the mechanochemical microenvironment—implications for regenerative medicine and drug delivery. Adv. Drug Deliv. Rev. 59: 1329–1339.

Renner, J.N., K.M. Cherry, R.S. Su and J.C. Liu. 2012. Characterization of resilin-based materials for tissue engineering applications. Biomacromolecules. 13: 3678–3685.

Rice, J.J., M.M. Martino, L. De Laporte, F. Tortelli, P.S. Briquez and J.A. Hubbell. 2013. Engineering the regenerative microenvironment with biomaterials. Adv. Healthc. Mater. 2: 57–71.

Rodell, C.B., J.W. MacArthur, S.M. Dorsey, R.J. Wade, Y.J. Woo and J.A. Burdick. 2015a. Shear-thinning supramolecular hydrogels with secondary autonomous covalent crosslinking to modulate viscoelastic properties. Adv. Funct. Mater. 25: 636–644.

Rodell, C.B., J.E. Mealy and J.A. Burdick. 2015b. Supramolecular guest-host interactions for the preparation of biomedical materials. Bioconjug. Chem. 26: 2279–2289.

Salinas, C.N. and K.S. Anseth. 2008. Mixed mode thiol-acrylate photopolymerizations for the synthesis of PEG-peptide hydrogels. Macromolecules. 41: 6019–6026.

Schwartz, M.P., B.D. Fairbanks, R.E. Rogers, R. Rangarajan, M.H. Zaman and K.S. Anseth. 2010. A synthetic strategy for mimicking the extracellular matrix provides new insight about tumor cell migration. Integr. Biol. 2: 32–40.

Sen, S., A.J. Engler and D.E. Discher. 2009. Matrix strains induced by cells: computing how far cells can feel. Cell Mol. Bioeng. 2: 39–48.

Shao, H. and J.R. Parquette. 2010. A pi-conjugated hydrogel based on an Fmoc-dipeptide naphthalene diimide semiconductor. Chem. Commun. (Camb.). 46: 4285–4287.

Shih, H. and C.C. Lin. 2012. Cross-linking and degradation of step-growth hydrogels formed by thiol-ene photoclick chemistry. Biomacromolecules. 13: 2003–2012.

Shih, H. and C.C. Lin. 2013. Visible-light-mediated thiol-ene hydrogelation using eosin-y as the only photoinitiator. Macromol. Rapid Commun. 34: 269–273.

Shih, H., A.K. Fraser and C.C. Lin. 2013. Interfacial thiol-ene photoclick reactions for forming multilayer hydrogels. ACS Appl. Mater. Interfaces. 5: 1673–1680.

Stephens-Altus, J.S., P. Sundelacruz, M.L. Rowland and J.L. West. 2011. Development of bioactive photocrosslinkable fibrous hydrogels. J. Biomed. Mater. Res. A. 98: 167–176.

Strehin, I., D. Gourevitch, Y. Zhang, E. Heber-Katz and P.B. Messersmith. 2013. Hydrogels formed by oxo-ester mediated native chemical ligation. Biomater. Sci. 1: 603–613.

Su, J., B.H. Hu, W.L. Lowe, D.B. Kaufman and P.B. Messersmith. 2010. Anti-inflammatory peptide-functionalized hydrogels for insulin-secreting cell encapsulation. Biomaterials. 31: 308–314.

Su, R.S., Y. Kim and J.C. Liu. 2014. Resilin: protein-based elastomeric biomaterials. Acta Biomater. 10: 1601–1611.

Tibbitt, M.W. and K.S. Anseth. 2009. Hydrogels as extracellular matrix mimics for 3D cell culture. Biotechnol. Bioeng. 103: 655–663.

Wade, R.J., E.J. Bassin, C.B. Rodell and J.A. Burdick. 2015. Protease-degradable electrospun fibrous hydrogels. Nat. Commun. 6: 6639.

Wang, C., R.J. Stewart and J. Kopecek. 1999. Hybrid hydrogels assembled from synthetic polymers and coiled-coil protein domains. Nature. 397: 417–420.

Wang, H., L. Cai, A. Paul, A. Enejder and S.C. Heilshorn. 2014. Hybrid elastin-like polypeptide-polyethylene glycol (ELP-PEG) hydrogels with improved transparency and independent control of matrix mechanics and cell ligand density. Biomacromolecules. 15: 3421–3428.

Wang, H. and S.C. Heilshorn. 2015. Adaptable hydrogel networks with reversible linkages for tissue engineering. Adv. Mater. 27: 3717–3736.

Webber, M.J., E.A. Appel, E.W. Meijer and R. Langer. 2015. Supramolecular biomaterials. Nat. Mater. 15: 13–26.

West, J.L. and J.A. Hubbell. 1995. Photopolymerized hydrogel materials for drug-delivery applicaitons. Reactive Polymers. 25: 139–147.

West, J.L. and J.A. Hubbell. 1999. Polymeric biomaterials with degradation sites for proteases involved in cell migration. Macromolecules. 32: 241–244.

Willerth, S.M., P.J. Johnson, D.J. Maxwell, S.R. Parsons, M.E. Doukas and S.E. Sakiyama-Elbert. 2007. Rationally designed peptides for controlled release of nerve growth factor from fibrin matrices. Journal of Biomedical Materials Research Part A. 80A: 13–23.

Wong Po Foo, C.T., J.S. Lee, W. Mulyasasmita, A. Parisi-Amon and S.C. Heilshorn. 2009. Two-component protein-engineered physical hydrogels for cell encapsulation. Proc. Natl. Acad. Sci. USA. 106: 22067–22072.

Woolfson, D.N. 2010. Building fibrous biomaterials from alpha-helical and collagen-like coiled-coil peptides. Biopolymers. 94: 118–127.

Yang, C., P.D. Mariner, J.N. Nahreini and K.S. Anseth. 2012. Cell-mediated delivery of glucocorticoids from thiol-ene hydrogels. J. Control. Release. 162: 612–618.

Yang, C., M.W. Tibbitt, L. Basta and K.S. Anseth. 2014. Mechanical memory and dosing influence stem cell fate. Nature Materials. 13: 645–652.

Zanuy, D., J. Poater, M. Sola, I.W. Hamley and C. Aleman. 2016. Fmoc-RGDS based fibrils: atomistic details of their hierarchical assembly. Phys. Chem. Chem. Phys. 18: 1265–1278.

Zhang, H., K.T. Dicker, X. Xu, X. Jia and J.M. Fox. 2014. Interfacial bioorthogonal cross-linking. Acs Macro. Letters. 3: 727–731.

Zhang, Y.N., R.K. Avery, Q. Vallmajo-Martin, A. Assmann, A. Vegh, A. Memic et al. 2015. A highly elastic and rapidly crosslinkable elastin-like polypeptide-based hydrogel for biomedical applications. Adv. Funct. Mater. 25: 4814–4826.

Zhou, M., A.M. Smith, A.K. Das, N.W. Hodson, R.F. Collins, R.V. Ulijn et al. 2009. Self-assembled peptide-based hydrogels as scaffolds for anchorage-dependent cells. Biomaterials. 30: 2523–2530.

Zhou, M., R.V. Ulijn and J.E. Gough. 2014. Extracellular matrix formation in self-assembled minimalistic bioactive hydrogels based on aromatic peptide amphiphiles. J. Tissue Eng. 5: 2041731414531593.

Index